# Frontiers In Medicinal Chemistry

# (Volume 10)

### Edited By

**Ashok Kumar Jha**
*Department of Chemistry*
*T.M. Bhagalpur University*
*Bhagalpur, Bihar*
*India*

&

**Ravi S. Singh**
*Bihar Agriculture University*
*Sabour, Bihar*
*India*

# Frontiers In Medicinal Chemistry

*(Volume 10)*

Editors: Ashok Kumar Jha & Ravi S. Singh

ISSN (Online): 1875-5763

ISSN (Print): 1567-2042

ISBN (Online): 978-981-5165-04-3

ISBN (Print): 978-981-5165-05-0

ISBN (Paperback): 978-981-5165-06-7

need for a court order if at any point you breach any terms of this License Agreement. In no event will any delay or failure by Bentham Science Publishers in enforcing your compliance with this License Agreement constitute a waiver of any of its rights.

3. You acknowledge that you have read this License Agreement, and agree to be bound by its terms and conditions. To the extent that any other terms and conditions presented on any website of Bentham Science Publishers conflict with, or are inconsistent with, the terms and conditions set out in this License Agreement, you acknowledge that the terms and conditions set out in this License Agreement shall prevail.

**Bentham Science Publishers Pte. Ltd.**
80 Robinson Road #02-00
Singapore 068898
Singapore
Email: subscriptions@benthamscience.net

**BENTHAM
SCIENCE**

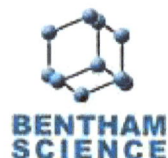

# CONTENTS

# FOREWORD

I am extremely happy to find that Dr. Ashok Kumar Jha, Department of Chemistry, Tilka Manjhi Bhagalpur University, Bhagalpur, has ventured to edit a book titled **"Frontiers in Medicinal Chemistry"**. Such a treatise is a long-standing requirement for those engaged in research and teaching the subject.

Medicinal Chemistry in Chemical Science has been serving humankind from the very beginning by way of the discovery of potentially bioactive molecules in the treatment of various ailments. Everybody would agree that the role of medicinal chemists is pivotal in the medical sciences. The development of recent therapeutic agents, secondary metabolites from plants and nano drugs, along with drug delivery targets, has added a new dimension to the field of medicinal chemistry. Methods of computational approaches in drug repositioning have emerged as effective techniques recently to cope with the devastating effects of mysterious diseases and pandemics, too. Different databases such as DrugBank, OMIM, ChemBank, and PubMed are worth mentioning in many drug repositioning prospects. A few discoveries have also taken place on isoxazole derivatives as a potential pharmacophore for new drug development. A lot of biological activities such as antimicrobial, antitubercular, antiepileptic, anthelmintic, and antimalarial have been found in heterocyclic compounds.

Cancer, arising from uncontrolled cell division, has emerged as a prominent cause of death around the globe. Carcinogenic agents and toxic heavy metals cause lung, breast and liver cancer in general, and cases of lung cancer among workers in chromium-related industries have already been established due to the ingestion of hexavalent chromium. Different types of chemotherapeutic agents and phytochemicals have been investigated for anticancerous activities.

In addition, nature has a vast treasure of medicinal plants that have not been explored for their therapeutic values till now, and so the mystery has to be unveiled for their medicinal value. From time immemorial, people have been using them as folk medicines to treat ailments. Intensive research is required to characterize the phytochemicals, which are instrumental in the cure of diseases. Some of the chapters on cancer treatment and causative agents, along with the mechanism of uncontrolled cell growth due to metal toxicity, will prove very beneficial for scientists who want to pursue advanced research in the field. Articles in the book "Frontiers in Medicinal Chemistry" have been contributed by experienced and recognized experts in the area of medicinal chemistry with a view to enrich the existing knowledge of those who are engaged in teaching and research in the field.

I do hope that this book will be appreciated by the faculties, researchers as well as students.

**D.C. Mukherjee**
Former President and Advisor
Indian Chemical Society
Kolkata
India

# PREFACE

In recent times, Medicinal Chemistry has emerged in Chemistry as a very fascinating and challenging area to cope with mysterious diseases, as a result of which this branch of Chemistry has attained prime importance. From the beginning of civilization in ancient times, Chemistry has been designed to serve humankind through Ayurveda, herbal medicines and metals in nano-size for drug delivery. In the Himalayas, there were very good and well-known plants used for the treatment of severe ailments. The ancient concept of Swarna bhasma, iron bhasma, and other bhasmas is nothing but modern time nano drugs. Lead and silver bhasmas were also in practice. There is no doubt that Medicinal Chemistry plays a significant role in the discovery of therapeutic agents or bioactive molecules for use in the treatment of various human ailments. It generally involves chemical, synthetic and computational aspects of identification and modification of molecules known as drugs either from natural or synthetic products.

This book, titled "Frontiers in Medicinal Chemistry," contains diverse topics from different areas of Medicinal Chemistry, including developments in drug discovery and design, identifying new targets for existing drugs through drug repurposing, along screening new and emerging drug targets. In addition, carcinogenicity due to hexavalent chromium and arsenic with a probable mechanism of mismatch DNA repair and proteotoxic stress have been discussed in the chapter of the book. Biosynthetic pathways, biotechnology, biochemistry, molecular biology and related topics from food science have also been incorporated in the book.

I do hope that this book will serve as an important repository of scientific information on Medicinal Chemistry to students, researchers and a broad scientific spectrum. We had long sittings in the calmness of the night and even under the fading stars of dawn, completely away from the din and bustle to complete this monumental treatise. We express our sincere thanks to Senior Research Fellow Sri Sachin Verma "Heavy Metal Remediation Laboratory'' for providing his computer skills and expertise. I also express my thanks to Dr. Ujjwal Kumar, AIIMS Patna, for showing interest in the present book.

Last but not least, we express our deep sense of gratitude to Prof. D.C Mukherjee for constant encouragement. We sincerely thank and appreciate Bentham Science Publishers for providing an opportunity to complete this project. Finally, we bow before the Almighty, Creator of the Universe, for instilling inner strength in us to complete this arduous task.

**Ashok Kumar Jha**
Department of Chemistry
T.M. Bhagalpur University
Bhagalpur, Bihar
India

**Ravi S. Singh**
Bihar Agriculture University
Sabour, Bihar
India

# List of Contributors

| | |
|---|---|
| **Abhishek Tiwari** | Faculty of Pharmacy, IFTM University, Moradabad-244102, Uttar Pradesh, India |
| **Asim Kumar** | Amity Institute of Pharmacy, Amity University Haryana, Manesar, Panchgaon-122412, India |
| **Anil Kumar Singh** | Department of Chemistry, School of Physical Sciences, Mahatma Gandhi Central University, Motihari, Bihar-845401, India |
| **Abhijeet Kumar** | Department of Chemistry, School of Physical Sciences, Mahatma Gandhi Central University, Motihari, Bihar-845401, India |
| **Ashok Kumar Jha** | University Department of Chemistry, Tilka Manjhi Bhagalpur University, Bhagalpur-812007, Bihar, India |
| **Aakansha Singh** | Department of Bioengineering and Biotechnology, Birla Institute of Technology, Mesra, Ranchi- 835215, Jharkhand, India |
| **Anjani Kumar** | ICAR-RCER, Farming System Research Centre for Hill & Plateau Region, Ranchi-834010, Jharkhand, India |
| **Biswa Mohan Sahoo** | Roland Institute of Pharmaceutical Sciences (Affiliated to Biju Patnaik University of Technology), Berhampur-760010, Odisha, India |
| **Bera Venkata Varaha Ravi Kumar** | Roland Institute of Pharmaceutical Sciences (Affiliated to Biju Patnaik University of Technology), Berhampur-760010, Odisha, India |
| **Bimal Krishna Banik** | Department of Mathematics and Natural Sciences, College of Sciences and Human Studies, Prince Mohammad Bin Fahd University, Al Khobar, Kingdom of Saudi Arabia |
| **Dina Nath Singh** | K.S. Saket PG College, Dr. Ram Manohar Lohia Avadh University, Ayodhya-224001, India |
| **Gaurav Joshi** | School of Pharmacy, Graphic Era Hill University, Dehradun-248002, India |
| **Garima Tripathi** | Department of Chemistry, T.N. B. College, TMBU, Bhagalpur, Bihar, India |
| **Ghanshyam Kumar Satyapal** | Department of Biotechnology, School of Earth Biological & Environmental Sciences, Central University of South Bihar, Gaya, India |
| **Krishna Chandra Panda** | Roland Institute of Pharmaceutical Sciences (Affiliated to Biju Patnaik University of Technology), Berhampur-760010, Odisha, India |
| **Kishan Singh** | Phytochemistry Division, CSIR-Central Institute of Medicinal and Aromatic Plants, Lucknow- 226015, India <br> Academy of Scientific and Innovative Research, Ghaziabad-201002, India |
| **Kapil Dev** | Phytochemistry Division, CSIR-Central Institute of Medicinal and Aromatic Plants, Lucknow- 226015, India <br> Academy of Scientific and Innovative Research, Ghaziabad-201002, India |
| **Lovely Sinha** | Department of Pulmonary Medicine, All India Institute of Medical Sciences, Patna-801507, Bihar, India |
| **Manish Kumar** | M.M. College of Pharmacy, Maharishi Markandeshwar (Deemed to Be University), Mullana-Ambala-133207, Haryana, India |
| **Manju Singh** | Phytochemistry Division, CSIR-Central Institute of Medicinal and Aromatic Plants, Lucknow- 226015, India |

| Nisha Verma | K.S. Saket PG College, Dr. Ram Manohar Lohia Avadh University, Ayodhya-224001, India |
| Neerja Tiwari | Phytochemistry Division, CSIR-Central Institute of Medicinal and Aromatic Plants, Lucknow- 226015, India |
| Namita Gupta | Phytochemistry Division, CSIR-Central Institute of Medicinal and Aromatic Plants, Lucknow- 226015, India |
| Pallavi Kumari | University Department of Chemistry, Tilka Manjhi Bhagalpur University, Bhagalpur-812007, Bihar, India |
| Ravi S. Singh | Department of Plant Breeding and Genetics, Bihar Agricultural University, Sabour, Bhagalpur, Bihar-813 210, India |
| Ruchi Kumari | University Department of Home Science-Food and Nutrition, Tilka Manjhi Bhagalpur University, Bhagalpur-812 007, Bihar, India |
| Sunil Singh | Department of Pharmaceutical Chemistry, Shri Sai College of Pharmacy, Handia, Prayagraj, U.P., 221503, India |
| Srikant Bhagat | Deppartment of Medicinal Chemistry, National Institute of Pharmaceutical Education and Research (NIPER), S.A.S. Nagar (Mohali), Punjab-160062, India |
| Sachin Verma | University Department of Chemistry, Tilka Manjhi Bhagalpur University, Bhagalpur-812007, Bihar, India |
| Shailesh Kumar | University Department of Chemistry, Tilka Manjhi Bhagalpur University, Bhagalpur-812007, Bihar, India |
| Sanjay Kumar | CSIR-Institutes of Himalyan Bioresource Technology, Palampur, Himachal Pradesh-176 061, India |
| Ujjwal Kumar | Research Associate, Department of Psychatry & Department of CFM, All India Institute of Medical Sciences, Deoghar - 814152, Jharkhand, India |
| Shailendra Kumar | Human Molecular Genetics Laboratory, Department of Pathology/Lab Medicine, All India Institute of Medical Sciences, Patna, India |
| Varsha Tiwari | Faculty of Pharmacy, IFTM University, Moradabad-244102, Uttar Pradesh, India |

*Frontiers In Medicinal Chemistry, 2023, Vol. 10, 1-49* 1

# CHAPTER 1

# Isoxazole Derivatives as Potential Pharmacophore for New Drug Development

**Biswa Mohan Sahoo[1,*], Bera Venkata Varaha Ravi Kumar[1], Krishna Chandra Panda[1], Bimal Krishna Banik[2,*], Abhishek Tiwari[3], Varsha Tiwari[3], Sunil Singh[4]** and **Manish Kumar[5]**

[1] *Roland Institute of Pharmaceutical Sciences (Affiliated to Biju Patnaik University of Technology), Berhampur-760010, Odisha, India*

[2] *Department of Mathematics and Natural Sciences, College of Sciences and Human Studies, Prince Mohammad Bin Fahd University, Al Khobar, Kingdom of Saudi Arabia*

[3] *Faculty of Pharmacy, IFTM University, Moradabad-244102, Uttar Pradesh, India*

[4] *Department of Pharmaceutical Chemistry, Shri Sai College of Pharmacy, Handia, Prayagraj, U.P., 221503, India*

[5] *M.M. College of Pharmacy, Maharishi Markandeshwar (Deemed to Be University), Mullana-Ambala-133207, Haryana, India*

**Abstract:** Isoxazoles are five-membered aromatic heterocyclic compounds in which oxygen and nitrogen atoms are present at positions 1 and 2 of the ring system. Isoxazole derivatives play a vital role due to their diverse biological activities, such as antimicrobial, antifungal, anti-viral, anti-tubercular, anti-epileptic, anti-diabetic, anticancer, anthelmintic, antioxidant, antipsychotic, antimalarial, analgesic, anti-inflammatory, *etc*. Isoxazole scaffold is present in various drug molecules, such as leflunomide (antirheumatic), valdecoxib (non-steroidal anti-inflammatory drug), and zonisamide (anti-convulsant). Similarly, isoxazole derivatives such as isocarboxazid act as monoamine oxidase inhibitors. It is used to treat symptoms of depression that may include anxiety, panic, or phobias. Whereas the isoxazole derivatives, including sulfamethoxazole, sulfisoxazole, and oxacillin, are used clinically for the treatment of bacterial infections. Isoxazole pharmacophore is also present in $\beta$-lactamase resistant antibiotics such as cloxacillin, dicloxacillin, and flucloxacillin. Cycloserine is a naturally occurring antibiotic that possesses isoxazole moiety with anti-tubercular, activity. This study focuses on the therapeutic potentials of isoxazole derivatives in new drug development.

* **Corresponding authors Biswa Mohan Sahoo and Bimal Krishana Banik:** Roland Institute of Pharmaceutical Sciences (Affiliated to Biju Patnaik University of Technology), Berhampur-760010, Odisha, India & Department of Mathematics and Natural Sciences, College of Sciences and Human Studies, Prince Mohammad Bin Fahd University, Al Khobar, Kingdom of Saudi Arabia; E-mails: drbiswamohansahoo@gmail.com; bimalbanik10@gmail.com

**Keywords:** Biological activity, Disease, Drug, Isoxazoles, Pharmacophore, synthesis.

## 1. INTRODUCTION

Heterocyclic compounds containing nitrogen and oxygen atoms play a significant role as medicinal agents due to their wide range of therapeutic activities [1]. Heterocycles are the common structural moiety present in various clinically available drugs [2]. The cyclic compound with at least two different atoms (one is carbon and the others are heteroatoms such as nitrogen, oxygen, and sulfur) in the ring system is called a heterocyclic compound [3]. Depending on the presence of a type of heteroatoms (N, O, or S), and ring size, the heterocyclic compounds are of different types, including three-membered (oxirane, thiirane, aziridine), four-membered (oxetane, thietane, azetidine), five-membered (oxolane, thiolane, azolidine, triazole, oxadiazole, thiazole, pyrrole, furan, thiophene, imidazole, oxazole, isoxazole), six-membered (pyridine, pyrimidine), seven-membered (azepine), eight-membered (azocine), *etc* [4]. In addition to this, fused heterocyclic compounds are present such as quinoline, isoquinoline, indole, benzofuran, benzothiophene, coumarin, purine, benzimidazole, *etc* [4]. Due to the structural diversity of the heterocycles, these compounds possess a wide spectrum of therapeutic applications such as anti-bacterial, anti-malarial, anti-viral, anti-psychotic, anti-fungal, anti-tumor, anticonvulsant, anti-oxidant, antilipidemic, analgesic, and anti-inflammatory [5].

### 1.1. Isoxazoles

Nitrogen-containing heterocycles are considered a major class of compounds in medicinal research [6]. Among these, isoxazole derivatives play a vital role due to their diverse pharmacological activities such as antimicrobial, antifungal, anti-viral, anti-tubercular, anti-diabetic, anticancer, anthelmintic, antioxidant, anti-epileptic, antipsychotic, antimalarial, analgesic, anti-inflammatory, *etc* [7]. Isoxazoles (**1**) are unsaturated five-membered heterocyclic aromatic compounds containing three carbon atoms, one oxygen atom, and one nitrogen atom in a ring system, as presented in Fig. (**1**) [8].

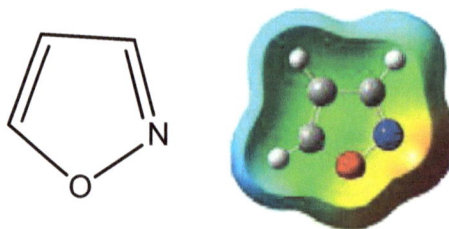

**Fig. (1).**  Structure of isoxazole.

It is an azole in which oxygen and nitrogen atoms are present at positions 1 and 2 of the ring system [9], as presented in Fig. (2). The partially saturated analogs of isoxazole (**1**) are named isoxazolines (**2**) and the completely saturated analog is called isoxazolidine (**3**) [10].

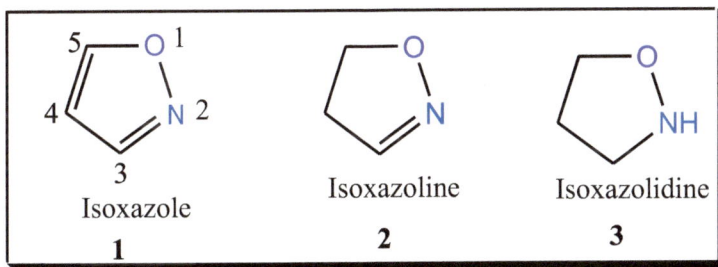

**Fig. (2).** Structure and nomenclature of isoxazole moiety.

## 1.1.1. General Methods of Synthesis

The chemistry of isoxazole and its derivatives have been developed extensively due to their diverse synthetic methodologies and potential pharmacological properties. The synthesis of isoxazole derivatives can be performed by the following methods.

The synthesis of isoxazole and its derivatives involves the cyclization of β-keto esters (**4**) with hydroxylamine (**5**) to produce 3-hydroxy-isoxazoles (3-isoxazolyl) (**6**). This method is called Claisen isoxazole synthesis (Fig. **3**) [11].

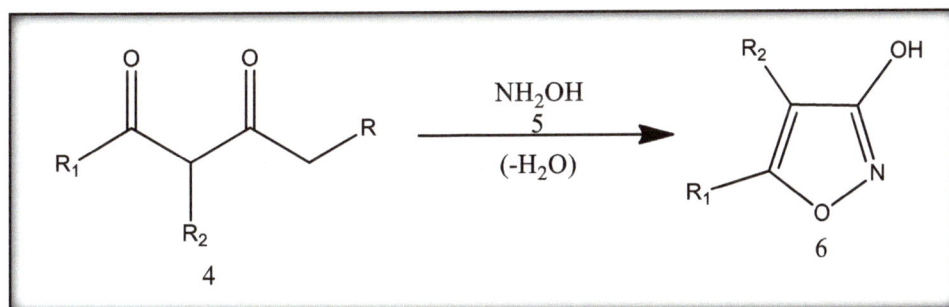

**Fig. (3).** Claisen isoxazole synthesis.

The synthesis of isoxazole derivatives (**8**) involves the cyclization of O-propioloyloxime (**7**) *(via* intermolecular arylidene group transfer using gold as a catalyst (Fig. **4**) [12].

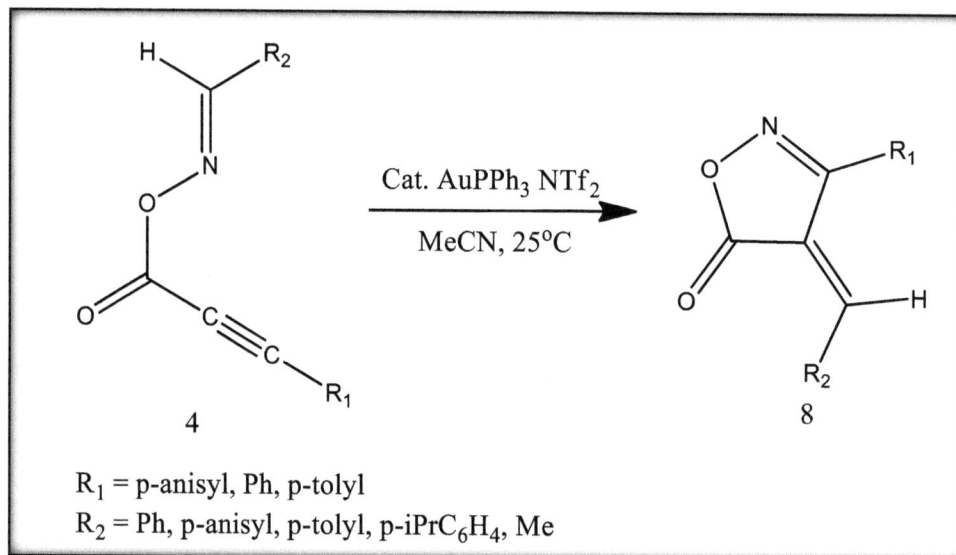

**Fig. (4).** Synthesis of isoxazole derivatives *via* cyclization of O-propioloyloxime.

3-phenylisoxazol-5-one (**10**) is prepared by condensation of ethyl-benzoyl acetate (**9**) with hydroxylamine (**5**) in the presence of ethanol (Fig. **5**) [13].

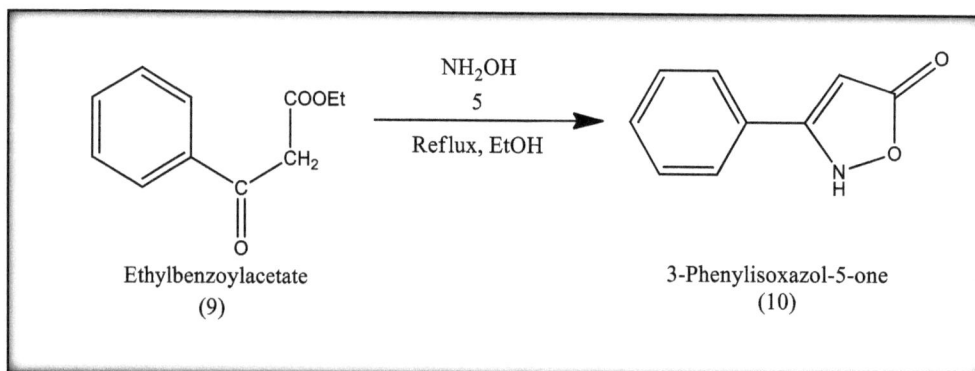

**Fig. (5).** Synthesis of 3-phenylisoxazol-5-one.

The synthesis of isoxazole derivatives (**12**) involves the condensation reaction of β-ketoesters (**11**) with hydroxylamine (**5**) in the presence of sodium hydroxide (Fig. **6**) [14].

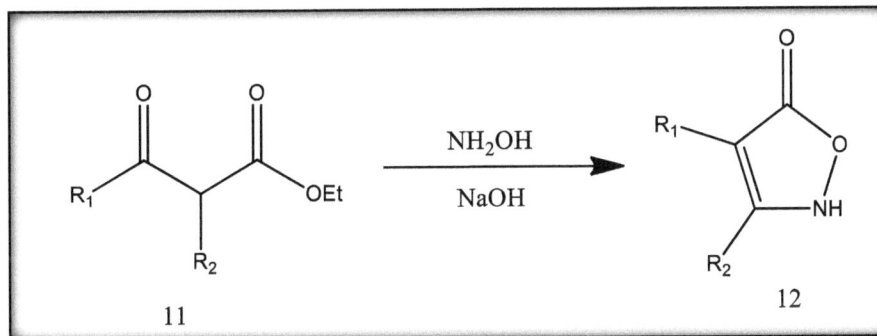

**Fig. (6).** Synthesis ofisoxazole derivatives from $\beta$-ketoesters.

The most common method for the synthesis of isoxazoles (**15**) involves one-pot three-component reactions of benzaldehydes (**13**), hydroxylamine hydrochlorides (**5**), and ethyl acetoacetate (**14**) using various catalysts such as 2-hydroxy-5-sulfo-benzoic acid (2-HSBA), sodium tetraborate, sodium saccharin, boric acid, sodium silicate, sodium benzoate, sodium azide, DABCO, potassium phthalimide, tartaric acid N-bromosuccinimide (NBS), zinc chloride, citric acid, starch solution and potassium hydrogen phthalate (Fig. **7**) [15].

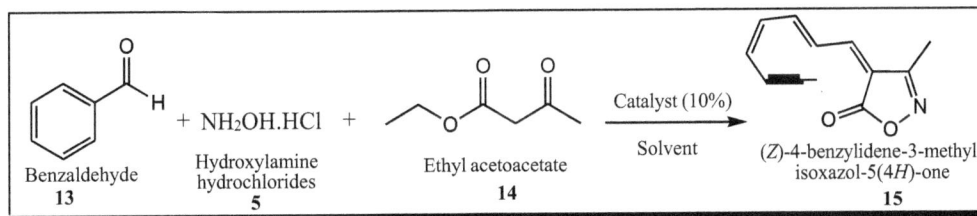

**Fig. (7).** Synthesis of isoxazoles *via* one-pot three-component reactions.

## 1.1.2. Green Synthesis of Isoxazoles

The cycloaddition of ethyl 2-nitroacetate or benzoylnitromethane (**16**) with terminal alkynes (**17**) leads to the production of isoxazoles (**18**) under green conditions. The methodology is free from the use of any base, catalyst, dehydrating agent, or hazardous solvent [16]. The mixture of water-polyethylene glycol (1:1) facilitates this synthetic process (Fig. **8**).

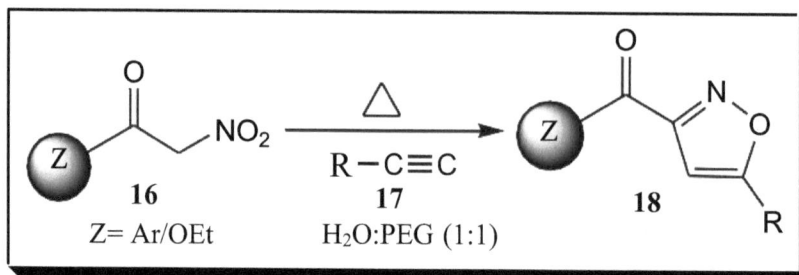

**Fig. (8).** Synthesis of isoxazole derivatives under green conditions.

Shaikh *et al.* demonstrated the synthesis of 3-methyl-4-arylmethylene isoxazole-5(4*H*)-ones (**20**) *via* multi-component reaction of substituted arylaldehydes (**19**), ethyl acetoacetate (**14**), and hydroxylamine (**5**) by using sodium acetate as a catalyst in ethanol. The reaction mixture was subjected to irradiation under visible light (tungsten lamp) at 150W for 4-18min (Fig. **9**) [17].

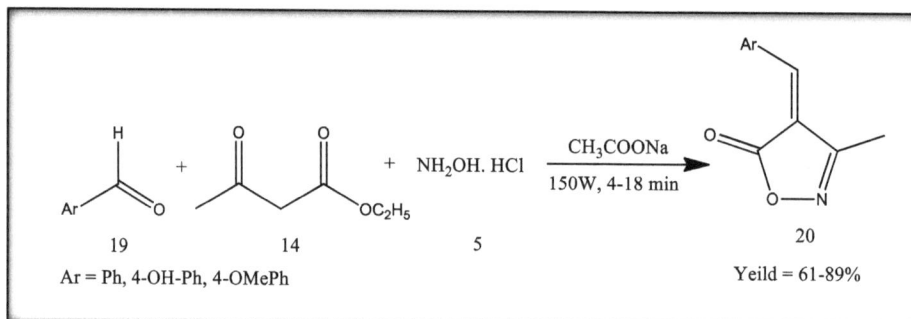

**Fig. (9).** Synthesis of 3-methyl-4-arylmethylene isoxazole-5(4*H*)-ones.

A mild and convenient route for the synthesis of isoxazole derivatives (**21**) has been developed using ZSM-5 as a heterogeneous catalyst. The reaction was carried out under a solvent-free condition to afford the desired products in good yields. A variety of functional groups was tolerated under the reaction conditions employed. Moreover, the heterogeneous catalyst (ZSM-5) was recovered and reused several times without significant loss of its catalytic activity (Fig. **10**) [18].

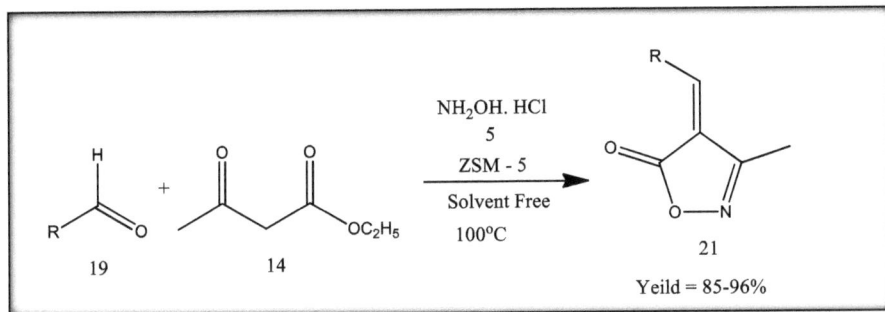

**Fig. (10).** Synthesis of isoxazole derivatives using ZSM-5 as catalyst.

Bharti *et al.* reported the different synthetic pathways for the production of 3,4-disubstituted isoxazole. It is based on a one-pot multicomponent reaction (MCR) using different catalysts. MCRs involve the single pot operation in which more than two reactants undergo a reaction in a single vessel to produce the final product without the formation of any by-product. The use of each catalyst exhibits its effect on the rate of synthetic reaction, product yield, and reaction time of the synthetic process. The significant features of the multicomponent reaction include eco-friendly, fewer reaction steps, atom economy, easy work-up, minimum formation of waste product, time-saving, waste reduction, efficient and energy-saving technique, *etc.* Kiyani *et al.* performed the multi-component synthesis of disubstituted-isoxazolone derivatives (**22**) in the presence of 2-hydroxy-5-sulfobenzoic acid (2-HSBA) as an organo-catalyst at room temperature. It involves the three-component reaction between ethyl acetoacetate (**14**), substituted aryl aldehydes (**19**), and hydroxylamine hydrochloride (**5**) in an aqueous medium. In addition to water, other solvents like DMSO, ethanol, dioxane, dichloromethane, hexane, and acetone were also used for the synthesis of isoxazole derivatives (Fig. **11**) [19].

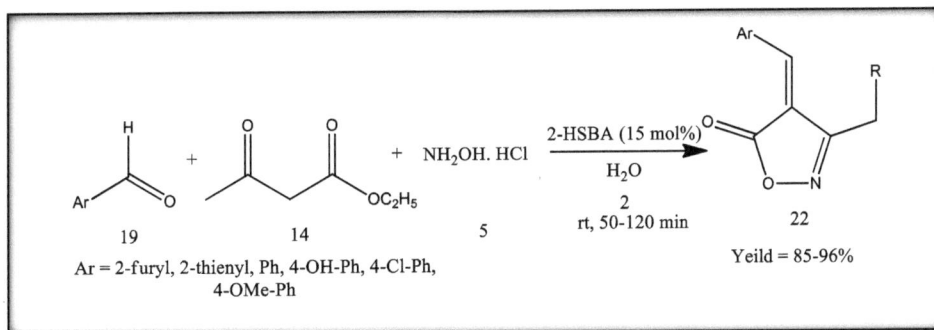

**Fig. (11).** Synthesis of disubstituted-isoxazolone derivatives.

Kiyani *et al.* described the protocol for the synthesis of disubstituted-isoxazolones (**23**) *via* one-pot reaction of various substituted arylaldehydes (**19**), ethyl acetoacetate (**14**), and hydroxylamine hydrochloride (**5**) by using a catalytic amount of N-bromosuccinimide (NBS) in an aqueous medium at room temperature (Fig. **12**). Various solvents were used for this synthesis include cyclohexane, ethanol, 1,4-dioxane, hexane, and acetone [20].

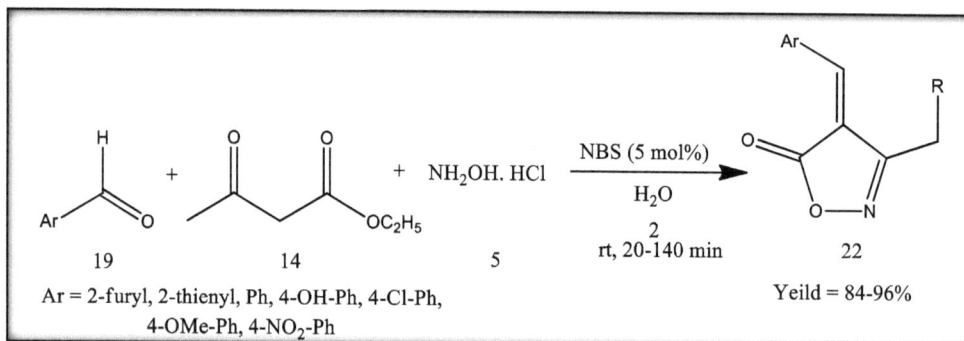

**Fig. (12).** Synthesis of disubstituted-isoxazolones *via* one-pot reaction.

Liu *et al.* described the efficient and green methodology for the synthesis of isoxazole derivatives (**24**). It involves the reaction of ethyl acetoacetate (**14**), substituted aryl aldehyde (**19**), and hydroxylamine hydrochloride (**5**) by using sodium benzoate as a catalyst in an aqueous medium at low temperature (Fig. **13**). Sodium benzoate was used as an efficient, novel, and green catalyst for the knoevenagel condensation of aryl aldehydes with active methylene compounds such as ethyl acetoacetate and malononitrile to afford substituted olefins. Various solvents used for this synthesis include water, ethanol, dioxane, cyclohexane, and acetone. But the best results were observed by using water as solvent [21].

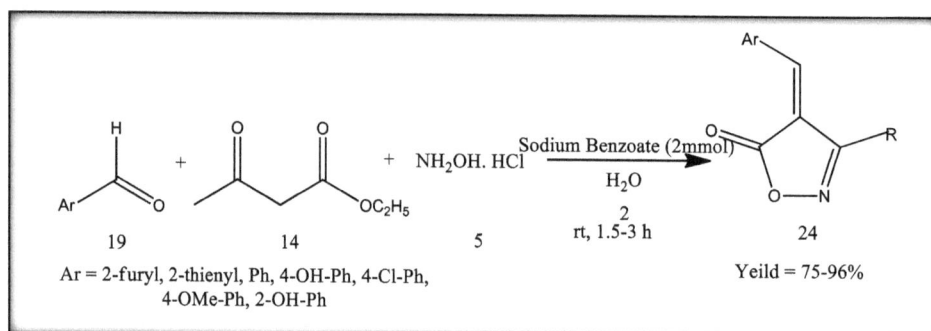

**Fig. (13).** Synthesis of isoxazole derivatives using sodium benzoate as a catalyst.

Kiyani *et al.* described the eco-friendly and efficient synthesis of 3,4-disubstituted isoxazole-5(4*H*)-ones by using a potassium phthalimide (PPI) as an organocatalyst (Fig. **14**). It involves the single pot reaction of substituted arylaldehydes (**19**), ethyl acetoacetate (**14**) with hydroxylamine hydrochloride (**5**) in water under mild reaction conditions to obtain isoxazole derivative (**25**) in good yield. In addition to water, other solvents were also used, such as ethanol, 1,4-dioxane, cyclohexane, hexane, and acetone (Table **1**). In this synthesis, PPI played a key role and the advantages of this method include green, efficient, clean, easy work-up, high product yields, shorter reaction time, inexpensive, *etc* [22].

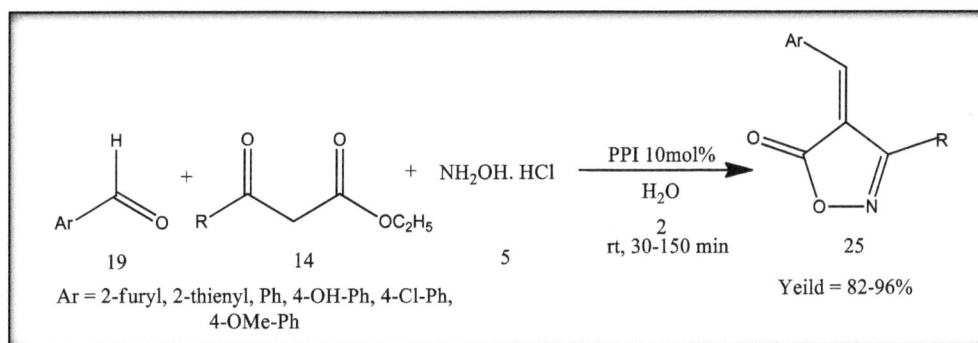

**Fig. (14).**  Synthesis of 3,4-disubstituted isoxazole-5(4*H*)-ones.

**Table 1. Optimised reaction condition for the synthesis of 3,4-disubstituted isoxazole-5(4*H*)-ones.**

| Entry | Solvent | PPI (mol%) | Time (min) | Yield (%) |
|-------|---------|------------|------------|-----------|
| 1 | $H_2O$ | 5 | 89 | 89 |
| 2 | $H_2O$ | 10 | 70 | 95 |
| 3 | $H_2O$ | 15 | 70 | 96 |
| 4 | $H_2O$ | 20 | 120 | 95 |
| 5 | $C_2H_5OH$ | 10 | 120 | 55 |
| 6 | Acetone | 10 | 120 | 10 |
| 7 | Hexane | 10 | 120 | 21 |
| 8 | $H_2O/C_2H_5OH$ (1:1) | 10 | 120 | 70 |
| 9 | $H_2O/Acetone$ (1:1) | 10 | 120 | 15 |
| 10 | $H_2O/Dioxane$ (1:1) | 10 | 120 | 10 |

Khandebharad *et al.* reported the synthesis of 3-methyl-4-arylmethylene-isoxazol-5(4*H*)-ones (**26**) *via* multi-component transformation of various aromatic aldehyde (**19**), ethyl acetoacetate (**14**), and hydroxylamine hydrochloride (**5**) by using different biodegradable organocatalyst in the presence of water as solvent at room temperature (Fig. **15**). It was observed that there was good product yield in less reaction time by using dl-tartaric acid as a catalyst (Tables **2** and **3**) [23].

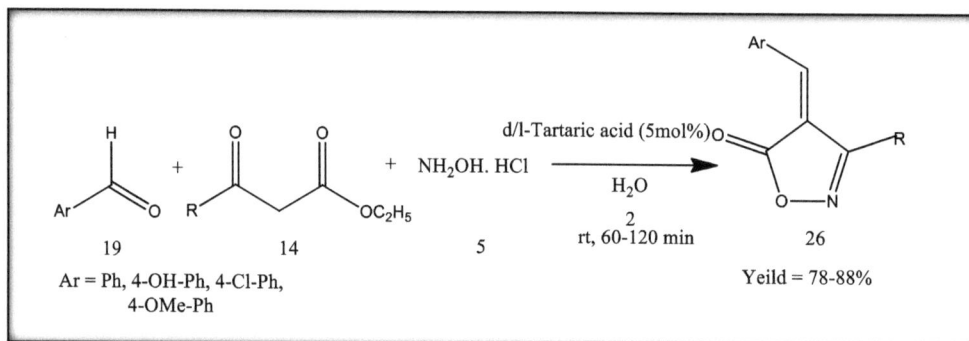

**Fig. (15).**  Synthesis of 3-methyl-4-arylmethylene-isoxazol-5(4*H*)-ones.

**Table 2. Effect of catalyst.**

| Entry | Catalyst | Reaction time (min) | Yield (%) |
|-------|----------|---------------------|-----------|
| 1 | Sodium citrate | 120 | 85 |
| 2 | Sodium saccharin | 100 | 90 |
| 3 | Sodium benzoate | 150 | 88 |
| 4 | dl-Tartaric acid | 100 | 88 |

**Table 3. Effect of mole % of dl -Tartaric acid.**

| Entry | dl-tartaric Acid (mole%) | Reaction Time (min) | Yield (%) |
|-------|--------------------------|---------------------|-----------|
| 1 | 2 | 135 | 65 |
| 2 | 5 | 120 | 80 |
| 3 | 7 | 100 | 82 |
| 4 | 10 | 100 | 85 |
| 5 | 15 | 100 | 88 |
| 6 | 20 | 100 | 88 |

## 1.2. Properties of Isoxazoles

### 1.2.1. Physical Properties

Isoxazole is a colorless liquid with a boiling point of 94.5°C. It is soluble in various organic solvents with a pyridine-like odor. It is a very weak base with a pKa of 1.3. It is less aromatic as compared to other five-membered heterocyclic compounds. Its dipole moment in benzene is 3.3 D [24]. The spectral property of isoxazole is presented in Table **4**.

**Table 4. Spectral data of Isoxazole.**

| UV ($H_2O$), $\lambda_{max}$ (nm) ($\varepsilon$) | $^1$H NMR (CCl$_4$), $\delta$ (ppm) | $^{13}$C (CDCl$_3$), $\delta$ (ppm) |
|---|---|---|
| 211 | C$_3$–H, 8.19; C$_4$–H, 6.32; C$_5$–H, 8.44 | C$_3$, 149.1; C$_4$, 103.7; C$_5$, 157.9 |

## 1.2.2. Chemical Properties

Isoxazole is a π-excessive heterocycle that contains typical properties of furan and pyridine. Isoxazole is an aromatic heterocycle, and its aromaticity is mainly influenced by the presence of heteroatoms (O and N) in the five-membered ring. It undergoes different reactions, including electrophilic substitution, nucleophilic substitution, oxidation, reduction, Diels-Alder reactions *etc* [25].

### 1.2.2.1. Electrophilic Substitution Reaction

In the case of isoxazole, electrophilic substitution occurs more readily than pyridine. Generally, the electrophilic attack occurs at the C$_4$ position of the isoxazole ring (**1**) due to the presence of high electron density at this atom. The common electrophilic reactions include nitration, sulfonation, chloromethylation, hydroxymethylation, halogenation (chlorination, iodination), *etc.* (Fig. **16**) [26].

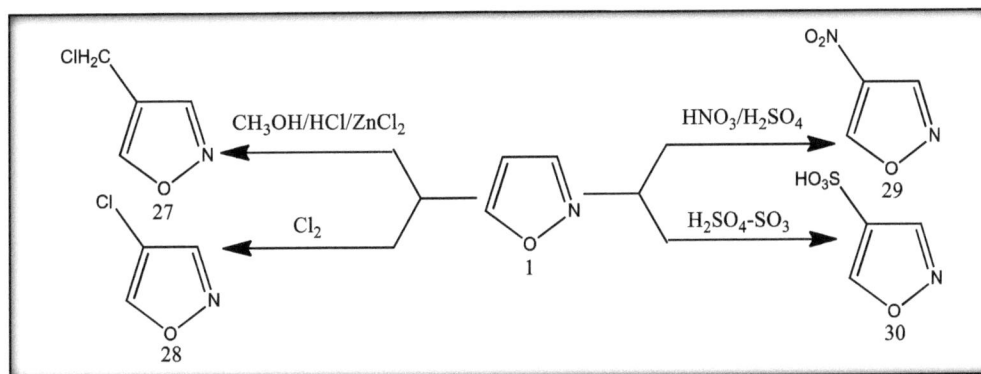

**Fig. (16).** Electrophilic substitution reaction.

## *1.2.2.2. Nucleophilic Substitution Reaction*

5-chloro-isoxazole (**31**) undergoes nucleophilic substitution reaction if there is the presence of activating substituent at the $C_4$-position (Fig. **17**) [27].

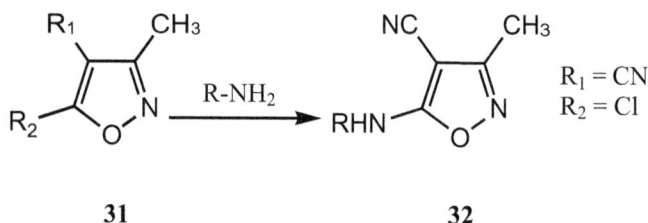

**Fig. (17).** Nucleophilic substitution reaction.

## *1.2.2.3. Oxidation Reactions*

Isoxazoles are less stable toward oxidizing agents.3,4,5-triphenyl-isoxazole (**34**) undergoes oxidation with $O_3$ to produce acyclic benzyl mono-oxime phenyl ester (**35**). Similarly, the oxidation of isoxazoles in the presence of $KMnO_4$, the unsaturated carbon side chain of isoxazoles is oxidized to the corresponding carboxylic acid derivatives (**33**) (Fig. **18**) [28].

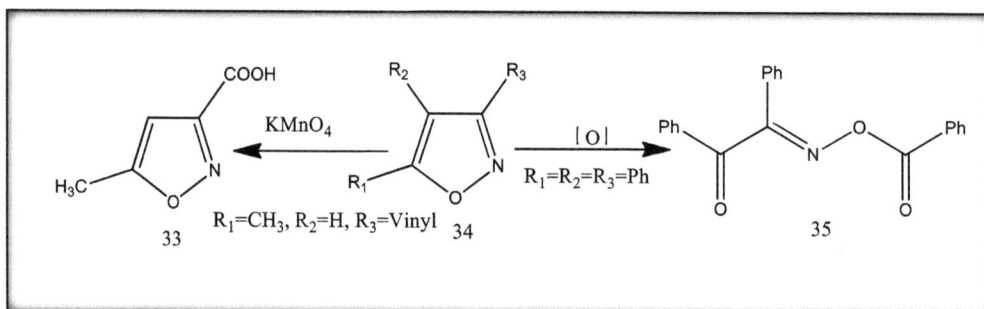

**Fig. (18).** Oxidation reactions.

## *1.2.2.4. Reduction Reactions*

Isoxazoles (**36**) readily undergo a reduction in the presence of reducing agents with cleavage of the weak O-N bond that produces acyclic products (**37**). The formation of the final products depends on the nature of the reducing agent involved in the reaction (Fig. **19**) [29].

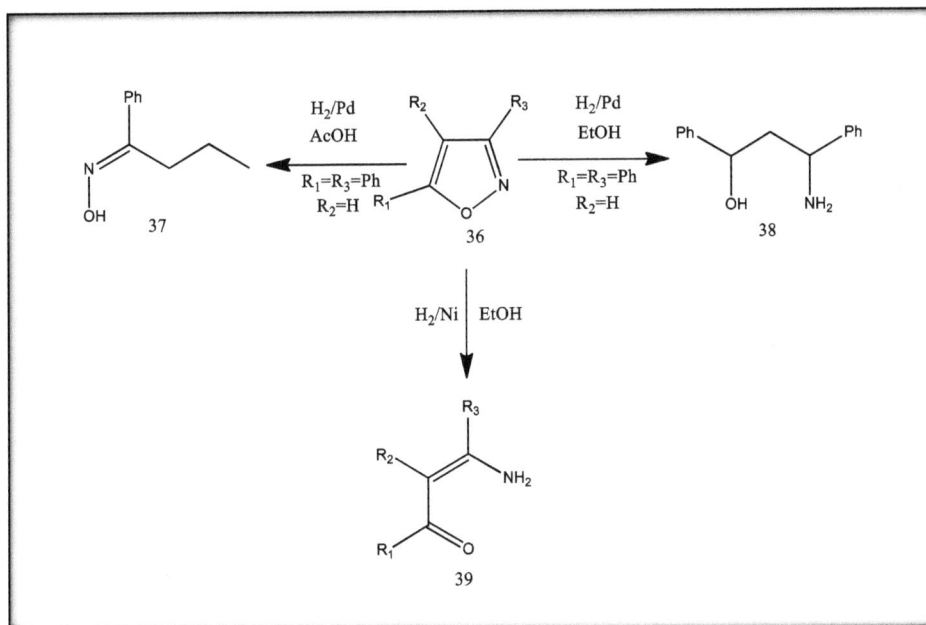

**Fig. (19).** Reduction reactions.

## *1.2.2.5. Diels-Alder Reactions*

Isoxazole (**40**) undergoes a cyclo-addition reaction as dienophiles and reacts with butadienes to produce the Diels-Alder adduct (**41**). The presence of electron-attracting groups on the isoxazole ring facilitates the reaction. This synthetic protocol is applied successfully to synthesize various pyridoisoxazoles (**42**) on the reaction of the 4-nitro-3-phenylisoxazole with a suitable diene (dimethylhydrazone or methacrolein) (Fig. **20**) [30].

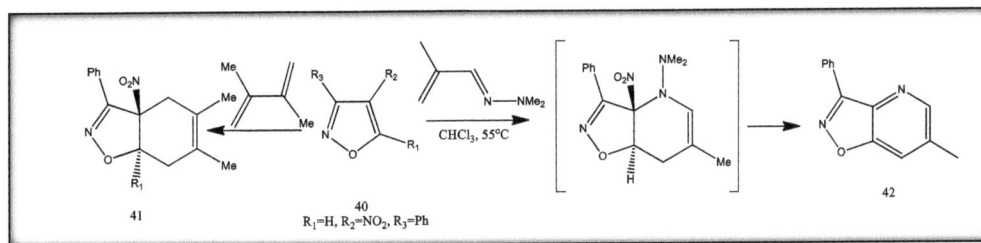

**Fig. (20).** Diels-Alder Reactions.

## 2. PHARMACOLOGICAL ACTIVITIES OF ISOXAZOLE DERIVATIVES

Isoxazole derivatives possess various promising pharmacological activities such as anti-bacterial, antifungal, diuretic, antiviral, anti-cancer, anti-tubercular, diuretic, muscle relaxant, anticonvulsant, analgesic and anti-inflammatory, *etc.* (Fig. **21**) [31, 32].

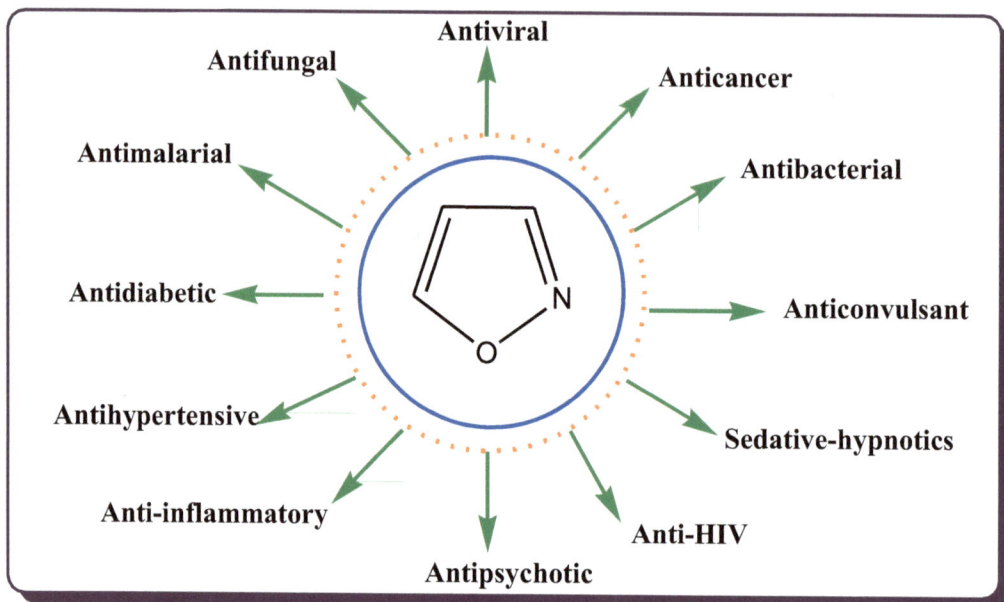

**Fig. (21).**  Pharmacological activities of Isoxazole derivatives.

Isoxazole forms the basis for different drug molecules such as leflunomide (antirheumatic drug), valdecoxib (non-steroidal anti-inflammatory drug), and zonisamide (anti-convulsant drug) [33]. Similarly, isoxazole derivatives, such as isocarboxazid, act as monoamine oxidase inhibitors. It is used to treat symptoms of depression that may include anxiety, panic, or phobias [34]. Whereas, the isoxazole derivatives, including sulfamethoxazole, sulfisoxazole, and oxacillin are used clinically to treat a wide variety of bacterial infections (Table **5**) [35].

**Table 5. List of drugs used clinically with Isoxazole scaffold.**

| Drug | Chemical Structure | Pharmacological Activity |
|---|---|---|
| Ibetonic acid |  | Brain-lesioning agent |

*(Table 5) cont.....*

| Drug | Chemical Structure | Pharmacological Activity |
|------|--------------------|--------------------------|
| Valdecoxib | | Non-steroidal anti-inflammatory drug (NSAID) |
| Flucloxacillin | | Antibiotic |
| Cloxacillin | | Antibiotic |
| Danazol | | Androgenic hormone |
| Risperidone | | Antipsychotic |
| Zonisamide | | Anticonvulsant |
| Cycloserine | | Antibiotic |

(Table 5) cont.....

| Drug | Chemical Structure | Pharmacological Activity |
|---|---|---|
| Acivicin | **51** | Antineoplastic agent |
| Sulfamethoxazo le | **52** | Antibiotic |
| Isoxaflutole | **53** | Herbicide |
| Isocarboxazid | **54** | Antidepressant |
| Teriflunomide | **55** | Immunomodulatory |

## 2.1. Isoxazoles as Antioxidants

Sherin *et al.* synthesized 3,5-bis(styryl)isoxazoles (**56**) derived from curcuminoids by mechanochemical grinding of the curcuminoids with hydroxylamine hydrochloride catalyzed by glacial acetic acid (Fig. **22**) and evaluated for antioxidant activity by DPPH, FRAP, and $\beta$-carotene assay methods. The presence of hydroxyl and methoxy groups on the terminal aryl moieties of 3,5-bis(styryl)isoxazoles improved the antioxidant activity [36].

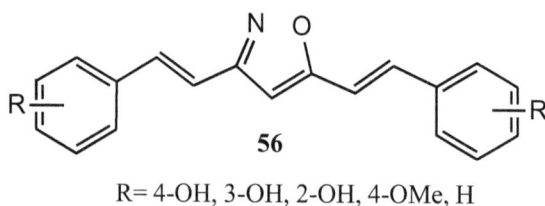

**56**

R= 4-OH, 3-OH, 2-OH, 4-OMe, H

**Fig. (22).** Isoxazole derivatives showing antioxidant activity.

## 2.2. Isoxazoles as Immunosuppressive Agents

Maczynski *et al.* reported the synthesis, immunosuppressive properties, and mechanism of action of a new series of isoxazole derivatives (**57**). It involves the reaction of 5-amino-N,3-dimethyl-1,2-oxazole-4-carbohydrazide with relevant carbonyl compounds (Fig. **23**). The tested compounds were found to inhibit phytohemagglutinin A (PHA)-induced proliferation of peripheral blood mononuclear cells (PBMCs). The cytotoxicity of the tested compounds was determined by measuring the growth of the human tumor epithelial lung A549 cell line. The results were presented as optical density (OD) values. The inhibition was significant at a concentration of 6.25 μM [37].

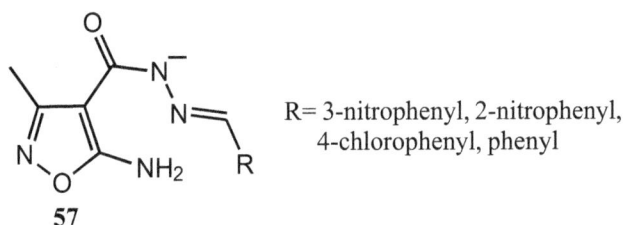

R= 3-nitrophenyl, 2-nitrophenyl, 4-chlorophenyl, phenyl

**Fig. (23).** Isoxazole derivatives showing immunosuppressive activity.

## 2.3. Isoxazoles with Hypolipidemic Activity

Mokale *et al.* synthesized a series of 2-methyl-2-(substituted phenyl isoxazole) phenoxyacetic acid derivatives (**58**) (Fig. **24**) and evaluated them for *in vivo* hypolipidemic activity by triton induced hyperlipidemia in rats. Most of the compounds could lower the elevated lipid levels, amongst which compounds **58a,** **58b,** and **58c** were found to be most active as compared to the standard drug Fenofibrate. Further, SAR studies revealed that the isoxazole ring is important for hypolipidemic activity [38].

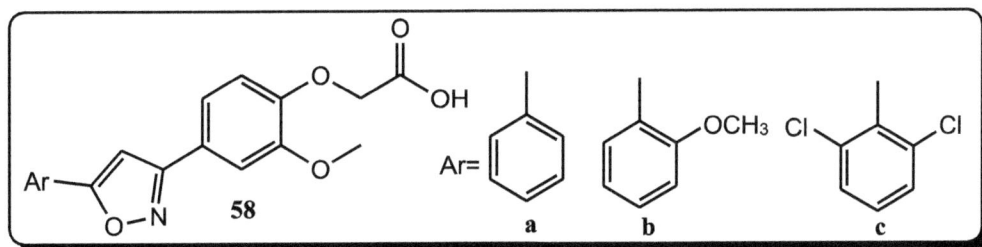

**Fig. (24).** Isoxazole derivatives showing hypolipidemic activity.

## 2.4. Isoxazoles as Anti-Microbial Agents

Saravanan *et al.* reported the synthesis, analgesic, anti-inflammatory, and *in vitro* antimicrobial activities of some novel isoxazole coupled quinazoline-4(3*H*)-one derivative (**60**). Target compounds were synthesized by adding hydroxylamine hydrochloride (**5**) infraction with the well-stirred mixture of 2-methyl-3-(4-(3-(substitutedphenyl)acryloyl)phenyl)quinazoline-4(3*H*)-one4a–4l (**59**) in ethanol (25 mL). To this catalytic quantity of sodium acetate and glacial acetic acid was added. The reaction mixture was then refluxed for a period of 10 h. Then the reaction mixture was cooled and poured into ice-cold water. The products were separated by filtration, washed, and vacuum dried. Finally, the products were recrystallized using ethanol to get pure form (Fig. **25**) [39].

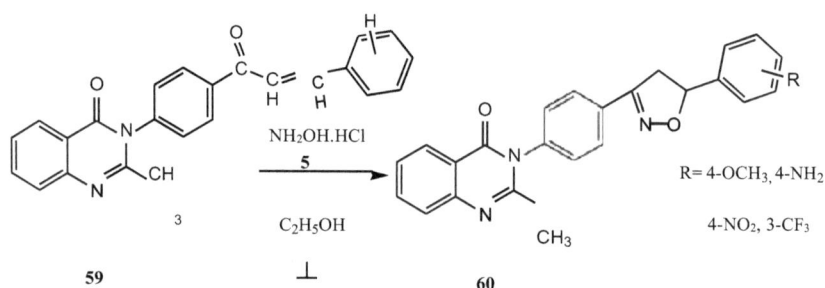

**Fig. (25).** Synthesis of isoxazole coupled quinazoline-4(3*H*)-one derivative.

Moreover, the electron-withdrawing group substituted derivatives showed remarkable antimicrobial properties than electron releasing group substituted compounds. Among several tested compounds, 2-methyl-3-(4-(5-(4-(trifluoro-methyl) phenyl) isoxazole-3-yl)phenyl)quinazoline-4(3*H*)-one **60e** showed better analgesic and anti-inflammatory activity which is more potent than reference standard Diclofenac (Fig. **26**) [40].

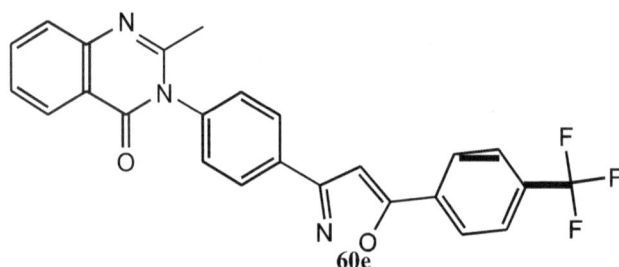

**Fig. (26).** Structure of isoxazole clubbed with quinazoline-4(3*H*)-one.

Esfahani *et al.* demonstrated the synthesis of some novel coumarin isoxazole-sulfonamide hybrid compounds (**61**). All of the synthesized products were evaluated for the antibacterial property against *Escherichia coli* (ATCC 25922) as Gram-negative and *Staphylococcus aureus* (ATCC 25923) as Gram-positive bacteria using the disk diffusion method. Derivatives, including halogen groups (Cl, Br) in *para* position (**61c, 61d**), showed higher antibacterial activity against *S. aureus* than *E coli* (Fig. **27**) [41].

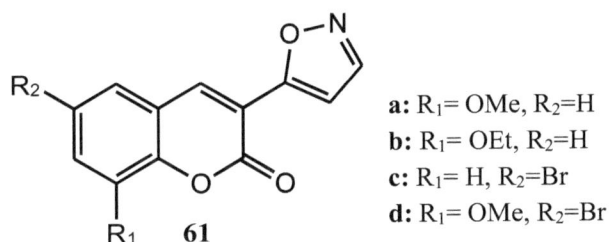

**a:** $R_1$= OMe, $R_2$=H
**b:** $R_1$= OEt, $R_2$=H
**c:** $R_1$= H, $R_2$=Br
**d:** $R_1$= OMe, $R_2$=Br

**Fig. (27).** Structure of biologically active coumarin-isoxazole hybrids.

Sahoo *et al.* performed the microwave-induced synthesis of substituted isoxazoles as potential anti-microbial agents. A series of isoxazole derivatives (**63**) were obtained by the reaction of Chalcones (**62**) with hydroxylamine hydrochloride in the presence of sodium acetate (Fig. **28**). Both microwave and conventional heating techniques are utilized to compare their product yields and reaction time. The antimicrobial activities of the synthesized compounds were evaluated *in vitro* against different bacterial and fungal strains. Ampicillin and Ketoconazole were used as reference drugs for antibacterial and antifungal activities, respectively. Various bacterial strains include *Staphylococcus aureus* (MTCC 87), *Escherichia coli* (MTCC 40), *Staphylococcus epidermidis* (MTCC 2639), *Pseudomonas aeruginosa*, whereas fungal stains include *Candida albicans* (MTCC 183) and *Aspergillus niger* (MTCC 281). All the tested compounds exhibited promising antimicrobial activity as compared to the standard drugs [42].

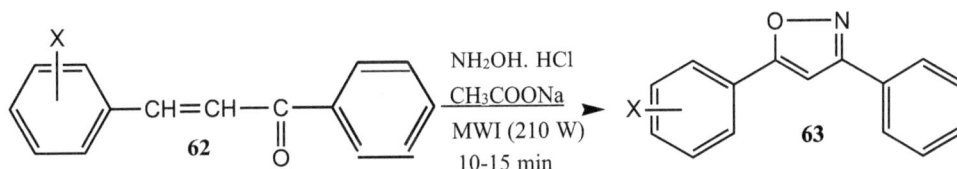

**Fig. (28).** Microwave-induced synthesis of substituted isoxazoles.

A series of chloro-substituted 4-aryl-isoxazoles (**65**) have been synthesized by the interaction of chloro-substituted-3-aroylflavones (**64**) with hydroxyl amine hydro chloride (**5**) (Fig. **29**). The reaction mixture was refluxed for two hours in the presence of ethanol and piperidine. The synthesized compounds were evaluated for their antifungal activity against different fungal strains of *Aspergillus niger, Rhizopus species, Curvularia lunata, Drechslera tetramera, Fusarium species, Bipolaris sorokeniana* by using the cup plate diffusion method. The tested compounds showed significant antifungal activity [43].

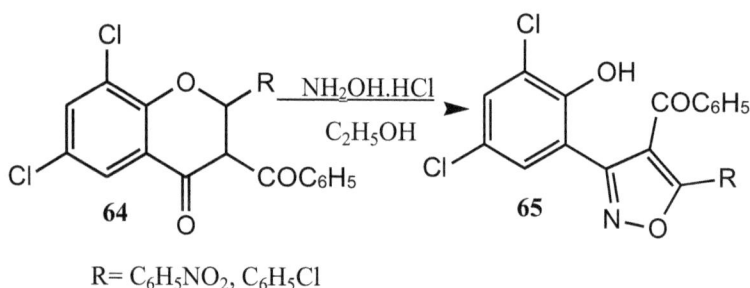

R= $C_6H_5NO_2$, $C_6H_5Cl$

**Fig. (29).** Synthesis of chloro-substituted 4-aryl-isoxazoles.

Murthy *et al.* reported the synthesis of novel 5-(heteroaryl)isoxazole derivatives (**67**). The synthetic process involves the [3+2] route of isoxazoles containing C-C-C and N=O fragments (Fig. **30**). In this case, 3- (dimethylamino)acryloalkanone was employed as C-C-C synthon and hydroxylamine hydrochloride or hydroxylamine-O-sulfonic acid as the N=O synthon. 3-(dimethylamino)acryloalkanone (**66**) undergoes a reaction with hydroxylamine hydrochloride in methanol to afford the required 5- (heteroaryl)isoxazole derivatives.

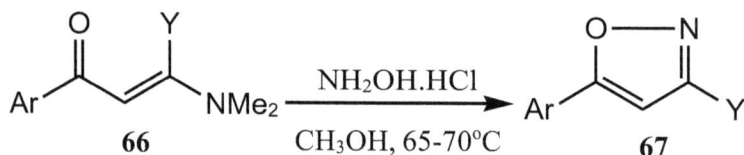

**Fig. (30).** Synthesis of novel 5-(heteroaryl)isoxazole derivatives.

Antibacterial activity of the 5-(heteroaryl)isoxazoles (**67a-n**) was evaluated against *E. coli* (NCIM 2065), *Staphylococcus aureus* (NCIM 2079), *Pseudomonas aeruginosa* (NCIM 2200) by the cup plate method. Among the tested compounds, Compounds **67a** and **67b** exhibited significant activity as compared to the reference standard (Sulfamethoxazole) (Fig. **31**), (Table **6**) [44].

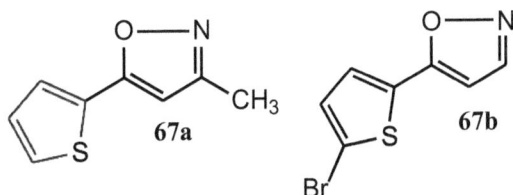

**Fig. (31).** Structure of compounds 67a and 67b.

**Table 6. Anti-bacterial activity of isoxazoles (200 mg/mL).**

| Compound | Zones of Inhibition | | |
|---|---|---|---|
| | *E. coli* | *Pseudomonas areginosa* | *Staphylococcus aureus* |
| **67a** | 15±0.2 | 18±0.2 | 30±0.2 |
| **67b** | 14±0.2 | 16±0.2 | 26±0.2 |
| Sulfamethoxazole (reference) | 28±0.2 | 30±0.2 | 40±0.2 |

## 2.5. Isoxazoles with Anti-Tubercular Activity

Substituted isoxazoline derivatives (**70**) were synthesized by using substituted acetophenones (**68**) and substituted benzaldehydes (**19**) *via* cyclization of substituted chalcone (**69**) in the presence of hydroxylamine hydrochloride (**5**) (Fig. **32**). The synthesized compounds were evaluated for *in vitro* anti-tubercular activity against *M. tuberculosis*. They exhibited promising anti-tubercular activity as compared to the standard drug Rifampicin [45].

Mao *et al.* performed the synthesis of mefloquine-isoxazole carboxylic esters and evaluated them for their anti-tubercular activity. Compound 71 (Fig. **33**) was found to possess promising activity and specificity against MTB $H_{37}Rv$ both intracellularly and extracellularly [46].

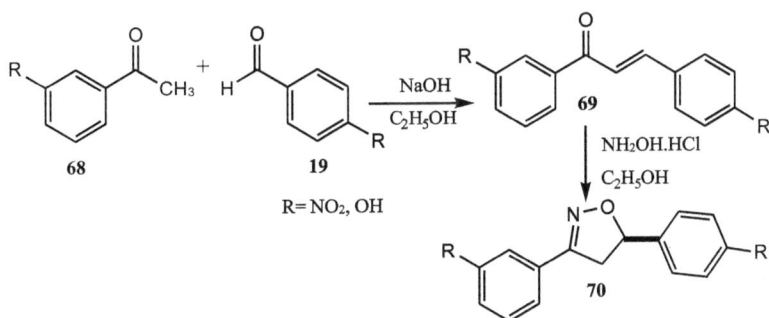

**Fig. (32).** Synthesis of substituted isoxazoline derivatives.

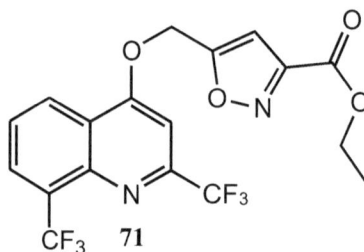

**Fig. (33).** Structure of mefloquine-isoxazole carboxylic esters.

Harinadha *et al.* demonstrated the synthesis and antitubercular activity of isoxazole incorporated 1,2,3-triazole derivatives. It involves cyclization of 1-azido-4- methoxy benzene (**72**) with acetylacetone (**73**) in the presence of sodium ethoxide to produce 1-(4-methoxyphenyl)-5-methyl-1H-1,2,3-triazole-4-yl) ethanone (**74**). Further, compound **74** undergoes Claisen-Schmidt condensation with different aromatic and heterocyclic aldehydes (**19**) to afford triazolyl Chalcones (**75**), which on refluxing with hydroxylamine hydrochloride (**5**) in glacial acetic acid produces 4-(5-(4-substituted phenyl)isoxazole-3- yl)-1-(4-methoxyphenyl)-5-methyl-1H- 1,2,3-triazoles (**76**) in good yields (Fig. **34**).

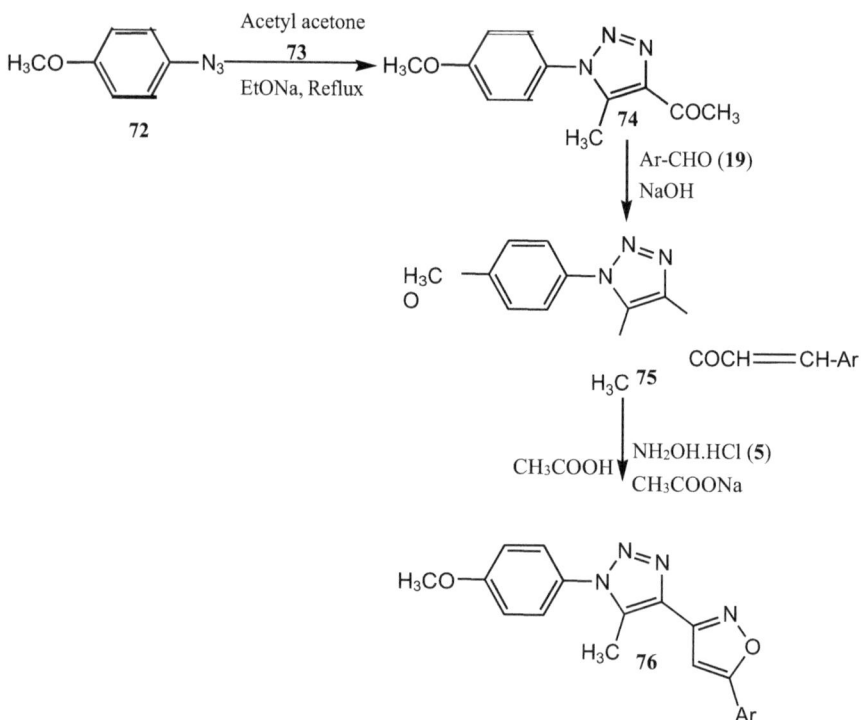

**Fig. (34).** Synthesis of isoxazole incorporated 1,2,3-triazole derivatives.

All the synthesized compounds were evaluated for anti-tubercular activity against *Mycobacterium tuberculosis* H37Rv and DKU 156 strains by using the broth dilution assay method. Some of the tested compounds exhibited good activity as compared to the standard drug, Isoniazid (Table **7**) [47].

**Table 7. Anti-tubercular activity of isoxazole incorporated 1,2,3-triazole derivatives.**

| Entry | Ar | MIC Values (µg/mL) *Mycobacterium tuberculosis* | |
|---|---|---|---|
| | | **H37Rv** | **DKU 156** |
| 76a | (phenyl, Cl) | 1.25 | 2.5 |
| 76b | (phenyl, F) | >10 | >10 |
| 76c | (phenyl, NO$_2$) | 5 | 5 |
| 76d | (phenyl, F) | 0.625 | 1.25 |
| 76e | (phenyl, Cl) | 0.625 | 1.25 |
| 76f | (phenyl, NO$_2$) | 2.5 | 5 |
| Isoniazid | - | 0.625 | 10 |

A series of 3-isoxazolecarboxylic acid esters derivatives (**77, 78**) was designed and evaluated for their activity against replicating and non-replicating *Mycobacterium tuberculosis* (Fig. **35**). These compounds exhibited good selectivity towards *Mtb* and displayed no cytotoxicity on Vero cells (IC$_{50}$> 128 M) [48].

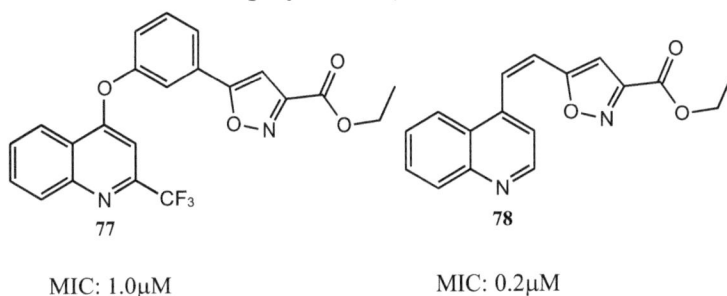

MIC: 1.0µM                MIC: 0.2µM

**Fig. (35).** Structure of 3-isoxazole carboxylic acid esters derivatives (77, 78).

A new series of 5-aryl-ethenyl isoxazole carboxylate derivatives were synthesized. The synthetic protocol involves the condensation of compound (**79**) and diethyl oxalate (**80**) to afford key intermediates (**81**) and transform into the final isoxazoles (**82**) by treatment with hydroxylamine hydrochloride (**5**) in ethanol and $H_2SO_4$ (Fig. **36**). The target compounds were evaluated for their *in vitro* activity against *Mycobacterium tuberculosis* H37Rv. The tested compounds exhibited minimum inhibitory concentrations in the low micro molar range (2.3-11.4 μM) [49].

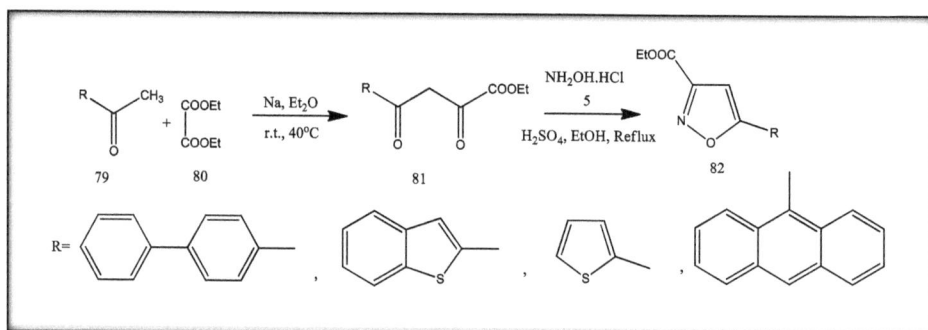

**Fig. (36).** Synthesis of 5-aryl-ethenyl isoxazole carboxylate derivatives.

Hamadi *et al.* reported the synthesis of carbohydrate-substituted isoxazoles (**83**). It involves the [3+2] cyclo-addition reaction of aromatic nitrile oxides with propargyl *O*-glycoside derivatives (Fig. **37**). The synthesized compounds were evaluated for their anti-tubercular activity against the *Mycobacterium tuberculosis H37Rv* strain (ATCC27294) using the agar dilution method. Several compounds significantly inhibit the growth of the bacterial strain with an MIC of 3.125 μg/mL in comparison with the standard drug, ethambutol [50].

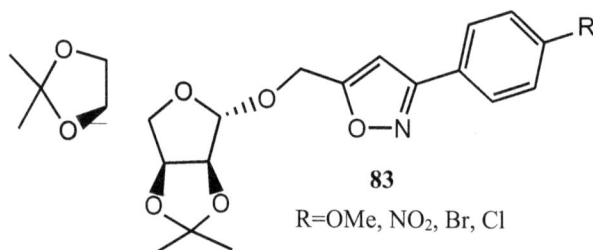

R=OMe, NO$_2$, Br, Cl

**Fig. (37).** Structure of carbohydrate-substituted isoxazoles.

A series of novel pyrimidine-linked isoxazole derivatives were synthesized that involve acid-catalyzed condensation of 4-substituted acetophenones (**85**) with isoxazole-3-carbaldehyde (**84**) to afford chalcones (**86**). Further, chalcones react with guanidine hydrochloride (**87**) in the presence of ethanolic potassium hydroxide solution to produce target compounds (**88**) (Fig. **38**).

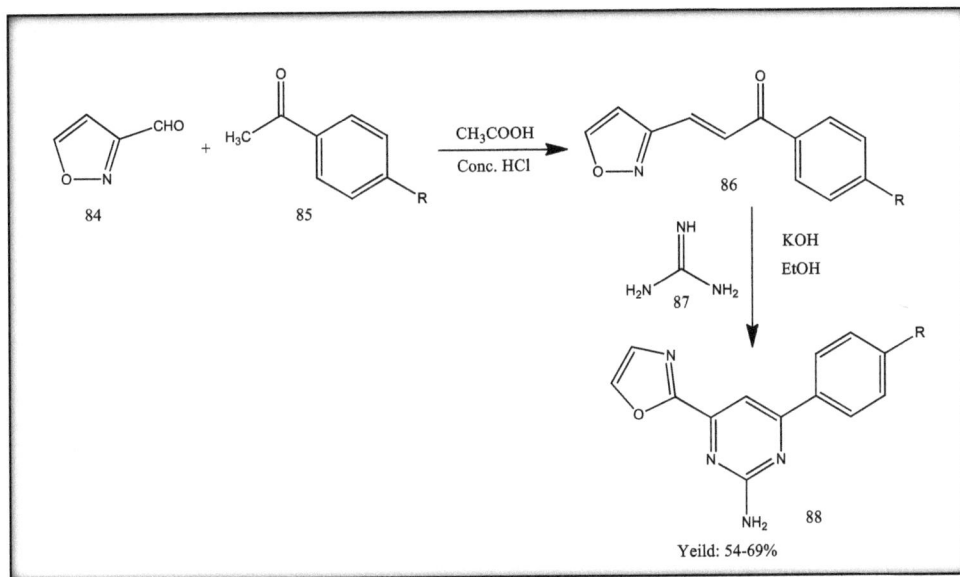

**Fig. (38).** Synthesis of clubbed isoxazole-pyrimidine derivatives.

The anti-tubercular activity of the target compounds was carried out against the strain of *Mycobacterium tuberculosis* H37Rv. Among the series, compounds **88h** and **88j** displayed promising anti-tubercular activity with an MIC of 0.78µg/ml and 1.562 µg/mL, respectively, than the reference drug (Pyrazinamide) (Fig. **39**), (Table **8**) [51].

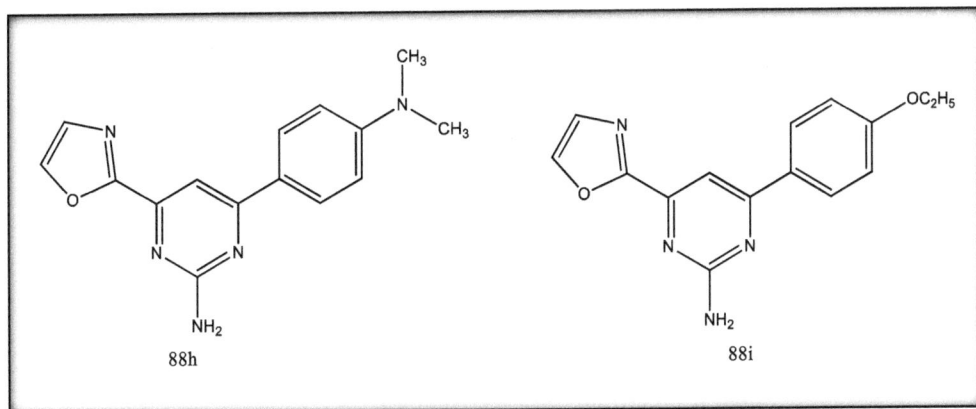

**Fig. (39).** Structure of compounds 88h and 88j.

Table 8. Anti-tubercular activity pyrimidine-linked isoxazole derivatives.

| Entry | R | MIC (μg/mL) *Mycobacterium tuberculosis* H37Rv |
|---|---|---|
| 88a | Bromo | 25 |
| 88b | Chloro | 50 |
| 88c | Fluoro | 50 |
| 88d | Trifluoromethyl | 100 |
| 88e | Methyl | 6.25 |
| 88f | Hydroxy | 3.125 |
| 88g | Amino | 3.125 |
| 88h | Dimethyl amino | 0.78 |
| 88i | Methoxy | 3.125 |
| 88j | Ethoxy | 1.562 |
| Standard drug | Pyrazinamide | 3.125 |

## 2.6. Isoxazoles with Anti-Stress Activity

Maurya *et al.* synthesized 3,5-disubstituted isoxazolines (**89**) and evaluated their anti-stress potential under acute stress conditions concerning peripheral and biochemical changes. Some compounds **89a and 89b** displayed protective effects against acute stress-induced elevation in gastric ulceration, adrenal hypertrophy, hyperglycemia, plasma creatine kinase activity, and corticosterone levels (Fig. **40**) [52].

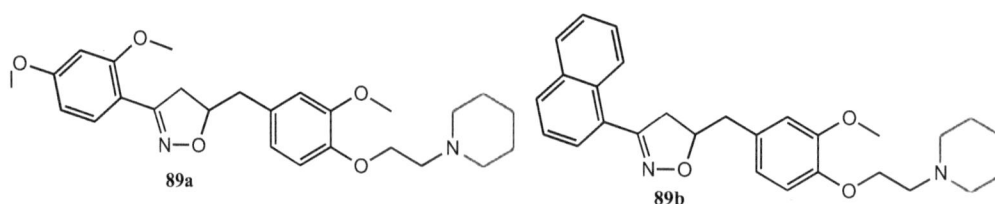

**Fig. (40).** Structure of 3,5-disubstituted isoxazolines.

Badru *et al.* synthesized a series of pyrroloisoxazole derivatives *via* 1,3-dipolar cycloaddition of azomethine N-oxides with N-(α-naphthyl) maleimide. Compound **90** (Fig. **41**) exhibited significant anti-stress activity in immobilization stress- induced increase in non-social behaviour [53].

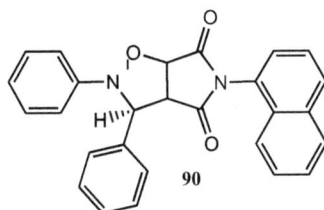

**Fig. (41).** Structure of pyrrolo isoxazole derivatives.

## 2.7. Isoxazoles as Anticancer Agents

Wang *et al.* demonstrated the design and synthesis of a series of isoxazole-naphthalene derivatives (**95**) as tubulin polymerization inhibitors (Fig. **42**). The synthesized compounds were evaluated for their antiproliferative activity against human breast cancer cell line MCF-7. Most of the tested compounds exhibited moderate to potent anti-proliferative activity ($IC_{50} < 10.0 \mu M$) as compared to the standard drug cisplatin ($15.24 \pm 1.27 \mu M$).

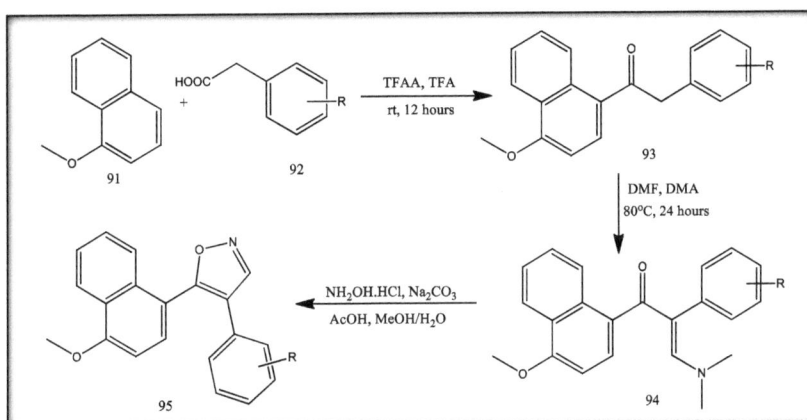

| Compound | R | Compound | R |
|----------|---|----------|---|
| 95a | 3,4,5-triOMe | 95f | 2-OMe |
| 95b | 4-OMe | 95g | 3-F-4-OMe |
| 95c | 4-Me | 95h | 3-OMe |
| 95d | 4-Cl | 95i | 3,4-diOMe |
| 95e | 2-Cl | 95j | 4-OEt |

**Fig. (42).** Scheme for the synthesis of isoxazole-naphthalene derivatives.

Among the tested compounds, compound **95j** containing 4-ethoxy substitution at the phenyl ring was found to be the most active compound with an $IC_{50}$ value of

$1.23 \pm 0.16\mu M$. Furthermore, the *in vitro* tubulin polymerization assay method reported that compound **95j** exhibited better inhibition activity on tubulin polymerization with $IC_{50}$ of 3.4μMas compared to standard drug colchicine ($IC_{50}$= 7.5μM) (Fig. **43**) [54].

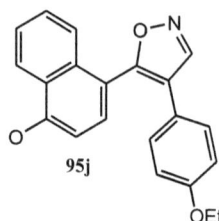

**95j**

| Compound | R | Compound | R |
|----------|---|----------|-----|
| 99a | H | 99f | 2-NO2 |

**Fig. (43).** Structure of compound 95j with 4-ethoxy substitution at the phenyl ring.

Burmaoglu *et al.* carried out the design, synthesis, and evaluation of 3,5-diaryl isoxazole derivatives (**99**) as potential anticancer agents. It involves the condensation of trimethoxy-acetophenone (**96**) with substituted benzaldehydes (**19**) in an aqueous solution of KOH afforded chalcone derivatives (**97**)(yield: 70-90%). Further, the chalcone derivatives (**97**) react with tosyl-hydroxylamine (TsNHOH) (**98**) in the presence of $K_2CO_3$ and $H_2O$ in MeOH afforded the isoxazole derivatives (**99**) in 60-78% yield (Fig. **44**).

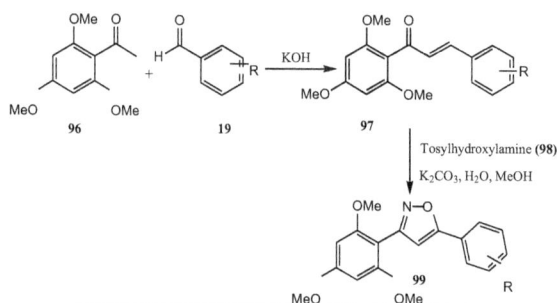

| 99b | 2-F | 99g | 3-Br |
|-----|-----|-----|-------|
| 99c | 3-F | 99h | 3-Cl |
| 99d | 4-F | 99i | 4-Cl |
| 99e | 4-Br | 99j | 3,4-F2 |

**Fig. (44).** Synthesis of 3,5-diaryl isoxazole derivatives.

The anticancer potential of target compounds was performed by using cancer PC3 cells and non-tumorigenic PNT1a cells. Within the tested compounds, compound **99c** exhibited high selectivity towards cancer cells (PC3 cancer cell line) with $IC_{50}$ of 15.893 µM as compared to standard drug 5-FU (Fig. **45**) [55].

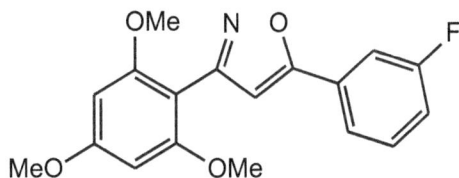

**Fig. (45).** Structure of compound 99c.

A series of isoxazole-piperazine analogs (**100**) were synthesized and evaluated for their antiproliferative activity against hepatocellular carcinoma (HCC; Huh7/Mahlavu) and breast (MCF-7) cancer cells. All the tested compounds displayed potent to moderate cytotoxicity on all cell lines with $IC_{50}$ values in the range of 0.09-11.7µM (Fig. **46**) [56].

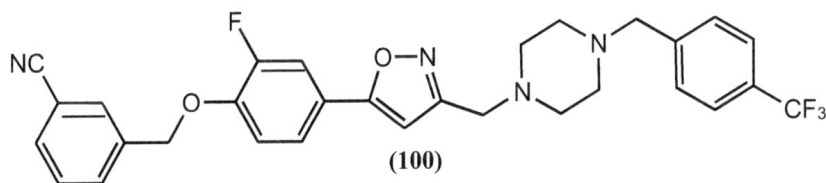

(100)

$IC_{50}$: 0.09µM(Huh7)

$IC_{50}$: 0.50µM(Mahlavu)

$IC_{50}$: 0.38µM(MCF-7)

**Fig. (46).** Structure of isoxazole-piperazine analogs.

A novel series of isoxazole-piperazine hybrids were synthesized. Hence, diethyloxalate (**101**) is treated with substituted acetophenones (**102**) in the presence of a base to get *β*-ketoesters (**103**). Theintermediates (**103**) were subsequently cyclized with hydroxylamine hydrochloride to provide isoxazole esters (**104**). Reduction of compound (**104**) with $LiAlH_4$ or $NaBH_4$ followed by bromination with $CBr_4$/PPh3 provided isoxazole methylbromides (**106**). Finally, these intermediate alkyl bromides were treated with 4-trifluoromethyl-benzylpiperazine (**107**) to achieve target compounds (**108**) (Fig. **47**).

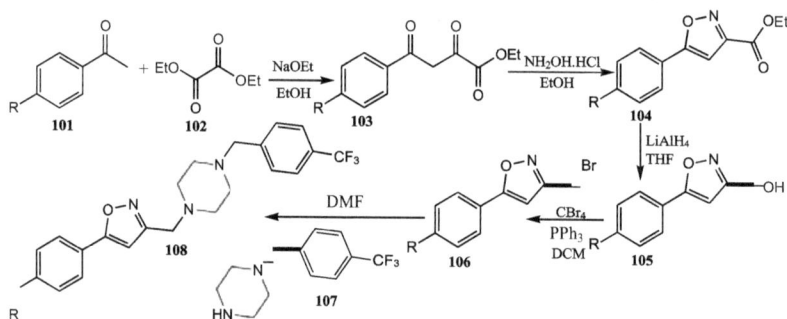

**Fig. (47).** Synthesis of isoxazole-piperazine hybrids.

| Compound | R | Compound | R |
|----------|-----|----------|---------|
| 108a | H | 108f | 4-iPr |
| 108b | 2-F | 108g | 4-OCF$_3$ |
| 108c | 3-Cl | 108h | 3-Cl |
| 108d | 4-CH$_3$ | 108i | 4-OH |
| 108e | 4-CF$_3$ | 108j | 4-OCH$_3$ |

The target compounds were evaluated for their cytotoxic activities against the human liver (Huh7 and Mahlavu) and breast (MCF-7) cancer cell lines. Among the series, compound (**108i**) exhibited potential cytotoxic activity on all cell lines with IC$_{50}$ values in the range of 0.3-3.7μM (Fig. **48**) [57].

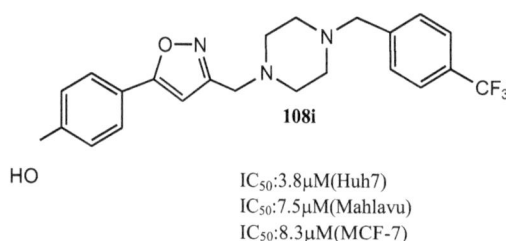

**108i**

HO

IC$_{50}$:3.8μM(Huh7)
IC$_{50}$:7.5μM(Mahlavu)
IC$_{50}$:8.3μM(MCF-7)

**Fig. (48).** Structure of compound (108i).

Thiriveedhi *et al.* synthesized a new series of isoxazole-chalcone conjugates (**108a-k**) by the Claisen-Schmidt condensation of the substituted acetophenones with isoxazole aldehydes (Fig. **49**). The synthesized compounds were evaluated for their *in vitro* cytotoxic activity against four different human cancer cell lines by using the sulforhodamine-B (SRB) method. Potential cytotoxic activity was observed for compounds **108a**, **108b**, and **108d** against the prostate DU-145 cancer cell line (Table **9**) [58].

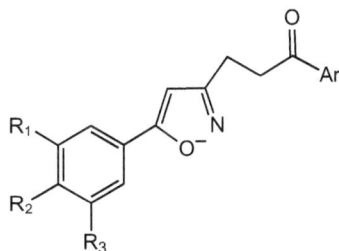

**Fig. (49).** Structure of isoxazole-chalcone conjugates.

**Table 9. Anticancer activity of isoxazole-chalcone conjugates (108a-d).**

| Compound | $R_1$ | $R_2$ | $R_3$ | Ar | $IC_{50}$ (µM) | | | |
|---|---|---|---|---|---|---|---|---|
| | | | | | DU- 145 | MDA MB- 231 | MCF-7 | A-549 |
| 108a | OCH$_3$ | OCH$_3$ | OCH$_3$ | 3,4,5-trimethoxy phenyl | 1.80 | 3.67 | 5.28 | 5.99 |
| 108b | OCH$_3$ | OCH$_3$ | OCH$_3$ | 3,4-dimethoxy phenyl | 1.72 | 3.15 | 4.25 | 6.35 |
| 108c | OCH$_3$ | OCH$_3$ | OCH$_3$ | 4-methoxy phenyl | 2.32 | 2.49 | 3.92 | 5.97 |
| 108d | OCH$_3$ | OCH$_3$ | OCH$_3$ | 4-fluorophenyl | 2.32 | 4.99 | 6.84 | 7.48 |

Narsaiah *et al.* demonstrated the synthesis of a series of novel 5-substituted isoxazole-3-carboxamide derivatives (Fig. **50**). The synthesis involves the coupling of 5-substituted isoxazole-3-carboxylic acids (**113**) with substituted-3-benzyloxy-aniline (**117**) by using DCC/HOBT as a coupling agent. The target compounds were evaluated for their cytotoxic activity on the A549 lung cancer cell line by the MTT assay method. Tested compounds exhibited moderate proliferative with low cytotoxicity [59].

## 2.8. Isoxazoles with Anti-Diabetic Activity

Duan *et al.* reported the anti-diabetic effects of novel isoxazole-based flavonoid (kaempferol) derivatives (**119**) (Fig. **51**). It was found to enhance glucose consumption at the nanomolar level ($EC_{50}$=0.8 nM) in insulin-resistant HepG2 cells as compared to that of metformin [60].

**Step-1**

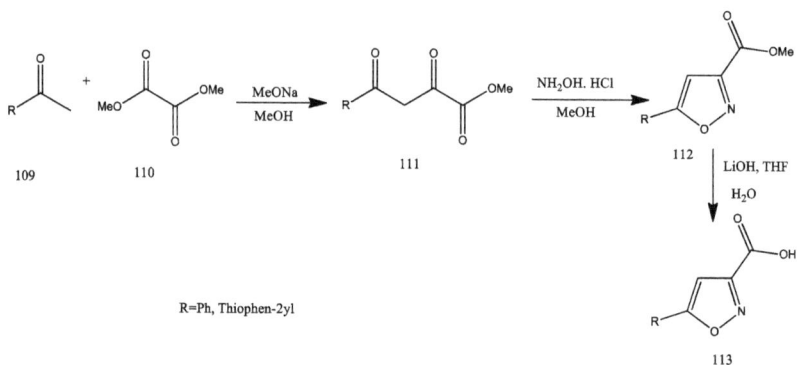

R=Ph, Thiophen-2yl

**Step-II**

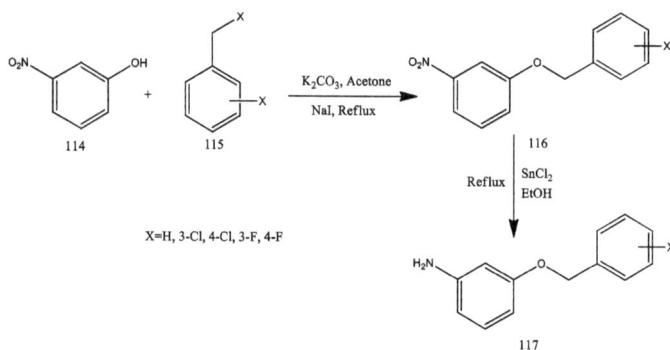

X=H, 3-Cl, 4-Cl, 3-F, 4-F

**Step-III**

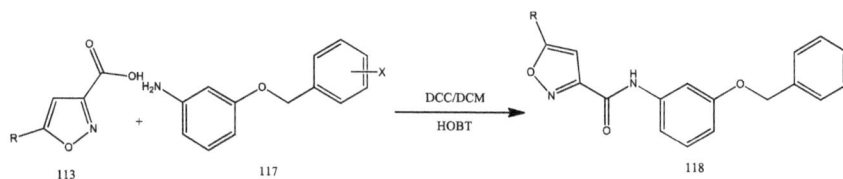

**Fig. (50).** Synthetic route to 5-substituted isoxazole-3-carboxamide derivatives.

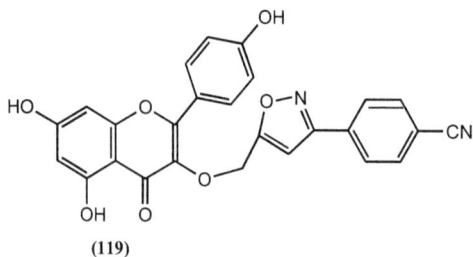

**(119)**

**Fig. (51).** Structure of isoxazole-based flavonoid (kaempferol).

Dacheng *et al.* performed the synthesis and preliminary evaluation of antidiabetic activity for β-amino ketone-containing isoxazole moiety (**122**). The β-amino ketones containing isoxazole moiety were synthesized through the Mannich reaction under mild reaction conditions with a product yield of 51.2-89.3%(Fig. **52**) [61].

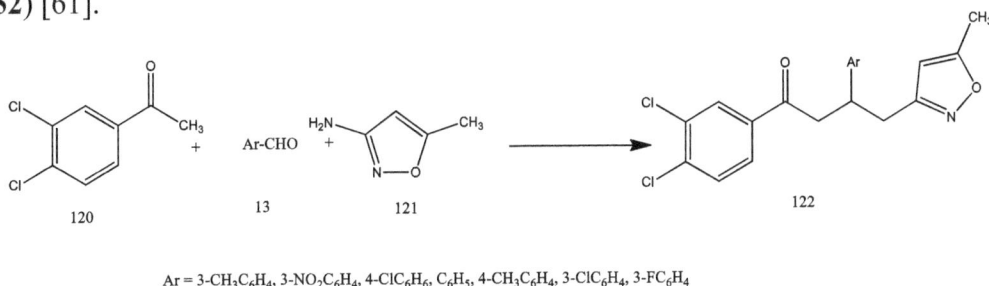

Ar = 3-CH₃C₆H₄, 3-NO₂C₆H₄, 4-ClC₆H₆, C₆H₅, 4-CH₃C₆H₄, 3-ClC₆H₄, 3-FC₆H₄

**Fig. (52).** Synthesis of β-amino ketone-containing isoxazole.

Preliminary bioassay indicated that most of the tested compounds possess weak α-glucosidase inhibitory activity and protein tyrosine phosphatase 1B inhibitory activity in low concentration. But the compound 1-(3,4-dichlorophenyl)-3-(6-methoxy-naphthalene-2-yl)-3-(5-methylisoxazole-3-ylamino)propane-1-one (**123**) has the strongest activity (75.3%) (Fig. **53**) [62].

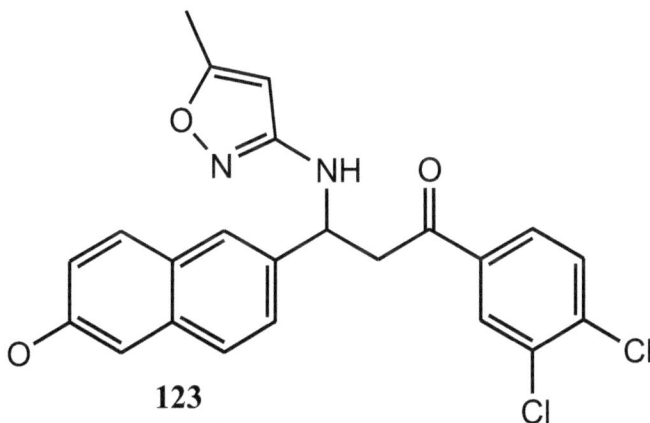

**Fig. (53).** Structure of tested compound (123) with α-glucosidase inhibitory activity.

## 2.9. Isoxazoles with Anti-Inflammatory Activity

Kapoor *et al.* reported the synthesis of new series of isoxazole derivatives *via* chalcone (**125**) (Fig. **54**). The newly synthesized compounds were evaluated for their anti-inflammatory activity *in vivo* by the carrageenan-induced paw edema method in rats. Among the series, **125c** and **125f** were found to be the most active compounds due to the presence of the methoxy group [63].

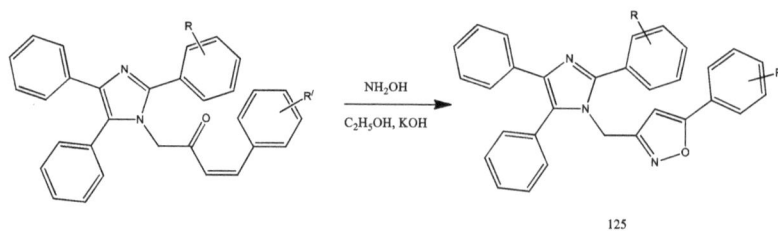

| Compound | R | R' |
|----------|---|-----|
| 125a | 4-OCH₃ | 4-CH₃ |
| 125b | 3,5-OCH₃ | 4-NO₂ |
| 125c | 4-OH, 3-OCH₃ | H |
| 125d | 4-N(CH₃)₂ | 4-CH₃ |
| 125e | 4-N(CH₃)₂ | 4-NO₂ |
| 125f | 3-OH | 3,4,5-OCH₃ |
| 125 | 3,5-OCH₃ | 3,4,5-OCH₃ |

**Fig. (54).** Synthesis of isoxazole derivatives *via* chalcone.

Fantappie *et al.* demonstrated the synthesis of 3-(3-chloro-phenyl)-5-(4-pyridyl)-4,5-dihydroisoxazole (**126**) (Fig. **55**). Both *in vitro* and *in vivo* anti-inflammatory effects of this compound were studied. It was observed that the target compound diminished the TNF-α and IL-6 release from LPS-stimulated macrophages in a dose-dependent manner. Also, it decreased the levels of COX-2 with subsequent inhibition of PGE2 production [64].

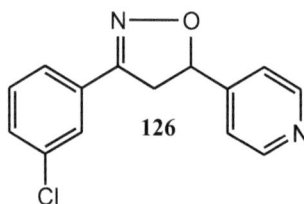

**Fig. (55).** Structure of 3-(3-chloro-phenyl)-5-(4-pyridyl)-4,5-dihydroisoxazole.

A series of novel coumarin isoxazoles (**128a-f**) and (**131a-f**) have been synthesized in good yield starting from 4-formyl-coumarins (Figs. **56** and **57**). All the synthesized compounds were screened for their antibacterial and anti-inflammatory activity. The tested compounds exhibited high selectivity against gram-positive bacterial strains as compared to gram-negative bacterial strains. Similarly, phenyl- sulphonamide substituted derivatives (**131a-f**) exhibited promising activity against bacterial strains [65].

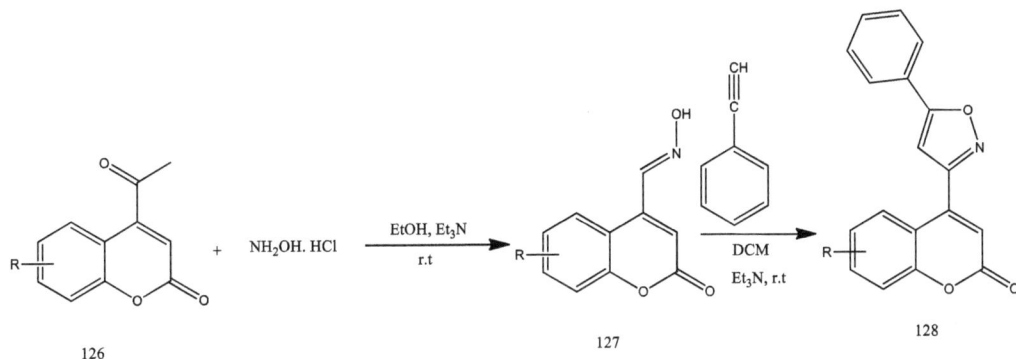

**Fig. (56).** Synthesis of coumarin isoxazole (128).

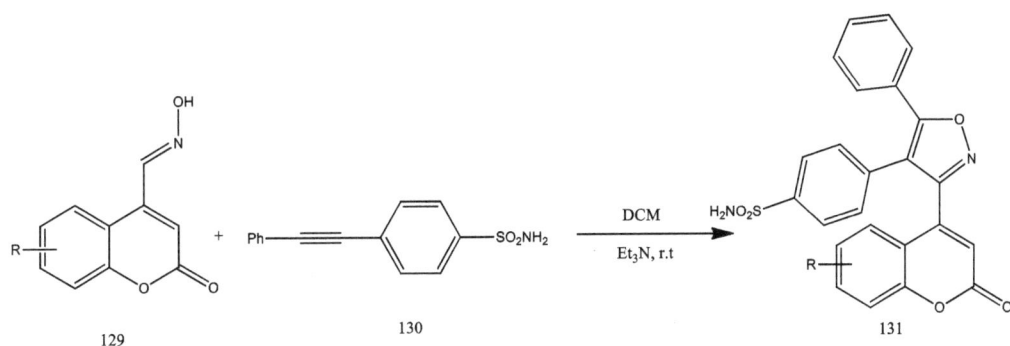

**Fig. (57).** Synthesis of coumarin isoxazole-phenyl sulphonamide (131).

## 2.10. Miscellaneous Activities

Solvent-free synthesis of 3-Aryl-1-(2-aryl-1H-indol-3-yl)prop-2-en-1-one has been accomplished in high yields (Fig. **58**) and lesser time by using green chemistry techniques (Grindstone chemistry and microwave irradiation). 3-Acetyl- 2-phenyl indoles on treatment with either acidic or basic catalyst generate the corresponding enolates, which react with aryl aldehydes affording the desired title products. They have also been screened for their antibacterial and anti-spermicidal activities and some of them have shown promising results against *Staphylococcus aureus*, *Escherichia coli*, and *Pseudomonas aeruginosa* [66].

Kalirajan *et al.* demonstrated the microwave irradiated synthesis of isoxazole substituted 9-anilino acridines (**139**) (Fig. **59**). The titled compounds were evaluated for their antibacterial activity by using the cup-plate method and also screened for their larvicidal activity by the larval bioassay method. The compounds 139d, 139e, 3139f, 139h, 139d, and 1394f exhibited significant antibacterial activity against Gram +ve bacteria like *Staphylococcus aureus* and *Bacillus megaterium*, and Gram −ve like   *Escherichia coli* and *Klebsiella pneumonia* at 25μg/ml. Similarly, compounds 139c, 139f, 4139a, and 139f displayed significant larvicidal activity against culex and anopheles species at an LC$_{50}$ value of 17-36ppm [67].

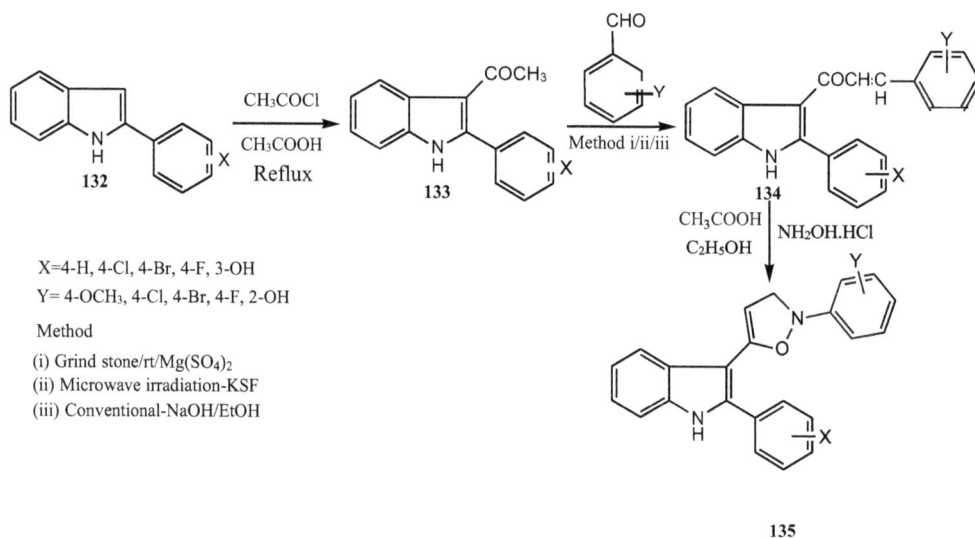

X=4-H, 4-Cl, 4-Br, 4-F, 3-OH

Y= 4-OCH₃, 4-Cl, 4-Br, 4-F, 2-OH

Method

(i) Grind stone/rt/Mg(SO₄)₂
(ii) Microwave irradiation-KSF
(iii) Conventional-NaOH/EtOH

**Fig. (58).**   Solvent-free synthesis of 3-Aryl-1-(2-aryl-1H-indol-3-yl)prop-2-en-1-one.

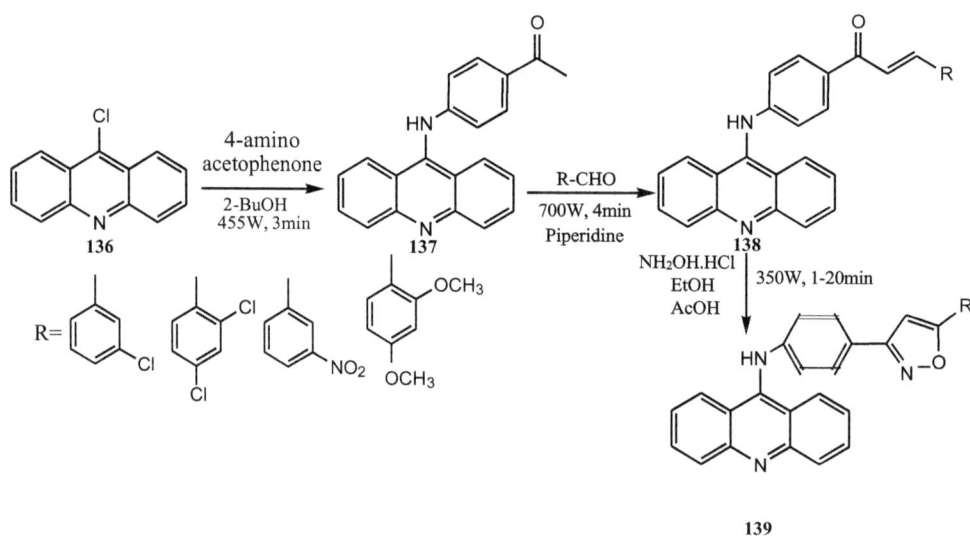

**Fig. (59).**   Microwave irradiated synthesis of isoxazole substituted 9-anilino acridines.

Multicomponent reaction (MCR) is considered a potential chemical tool in which three or more starting materials react to a single reaction vessel to produce a product. MCR is an environmentally friendly synthetic approach for the efficient generation of highly functionalized heterocycles in a one-pot one-step method. Different name reactions involved during preparation of various heterocyclic compounds *via* MCRs include Michael reaction, Mannich reaction, Knovenagel reaction, Aldol reaction, Wittig reaction, *etc*. MCRs is advantageous over multistep reaction in terms of high efficiency, atom economy, reduced waste production, short reaction time, and energy-efficient [68].

Based on this concept, a series of novel 5-amino-isoxazole-4-carbonitriles (**141**) are synthesized *via* green and efficient multicomponent reaction between malononitrile (**140**), hydroxylamine hydrochloride (**5**), and different aryl or heteroaryl aldehydes (**19**) with good product yields in short reaction time (Fig. **60**). Glycerol and $K_2CO_3$ (4:1 molar) were used as green catalytic media for optimal reaction conditions. All synthesized compounds were evaluated for their *in vitro* inhibitory activity against different pathogenic bacteria, such as Gram-negative and Gram-positive strains as well as fungal strains. In addition, these compounds were assessed for their free radical scavenging activities against DPPH. Broad-spectrum antimicrobial activities were observed with isoxazoles. It was observed that the *in vitro* antioxidant activity of compound **141i** with pyridine-4yl substituent was presented with an $IC_{50}$ of 67.51 µg ml$^{-1}$ (Table **10**) [69].

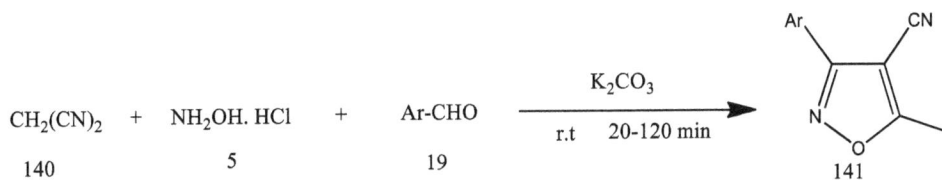

| Compound | Ar | Compound | R |
|---|---|---|---|
| 141a | 4-CH$_3$-C$_6$H$_4$ | 141f | 2-OH-2-OCH$_3$-C$_6$H$_3$ |
| 141b | 4-OH-C$_6$H$_4$ | 141g | Furan-2yl |

**Fig. (60).** Multicomponent synthesis of 5-amino-isoxazole-4-carbonitriles.

**Table 10. Reaction conditions for the synthesis of isoxazole derivatives *via* MCR.**

| Entry | Conditions | Catalyst | Time (min) | Yield (%) |
|-------|-----------|----------|-----------|-----------|
| 1 | EtOH, reflux | DABCO | 1.5–15 | 65–85 |
| 2 | aq. EtOH, hv | CH₃COONa | 5–10 | 61–89 |
| 3 | H2O, rt | Potassium phthalimide | 30–150 | 85–96 |
| 4 | H2O, rt | Boric acid | 50–1440 | 82–95 |

Kalirajan *et al.* reported the convenient synthesis of novel isoxazole-substituted 9-anilinoacridine derivatives (**143**) (Fig. **61**). The compounds were screened for *in vitro* antioxidant activity by the DPPH method, reducing power assay, and total antioxidant capacity method. The cytotoxic activity of the compounds was also studied in the HEp-2 cell line [70].

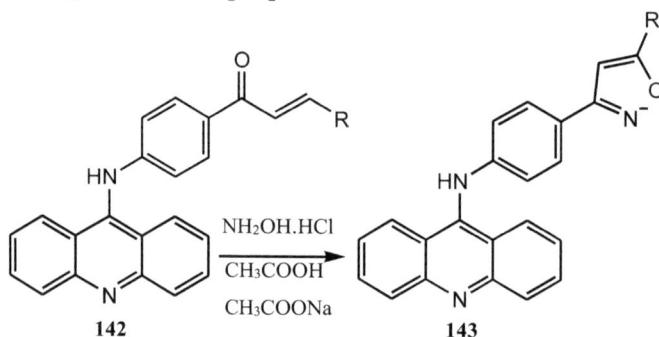

**Fig. (61).** Synthesis of novel isoxazole-substituted 9-anilino acridine derivatives.

A novel series of 3-methyl-4-nitro-5-(substituted styryl) isoxazoles (**147**) were synthesized (Fig. **62**) and subjected for evaluation for antioxidant, anti-inflammatory, and analgesic activities. Compounds with sterically hindered phenolic groups displayed promising anti-inflammatory properties with significant antioxidant activity. These compounds were found to have low ulcerogenic at a dose of 100mg/kg, p.o. and found to be less toxic [71].

A series of substituted benzofuran chalcones were prepared by the reaction of 2-acetyl benzofuran (**148**) with different aromatic aldehydes (**19**) in the presence of a strong base. Further, benzofuran chalcones (**149**) on cyclo-condensation with hydroxylamine hydrochloride (**5**) in the presence of sodium acetate furnished various 3-(1-benzofuran-2-yl)-5-phenylisoxazoles (**150**) (Fig. **63**). The benzofuran isoxazoles were evaluated for their, antitubercular, antimicrobial, and anti-inflammatory activities. Some of the compounds have shown promising antitubercular and antibacterial activity [72].

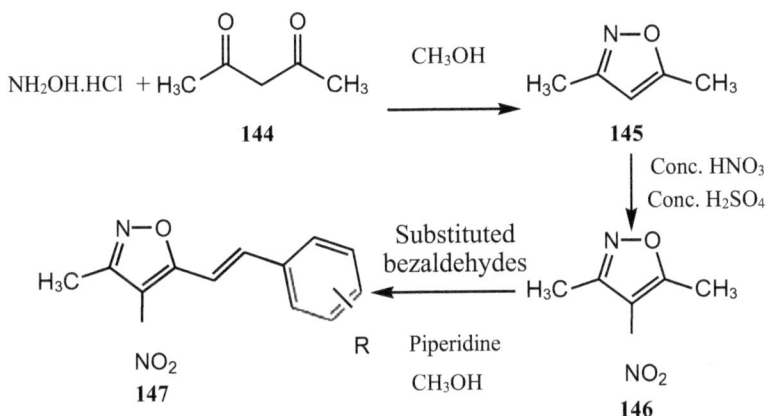

**Fig. (62).** Synthesis of 3-methyl-4-nitro-5-(substituted styryl)isoxazoles.

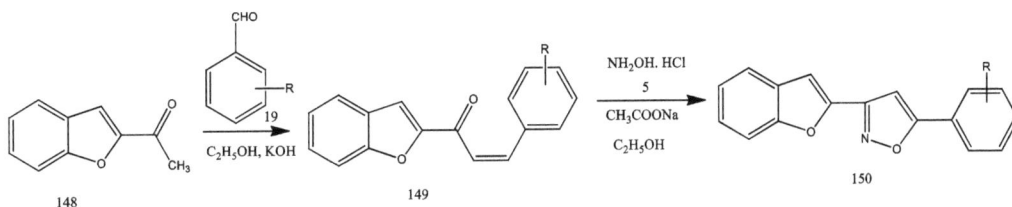

**Fig. (63).** Synthesis of 3-(1-benzofuran-2-yl)-5-phenyl isoxazoles.

Bhalgat *et al.* also performed the *in vitro* cytotoxic activity on HeLa cell lines of 3- (1-benzofuran-2-yl)-5-(substituted phenyl)isoxazole. Among these derivatives, 4- hydroxy benzaldehyde (**151**), 3-ethoxy,4-hydroxy benzaldehyde substituted derivative (**152**) showed good cytotoxic activity (Fig. **64**) [73].

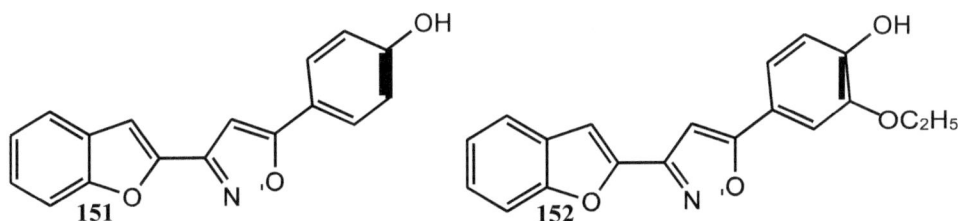

**Fig. (64).** Structure of 3-(1-benzofuran-2-yl)-5-(substituted phenyl)isoxazole.

Joseph *et al.* reported the syntheses of novel isoxazole derivatives *via* chalcones. First of all, chalcones (**155**) are prepared by a reaction between aromatic aldehydes (**153**) and aromatic ketones (**154**) in the presence of aqueous-alcoholic alkali solution. Then chalcones react with hydroxylamine hydrochloride (**5**) in the presence of sodium acetate to produce title compounds (Fig. **65**). The prepared compounds were subjected to anti-bacterial and *in-vitro* antidiabetic activities. The antibacterial activity was determined by using the agar disc diffusion method. Similarly, the evaluation of antidiabetic activity was carried out by yeast and enzymatic method. Several tested compounds displayed potential anti-bacterial activity as compared to standard drug ciprofloxacin. Whereas isoxazole derivatives with halogen and nitro substitution on phenyl ring exhibited promising antidiabetic activity [74].

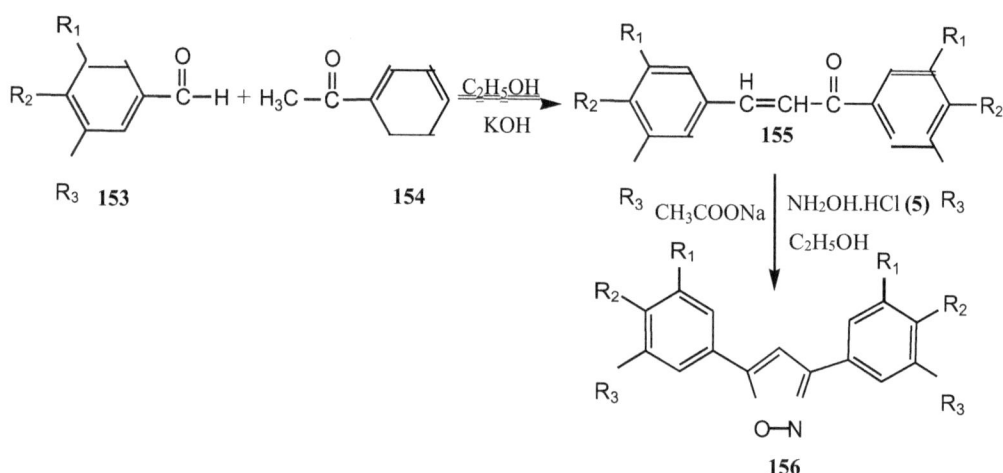

**Fig. (65).** Syntheses of isoxazole derivatives *via* chalcones.

Aisa *et al.* performed the design and synthesis of a new series of chalcone derivatives (**157a-f**), bearing isoxazole scaffold (Fig. **66**). The target compounds were evaluated for their anti-vitiligo activity on mushroom tyrosinase and melanin synthesis in murine B16 cells. Among the series, compounds **157b, d,** and **f** demonstrated significant activity with an $EC_{50}$ of 11.9, 1.71, and 14.6 $\mu molL^{-1}$, respectively, as compared to the positive control 8-methoxy psoralen (8-MOP, $EC_{50} = 14.8 \mu molL^{-1}$) (Table **11**) [75].

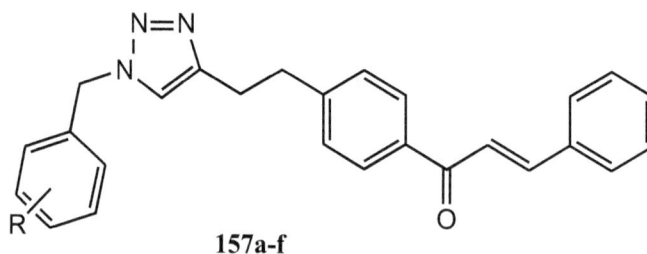

**157a-f**

**Fig. (66).** Structure of chalcone derivatives bearing an isoxazole scaffold.

**Table 11. Anti-vitiligo activity of titled compounds (157a-f).**

| Compound | Substituent (R) | $EC_{50}(\mu M)$ |
|---|---|---|
| 157a | 3-OCH₃ | 37.4±2.2 |
| 157b | 3-Cl | 11.9±0.9 |
| 157c | 4-Cl | 23.9±2.6 |
| 157d | 3,4-Cl₂ | 1.71±0.23 |
| 157e | 3-F | 5.6±0.5 |
| 157f | 4-F | 14.6±1.4 |
| 8-MOP (positive control) | - | 14.80±1.5 |

Bustos *et al.* reported the one-pot synthesis of 3,4,5-trisubstituted isoxazoles (**159**) in good yields by the treatment of *β*-diketo-hydrazones of the type (3-(2-(4-R-phenyl)hydrazinylidene)pentane2,4-dione (**158**) with hydroxyl ammonium chloride (**5**) in ethanol and acetic acid as a catalyst (Fig. **67**).

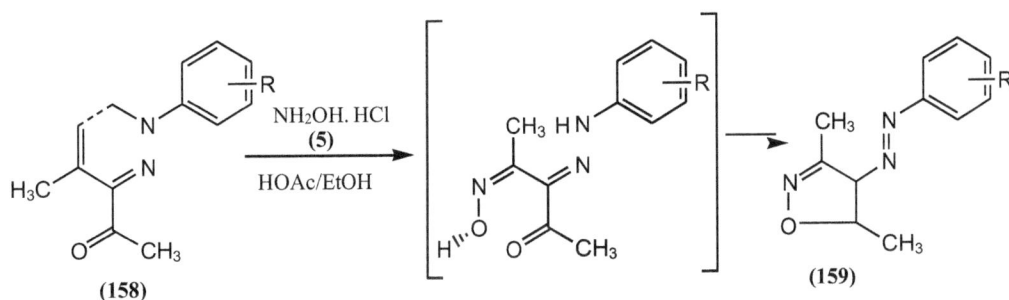

**Fig. (67).** One-pot synthesis of 3,4,5-trisubstituted isoxazoles.

The cytotoxic activity of the synthesized compounds was evaluated on human promyelocytic leukemia cells, HL-60 by using the MTT reduction method. Compounds (E)-3,5-dimethyl-4-(*p*-tolyldiazenyl)isoxazole **160** and (E)-4- ((4-chlorophenyl)diazenyl)-3,5-dimethylisoxazole **161** are the compounds that exhibit significant cytotoxic activity, with $IC_{50}$ values below 100 µM (Fig. **68**) [76].

Chalcones were synthesized by reacting indole-3-aldehyde (**163**), prepared by Vilsemeir Haack reaction with 4-substituted acetophenone (**164**) in ethanolic KOH solution. These chalcones were immediately reacted with hydroxylamine hydrochloride in the presence of glacial acetic acid as a reagent to obtain the corresponding isoxazole derivatives (Fig. **69**). These compounds were tested for acute anti-inflammatory activity and antibacterial activity using the carrageenan-induced rat paw edema method and cup-plate method, respectively. The tested compounds showed significant anti-inflammatory activity comparable to ibuprofen. Whereas the compounds 166b and 166j showed good activity against *S. aureus*. Compounds 166b, 166c, 166d, and 166j showed moderate activity against *P. aeruginosa* [77].

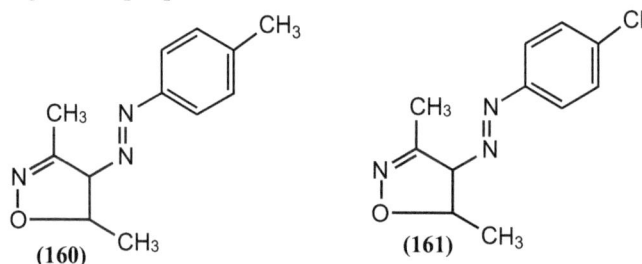

**Fig. (68).** Structure of compounds 160 and 161.

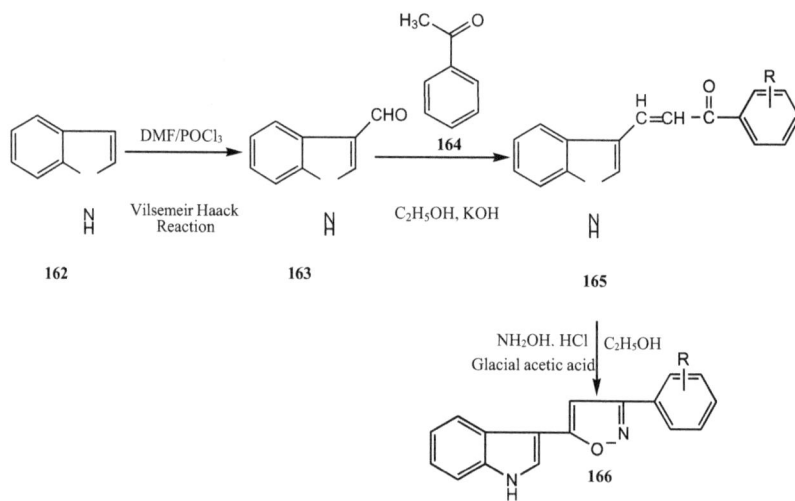

**Fig. (69).** Synthesis of isoxazole derivatives from indole-3-aldehyde.

## 3. SAR STUDY OF ISOXAZOLES

The structure-activity relationships (SAR) study of isoxazole moiety represents its structural properties responsible for different biological activities (Fig. **70**). The promising therapeutic potentials of the isoxazole derivatives may be due to the position (*ortho, meta,* and *para)* and type of substituents (electron-withdrawing and donating groups) on the isoxazole ring. The presence of an aryl ring on the isoxazole scaffold is responsible for the lipophilic or hydrophobic property of the drug molecules. It is observed that there is a wide range of pharmacological activities due to the derivatization of isoxazole with other moieties like sulphonamide, coumarin, chalcone, kaempferol, curcumin, piperazine, *etc* [78 - 80].

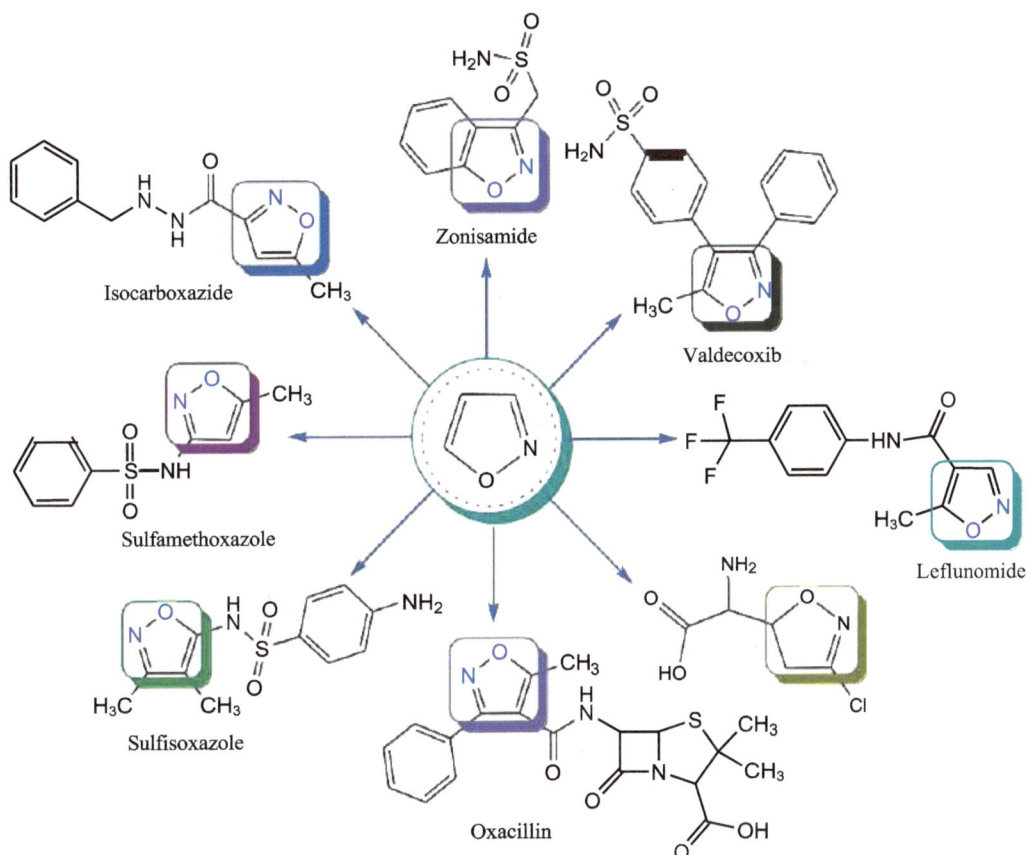

**Fig. (70).** SAR study of isoxazole scaffold.

## 4. FUTURE DEVELOPMENTS

Due to the increased occurrence of various disease states in human beings, there is a continuous requirement to develop novel therapeutic agents with promising pharmacokinetic and pharmacodynamic properties. For this purpose, researchers are focusing on the synthesis of isoxazole-containing compounds *via* different synthetic protocols. The implementation of the green chemistry approach also provides an eco-friendly strategy for the production of isoxazole analogs. Microwave-induced drug synthesis has gained popularity because this procedure offers features like clean, efficient, faster, and economical processes for the synthesis of compounds with diverse molecular structures. This heating method facilitates several chemical reactions to be completed under mild reaction conditions in shorter reaction times with higher product yield. In the future, many more microwave-induced chemical syntheses can be performed on industrial scales to increase the overall efficiency of the processes. So, the application of microwave-assisted drug synthesis looks bright because of its efficiency and potential to generate cleaner products [81, 82].

## CONCLUSION

The current study focuses on the different synthetic approaches of isoxazole derivatives and discusses their several pharmacological activities. Drugs containing isoxazole moiety are found to be effective in treating various disease states like cancer, epilepsy, cardiac disease, diabetes, inflammation, malaria, tuberculosis, bacterial, fungal, and viral infections, *etc*. Isoxazoles are considered a significant heterocyclic moiety as these are essential constituent of several marketed and clinically available drugs. Due to the wide spectrum of biological activities, isoxazoles have enormous potential to be investigated for determining their newer therapeutic activities. So it is utilized as a lead compound for the development of new chemical entities to treat various disease conditions of clinical importance.

## REFERENCES

[1]     Katritzky, A.R.; Rees, C.W. Comprehensive heterocyclic chemistry. pergamom Press, **1984**; p. 106.

[2]     Brown, D.J.; Mason, S.F. Chemistry of heterocyclic compounds: The pyrimidines. wiley, **2008**; pp. 31-81.

[3]     Agarwal, O.P. Organic chemistry reactions & reagents by krishna prakashan. Anu, **2008**; pp. 735-738.

[4]     Katritzky, A.R.; Ramsden, C.A.; Scriven, E.F.V.; Taylor, R.J.K. Comprehensive heterocyclic chemistry. Pergamon: Oxford, U.K., **2008**; pp. 1-13.

[5]     Ram, Ji Five-membered heterocycles. *Chem. Heterocyc.,* **2019**, 149-478.
[http://dx.doi.org/10.1016/B978-0-08-101033-4.00005-X]

[6]     Ajay Kumar, K.; Jayaroopa, P. Isoxazoles: Molecules with potential medicinal properties. *IJPCBS,* **2013**, *3*(2), 294-304.

[7]     Chikkula, K.V.; S, R. Isoxazole: A potent pharmacophore. *Int. J. Pharm. Pharm. Sci.,* **2017**, *9*(7), 13-24.
[http://dx.doi.org/10.22159/ijpps.2017.v9i7.19097]

[8]     Pradeep, K.Y.; Ruthu, M.; Chetty, C.M.; Prasanthi, G.; Reddy, V.J. Pharmacological activities of isoxazole derivatives. *J. Glob. Trends Pharm. Sci.,* **2011**, *2*(1), 55-62.

[9]     Barmade, M.A.; Murumkar, P.R.; Sharma, M.K.; Yadav, M.R. Medicinal chemistry perspective of fused isoxazole derivatives. *Curr. Top. Med. Chem.,* **2016**, *16*(26), 2863-2883.
[http://dx.doi.org/10.2174/1568026616666160506145700] [PMID: 27150366]

[10]    Renuka, S.; Rama, Krishna Kota. Medicinal and biological significance of isoxazole a highly important scaffold for drug discovery. *Asian J. Res. Chem,* **2011**, *4*(7), 1038-1042.

[11]    Li, J.J. Claisen isoxazole synthesis. *Name Reactions,* **2014**, *138–139*, 138-139.
[http://dx.doi.org/10.1007/978-3-319-03979-4_62]

[12]    Parikh, A.R.; Merja, B.C.; Joshi, A.M.; Parikh, K.A. Synthesis and biological evaluation of isoxazoline derivatives. *Indian J. Chem.,* **2004**, *43B*, 955-959.

[13]    Hamama, W.S.; Ibrahim, M.E.; Zoorob, H.H. Synthesis and biological evaluation of some novel isoxazole derivatives. *J. Heterocycl. Chem.,* **2017**, *54*(1), 341-346.
[http://dx.doi.org/10.1002/jhet.2589]

[14]    Zhu, J.; Mo, J.; Lin, H.; Chen, Y.; Sun, H. The recent progress of isoxazole in medicinal chemistry. *Bioorg. Med. Chem.,* **2018**, *26*(12), 3065-3075.
[http://dx.doi.org/10.1016/j.bmc.2018.05.013] [PMID: 29853341]

[15]    Agrawal, N.; Mishra, P. The synthetic and therapeutic expedition of isoxazole and its analogs. *Med. Chem. Res.,* **2018**, *27*(5), 1309-1344.
[http://dx.doi.org/10.1007/s00044-018-2152-6] [PMID: 32214770]

[16]    Gangadhara Chary, R.; Rajeshwar Reddy, G.; Ganesh, Y.S.S.; Vara Prasad, K.; Raghunadh, A.; Krishna, T.; Mukherjee, S.; Pal, M. Effect of aqueous polyethylene glycol on 1,3-dipolar cycloaddition of benzoylnitromethane/ethyl 2-nitroacetate with dipolarophiles: Green synthesis of isoxazoles and isoxazolines. *Adv. Synth. Catal.,* **2014**, *356*(1), 160-164.
[http://dx.doi.org/10.1002/adsc.201300712]

[17]    Saikh, F.; Das, J.; Ghosh, S. Synthesis of 3-methyl-4-arylmethylene isoxazole-5(4*H*)-ones by visible light in aqueous ethanol. *Tetrahedron Lett.,* **2013**, *54*(35), 4679-4682.
[http://dx.doi.org/10.1016/j.tetlet.2013.06.086]

[18]    Hatvate, N.T.; Ghodse, S.M. One-pot three-component synthesis of isoxazole using ZSM-5 as a heterogeneous catalyst. *Synth. Commun.,* **2020**, *50*(23), 3676-3683.
[http://dx.doi.org/10.1080/00397911.2020.1815786]

[19]    Kiyani, H.; Darbandi, H.; Mosallanezhad, A.; Ghorbani, F. 2-Hydroxy-5-sulfobenzoic acid: An efficient organocatalyst for the three-component synthesis of 1-amidoalkyl-2-naphthols and 3,4-disubstituted isoxazol-5(4H)-ones. *Res. Chem. Intermed.,* **2015**, *41*(10), 7561-7579.
[http://dx.doi.org/10.1007/s11164-014-1844-x]

[20]    Kiyani, H.; Kanaani, A.; Ajloo, D.; Ghorbani, F.; Vakili, M. N-bromosuccinimide (NBS)-promoted, three-component synthesis of α,β-unsaturated isoxazol-5(4H)-ones, and spectroscopic investigation and computational study of 3-methyl-4-(thiophen-2-ylmethylene)isoxazol-5(4H)-one. *Res. Chem. Intermed.,* **2015**, *41*(10), 7739-7773.
[http://dx.doi.org/10.1007/s11164-014-1857-5]

[21]    Liu, T.; Dong, X.; Xue, N.; Wu, R.; He, Q.; Yang, B.; Hu, Y. Synthesis and biological evaluation of 3,4-diaryl-5-aminoisoxazole derivatives. *Bioorg. Med. Chem.,* **2009**, *17*(17), 6279-6285.
[http://dx.doi.org/10.1016/j.bmc.2009.07.040] [PMID: 19665898]

[22]    Kiyani, H.; Ghorbani, F. Potassium phthalimide as efficient basic organocatalyst for the synthesis of 3,4-disubstituted isoxazol-5(4H)-ones in aqueous medium. *J. Saudi Chem. Soc.,* **2017**, *21*, S112-S119.
d
[http://dx.doi.org/10.1016/j.jscs.2013.11.002]

[23]    Khandebharad Amol, U.; Sarda, Swapnil R.; Gill, Charansingh; Agrawal, Brijmohan R. Synthesis of 3-Methyl-4-arylmethylene-isoxazol-5(4H)-ones catalyzed by Tartaric acid in aqueous media. *Res. J. Chem. Sci.,* **2015**, *5*(5), 1-6.

[24]    Ram, Ji Five-membered heterocycles. *Chem. Heteroc.,* **2019**, 149-478.
[http://dx.doi.org/10.1016/B978-0-08-101033-4.00005-X]

[25]    Zhu, Jie; Mo, Jun; Chen, Y The recent progress of isoxazole in medicinal chemistry. *Bioorg Med Chem.,* **2018**, *26*(12), 3065-3075.
[http://dx.doi.org/10.1016/j.bmc.2018.05.013]

[26]   Walunj, Y.; Mhaske, P.; Kulkarni, P. Application, reactivity and synthesis of isoxazole derivatives. *Mini Rev. Org. Chem.,* **2021**, *18*(1), 55-77.
[http://dx.doi.org/10.2174/1570193X17999200511131621]

[27]   Rajput, S.S.; Patel, S.N.; Jadhav, N.B. Cheminform abstract: Isoxazole : A basic aromatic heterocycle: Synthesis, reactivity and biological activity. *ChemInform,* **2016**, *47*(15), no.
[http://dx.doi.org/10.1002/chin.201615225]

[28]   Pinho e Melo, T. Recent advances on the synthesis and reactivity of isoxazoles. *Curr. Org. Chem.,* **2005**, *9*(10), 925-958.
[http://dx.doi.org/10.2174/1385272054368420]

[29]   Hu, F.; Szostak, M. Recent developments in the synthesis and reactivity of isoxazoles: Metal catalysis and beyond. *Adv. Synth. Catal.,* **2015**, *357*(12), 2583-2614.
[http://dx.doi.org/10.1002/adsc.201500319]

[30]   Chiranjit, Jana.; Subhasis, Banerjee. A brief insight into isoxazole analogues. *Pharm. Lett.,* **2016**, *8*(8), 121-136.

[31]   Sysak, A.; Obmińska-Mrukowicz, B. Isoxazole ring as a useful scaffold in a search for new therapeutic agents. *Eur. J. Med. Chem.,* **2017**, *137*, 292-309.
[http://dx.doi.org/10.1016/j.ejmech.2017.06.002] [PMID: 28605676]

[32]   Chikkula, K.V.; S, R. Isoxazole : A potent pharmacophore. *Int. J. Pharm. Pharm. Sci.,* **2017**, *9*(7), 13-24.
[http://dx.doi.org/10.22159/ijpps.2017.v9i7.19097]

[33]   Ryng, S.; Sonnenberg, Z.; Zimecki, M. RM-11, a new izoxasole derivative, is a potent stimulator of the humoral and cellular immune responses in mice. *Arch. Immunol. Ther. Exp.,* **2000**, *48*(2), 127-131.
[PMID: 10807054]

[34]   Alsalameh, S.; Burian, M.; Mahr, G.; Woodcock, B.G.; Geisslinger, G. The pharmacological properties and clinical use of valdecoxib, a new cyclo-oxygenase-2-selective inhibitor. *Aliment. Pharmacol. Ther.,* **2003**, *17*(4), 489-501.
[http://dx.doi.org/10.1046/j.1365-2036.2003.01460.x] [PMID: 12622757]

[35]   Vitaku, E.; Smith, D.T.; Njardarson, J.T. Analysis of the structural diversity, substitution patterns, and frequency of nitrogen heterocycles among U.S. FDA approved pharmaceuticals. *J. Med. Chem.,* **2014**, *57*(24), 10257-10274.
[http://dx.doi.org/10.1021/jm501100b] [PMID: 25255204]

[36]   Sherin, D.R.; Rajasekharan, K.N. Curcuminoid-derived 3,5-bis(styryl)isoxazoles : Mechanochemical synthesis and antioxidant activity. *J. Chem. Sci.,* **2016**, *128*(8), 1315-1319.
[http://dx.doi.org/10.1007/s12039-016-1119-8]

[37]   Mączyński, M.; Borska, S.; Mieszała, K.; Kocięba, M.; Zaczyńska, E.; Kochanowska, I.; Zimecki, M. Synthesis, immunosuppressive properties, and mechanism of action of a new isoxazole derivative. *Molecules,* **2018**, *23*(7), 1545.
[http://dx.doi.org/10.3390/molecules23071545] [PMID: 29949951]

[38]   Mokale, S.N.; Dube, P.N.; Nevase, M.C.; Sakle, N.S.; Shelke, V.R.; Bhavale, S.A.; Begum, A. Synthesis of some novel substituted phenylisoxazol phenoxy 2-methylpropanoic acids and there *in vivo* hypolipidemic activity. *Med. Chem. Res.,* **2016**, *25*(3), 422-428.
[http://dx.doi.org/10.1007/s00044-015-1498-2]

[39]   Saravanan, G.; Veerachamy, Alagarsamy; Pandurangan, Dineshkumar Synthesis, analgesic, anti-inflammatory and *in vitro* antimicrobial activities of some novel isoxazole coupled quinazoline-4(3H)-one derivative. *Arch. Pharm. Res.,* **2021**, *44*(8), 1-11.
[http://dx.doi.org/10.1007/s12272-013-0262-8] [PMID: 24155019]

[40]   Dannhardt, G.; Kiefer, W. Cyclooxygenase inhibitors : Current status and future prospects. *Eur. J. Med. Chem.,* **2001**, *36*(2), 109-126.

[http://dx.doi.org/10.1016/S0223-5234(01)01197-7] [PMID: 11311743]

[41] Esfahani, S.N.; Damavandi, M.S.; Sadeghi, P.; Nazifi, Z.; Salari-Jazi, A.; Massah, A.R. Synthesis of some novel coumarin isoxazol sulfonamide hybrid compounds, 3D-QSAR studies, and antibacterial evaluation. *Sci. Rep.,* **2021**, *11*(1), 20088.
[http://dx.doi.org/10.1038/s41598-021-99618-w] [PMID: 34635732]

[42] Biswa Mohan, S.; Binayani, S.; Jnyanaranjan, P.; Anjan, K. Microwave: Induced synthesis of substituted isoxazoles as potential antimicrobial agents. *Curr. Microw. Chem.,* **2017**, *4*(2), 1-6.

[43] Hushare, V.J.; Rajput, P.R. Synthesis, characterization and antimicrobial activity of some novel isoxazoles. *Rasayan J. Chem.,* **2012**, *5*(1), 121-126.

[44] RamaRao, R.J.; Rao, A.K.S.B.; Sreenivas, N.; Kumar, B.S.; Murthy, Y.L.N. Synthesis and antibacterial activity of novel 5-(heteroaryl)isoxazole derivatives. *J. Korean Chem. Soc.,* **2011**, *55*(2), 243-250.
[http://dx.doi.org/10.5012/jkcs.2011.55.2.243]

[45] Jain, D.K.; Goyal, N.; Bhadoriya, U. Synthesis, characterization and biological evaluation of some new isoxazoline derivatives. *Asian J. Chem.,* **2013**, *25*(2), 789-792.
[http://dx.doi.org/10.14233/ajchem.2013.12899]

[46] Mao, J.; Yuan, H.; Wang, Y.; Wan, B.; Pak, D.; He, R.; Franzblau, S.G. Synthesis and antituberculosis activity of novel mefloquine-isoxazole carboxylic esters as prodrugs. *Bioorg. Med. Chem. Lett.,* **2010**, *20*(3), 1263-1268.
[http://dx.doi.org/10.1016/j.bmcl.2009.11.105] [PMID: 20022500]

[47] Priyanka, G.; Naresh, K.; Nudrath, U.; Madhava Reddy, B.; Harinadha Babu, V. Synthesis and antitubercular activity of isoxazole incorporated 1,2,3-triazole derivatives.res. j of pharm, bio. *Chem. Sci.,* **2016**, *7*(2), 1167-1171.

[48] Lilienkampf, A.; Pieroni, M.; Franzblau, S.G.; Bishai, W.R.; Kozikowski, A.P. Derivatives of 3-isoxazolecarboxylic acid esters: A potent and selective compound class against replicating and nonreplicating *Mycobacterium tuberculosis. Curr. Top. Med. Chem.,* **2012**, *12*(7), 729-734.
[http://dx.doi.org/10.2174/156802612799984544] [PMID: 22283815]

[49] Vergelli, C.; Cilibrizzi, A.; Crocetti, L.; Graziano, A.; Dal Piaz, V.; Wan, B.; Wang, Y.; Franzblau, S.; Giovannoni, M.P. Synthesis and evaluation as antitubercular agents of 5-arylethenyl and 5-(hetero)aryl-3-isoxazolecarboxylate. *Drug Dev. Res.,* **2013**, *74*(3), 162-172.
[http://dx.doi.org/10.1002/ddr.21057]

[50] Hajlaoui, K.; Guesmi, A.; Hamadi, N.B.; Msaddek, M. Synthesis of carbohydrate-substituted isoxazoles and evaluation of their antitubercular activity. *Heterocycl. Commun.,* **2017**, *23*(3), 225-229.
[http://dx.doi.org/10.1515/hc-2016-0185]

[51] Nagaraju, Pappula; Ravichandra, Sharabu Synthesis, characterization, anti-mycobacterial evaluation and *in-silico* molecular docking of novel isoxazole clubbed pyrimidine derivatives. *J. Pharm. Res. Int.,* **2021**, *33*(26B), 69-79.

[52] Maurya, R.; Gupta, P.; Ahmad, G.; Yadav, D. K.; Chand, K.; Singh, A. B.; Tamrakar, A. K.; Srivastava, A. K. Synthesis of 3,5-disubstituted isoxazolines as protein tyrosine phosphatase 1B inhibitors. *Med Chem Res,* **2008**, *17*(2-7), 123-136.
[http://dx.doi.org/10.1007/s00044-007-9043-6]

[53] Badru, R.; Anand, P.; Singh, B. Synthesis and evaluation of hexahydropyrrolo[3,4-d]isoxazole-4-6-diones as anti-stress agents. *Eur. J. Med. Chem.,* **2012**, *48*, 81-91.
[http://dx.doi.org/10.1016/j.ejmech.2011.11.037] [PMID: 22178092]

[54] Wang, G.; Liu, W.; Huang, Y.; Li, Y.; Peng, Z. Design, synthesis and biological evaluation of isoxazole-naphthalene derivatives as anti-tubulin agents. *Arab. J. Chem.,* **2020**, *13*(6), 5765-5775.
[http://dx.doi.org/10.1016/j.arabjc.2020.04.014]

[55] Aktaş, D.A.; Akinalp, G.; Sanli, F.; Yucel, M.A.; Gambacorta, N.; Nicolotti, O.; Karatas, O.F.; Algul,

O.; Burmaoglu, S. Design, synthesis and biological evaluation of 3,5-diaryl isoxazole derivatives as potential anticancer agents. *Bioorg. Med. Chem. Lett.,* **2020,** *30*(19), 127427.
[http://dx.doi.org/10.1016/j.bmcl.2020.127427] [PMID: 32750679]

[56]    İbiş, K.; Nalbat, E.; Çalışkan, B.; Kahraman, D.C.; Cetin-Atalay, R.; Banoglu, E. Synthesis and biological evaluation of novel isoxazole-piperazine hybrids as potential anti-cancer agents with inhibitory effect on liver cancer stem cells. *Eur. J. Med. Chem.,* **2021,** *221,* 113489.
[http://dx.doi.org/10.1016/j.ejmech.2021.113489] [PMID: 33951549]

[57]    Çalışkan, B.; Sinoplu, E.; İbiş, K.; Akhan Güzelcan, E.; Çetin Atalay, R.; Banoglu, E. Synthesis and cellular bioactivities of novel isoxazole derivatives incorporating an arylpiperazine moiety as anticancer agents. *J. Enzyme Inhib. Med. Chem.,* **2018,** *33*(1), 1352-1361.
[http://dx.doi.org/10.1080/14756366.2018.1504041] [PMID: 30251900]

[58]    Thiriveedhi, A.; Nadh, R.V. Navuluri srinivasu1 and kishore kaushal, novel hybrid molecules of isoxazole chalcone derivatives: Synthesis and study of *in vitro* cytotoxic activities. *Lett. Drug Des. Discov.,* **2018,** *15,* 1-7.

[59]    Veeraswamy, B.; Kurumurthy, C Kumar.; Santhosh Rao, G.; Sambasiva Thelakkat, P.; Kavya, K.; Srigiridhar, K. Synthesis of novel 5-substituted isoxazole-3-carboxamide derivatives and cytotoxicity studies on lung cancer cell line. *Indian J. Chem.,* **2012,** *51B,* 1369-1375.

[60]    Nie, Jiang-Ping; Qu, Zhen-Ni; Chen, Ying; Chen, Jia-Hao; Jiang, Yue; Jin, Mei-Na; Yu, Yang; Niu, Wen-Yan; Duan, Hong-Quan; Qin, Nan Discovery and anti-diabetic effects of novel isoxazole based flavonoid derivatives *Fitoterapia,* **2020,** *142,* 104499.
[http://dx.doi.org/10.1016/j.fitote.2020.104499]

[61]    Zhou, Zuwen; Yan, Jufang; Tang, Xuemei; Zhang, Weiyu; Zhang, Yingxia; Chen, Xin; Su, Xiaoyan; Yang, Dacheng Synthesis and preliminary evaluation of antidiabetic activity for β-amino ketone containing isoxazole moiety. *Chin. J. Org. Chem.,* **2010,** *4*(30), 582-589.

[62]    Ali, M.; Kim, D.; Seong, S.; Kim, H.R.; Jung, H.; Choi, J. α-Glucosidase and protein tyrosine phosphatase 1b inhibitory activity of plastoquinones from marine brown alga sargassum serratifolium. *Mar. Drugs,* **2017,** *15*(12), 368.
[http://dx.doi.org/10.3390/md15120368] [PMID: 29194348]

[63]    Archana, K.; Renu, B. Anti-inflammatory evaluation of isoxazole derivatives. *Pharm. Lett.,* **2016,** *8*(12), 127-134.

[64]    Vicentino, A.R.R.; Carneiro, V.C.; Amarante, A.M.; Benjamim, C.F.; de Aguiar, A.P.; Fantappié, M.R. Evaluation of 3-(3-chloro-phenyl)-5-(4-pyridyl)-4,5-dihydroisoxazole as a novel anti-inflammatory drug candidate. *PLoS One,* **2012,** *7*(6), e39104.
[http://dx.doi.org/10.1371/journal.pone.0039104] [PMID: 22723938]

[65]    Esfahani, S.N.; Damavandi, M.S.; Sadeghi, P.; Nazifi, Z.; Salari-Jazi, A.; Massah, A.R. Synthesis of some novel coumarin isoxazol sulfonamide hybrid compounds, 3D-QSAR studies, and antibacterial evaluation. *Sci. Rep.,* **2021,** *11*(1), 20088.
[http://dx.doi.org/10.1038/s41598-021-99618-w] [PMID: 34635732]

[66]    Chawla, C.; Indoriya, S.; Jain, R.; Sharma, S. A highly efficient, simple, and ecofriendly microwave-induced synthesis of indolyl-chalcones and isoxazoles. *J. Chem. Pharm. Res.,* **2014,** *6*(7), 2097-2104.

[67]    Kalirajan, R; Jubie, S; Gowramma, B. Microwave irradated synthesis, characterization and evaluation for their antibacterial and larvicidal activities of some novel chalcone and isoxazole substituted 9-anilino acridines *Open J Chem,* **2015,** *1*(1), 001-007.

[68]    Sunderhaus, J.D.; Martin, S.F. Applications of multicomponent reactions to the synthesis of diverse heterocyclic scaffolds. *Chemistry,* **2009,** *15*(6), 1300-1308.
[http://dx.doi.org/10.1002/chem.200802140] [PMID: 19132705]

[69]    Beyzaei, Hamid; Deljoo, Kamali Green multicomponent synthesis, antimicrobial and antioxidant evaluation of novel 5-amino-isoxazole-4-carbonitriles *Chem. Cent. J.,* **2018,** *12*(1), 114.

[http://dx.doi.org/10.1186/s13065-018-0488-0]

[70]    Kalirajan, R.; MohammedRafick, M. H.; Sankar, S.; Jubie, S. Docking studies, synthesis, characterization, and evaluation of their antioxidant and cytotoxic activities of some novel isoxazole-substituted 9-anilino acridine derivatives *Sci. World J., ***2012**, *2012*, 1-6.
[http://dx.doi.org/10.1100/2012/165258]

[71]    Madhavi, K; Bharathi, K; Prasad, KVSRG Synthesis and evaluation of 3-methyl-4-nitro-5-(substituted styryl) isoxazoles for antioxidant and anti-inflammatory activities *RJPBCS,* **2010**, *1*(4), 1073.

[72]    Manna, K.; Agarwal, Y.K.; Srinivasan, K.K. Synthesis and biological evaluation of new benzofuranyl isoxazoles as antitubercular, antibacterial, and antifungal agents. *Indian J. Heterocycl. Chem.,* **2008**, *18*(1), 87-88.

[73]    Chetan, M.; Patil Sachin, L.; Chitale Sandeep, K.; Randive, K.; Patil Kumar, G.; Patil, S. Synthesis and cytotoxic studies of newer 3-(1-Benzofuran-2-Yl)-5-(substituted Aryl)isoxazole. *Research J. Pharm. and Tech.,* **2011**, *4*(1), 1-5.

[74]    Joseph, L.; George, M. Anti-bacterial and *in vitro* antidiabetic potential of novel isoxazole derivatives. *Br. J. Pharm. Res.,* **2016**, *9*(4), 1-7.
[http://dx.doi.org/10.9734/BJPR/2016/21926]

[75]    Niu, C.; Yin, L.; Nie, L.F.; Dou, J.; Zhao, J.Y.; Li, G.; Aisa, H.A. Synthesis and bioactivity of novel isoxazole chalcone derivatives on tyrosinase and melanin synthesis in murine B16 cells for the treatment of vitiligo. *Bioorg. Med. Chem.,* **2016**, *24*(21), 5440-5448.
[http://dx.doi.org/10.1016/j.bmc.2016.08.066] [PMID: 27622747]

[76]    Bustos, C.; Molins, E.; Cárcamo, J.G.; Aguilar, M.N.; Sánchez, C.; Moreno-Villoslada, I.; Nishide, H.; Mesías-Salazar, A.; Zarate, X.; Schott, E. New 3,4,5-trisubstituted isoxazole derivatives with potential biological properties. *New J. Chem.,* **2015**, *39*(6), 4295-4307.
[http://dx.doi.org/10.1039/C4NJ02427C]

[77]    Panda, S.S.; Chowdary, P.V.R.; Jayashree, B.S. Synthesis, antiinflammatory and antibacterial activity of novel indolyl-isoxazoles. *Indian J. Pharm. Sci.,* **2009**, *71*(6), 684-687.
[http://dx.doi.org/10.4103/0250-474X.59554] [PMID: 20376225]

[78]    Ratcliffe, P.; Abernethy, L.; Ansari, N.; Cameron, K.; Clarkson, T.; Dempster, M.; Dunn, D.; Easson, A.M.; Edwards, D.; Everett, K.; Feilden, H.; Ho, K.K.; Kultgen, S.; Littlewood, P.; Maclean, J.; McArthur, D.; McGregor, D.; McLuskey, H.; Neagu, I.; Nimz, O.; Nisbet, L.A.; Ohlmeyer, M.; Palin, R.; Pham, Q.; Rong, Y.; Roughton, A.; Sammons, M.; Swanson, R.; Tracey, H.; Walker, G. Discovery of potent, soluble and orally active TRPV1 antagonists. Structure–activity relationships of a series of isoxazoles. *Bioorg. Med. Chem. Lett.,* **2011**, *21*(15), 4652-4657.
[http://dx.doi.org/10.1016/j.bmcl.2011.01.051] [PMID: 21723725]

[79]    Arya, G.C.; Kaur, K.; Jaitak, V. Isoxazole derivatives as anticancer agent: A review on synthetic strategies, mechanism of action and SAR studies. *Eur. J. Med. Chem.,* **2021**, *221*, 113511.
[http://dx.doi.org/10.1016/j.ejmech.2021.113511] [PMID: 34000484]

[80]    Chithra, V.S.; Reji, T.F.A.F.; Brindha, J. Synthesis and structure-activity relationship study of novel isoxazole derivatives as promising antioxidants. *Asian J. Res. Chem,* **2018**, *11*(1), 65-68.
[http://dx.doi.org/10.5958/0974-4150.2018.00014.7]

[81]    Duc, D.X.; Dung, V.C. Recent progress in the synthesis of isoxazoles. *Curr. Org. Chem.,* **2021**, *25*(24), 2938-2989.
[http://dx.doi.org/10.2174/1385272825666211118104213]

[82]    Kakkar, S.; Narasimhan, B. A comprehensive review on biological activities of oxazole derivatives. *BMC Chem.,* **2019**, *13*(1), 16.
[http://dx.doi.org/10.1186/s13065-019-0531-9] [PMID: 31384765]

# CHAPTER 2

# Contemporary Trends in Drug Repurposing: Identifying New Targets for Existing Drugs

**Srikant Bhagat**[1,*,#], **Asim Kumar**[2,#] and **Gaurav Joshi**[3,#]

*¹ Department of Medicinal Chemistry, National Institute of Pharmaceutical Education and Research (NIPER), S.A.S. Nagar (Mohali), Punjab-160062, India*

*² Amity Institute of Pharmacy, Amity University Haryana, Manesar, Panchgaon-122412, India*

*³ School of Pharmacy, Graphic Era Hill University, Dehradun-248002, India*

**Abstract:** Drug repurposing or drug repositioning has emerged as an efficient, very popular and alternative technique in modern drug discovery to identify old drugs for new targets cost-effectively and dynamically. This concept gets a tremendous boost, especially in the century's most challenging healthcare concern of the Covid-19 pandemic across the globe. In this approach, scientists seek new indications and clinical use of the drugs at minimum risk, which have previously already been pharmacologically established and approved. The methods developed for drug repositioning include computational approaches and biological methodologies, and with the fast technological advancement, various new drug-target- diseases are discovered, and thereby immense information is now available in the different databases, such as DrugBank, OMIM, ChemBank, KEGG, Pubmed, Genecard, and many more. The information available on all the above public domain databases has been utilized successfully in many drug repositioning projects. The present chapter discusses the concept of drug repurposing and its impact on academia, industries and, of course, their social implications. Besides this, the chapter will also cover details on tools and techniques to identify drugs for repositioning and their application in identifying drugs for various diseases and disorders. The current work will also foresee the recent market analysis and updates on the cost of drug discovery and development by drug repurposing, its comparison with traditional drug discovery approaches, challenges involved with drug repurposing, and future perspectives.

**Keywords:** Case studies, Drug repositioning, Drug repurposing, *in silico* approaches, Polypharmacology, Pharmacological approaches.

---
**\* Corresponding authors Srikant Bhagat, Asim Kumar and Gaurav Joshi:** Dept. of Medicinal Chemistry, National Institute of Pharmaceutical Education and Research, Mohali; E-mails: srikantbhagat@gmail.com, asimniper02@gmail.com, gauravpharma29@gmail.com
\# *All authors have equally contributed*

**Ashok Kumar Jha & Ravi S. Singh (Eds.)**

# 1. INTRODUCTION

Drug repurposing or repositioning, or reprofiling, is an alternative and modern drug discovery approach that involves identifying the role of older drugs for newer targets or diseases. It is a cheaper and faster way of drug development for the disease [1]. The first example of drug repurposing goes back to the 1920s, when serendipitous incidents usually developed the drugs, and their history has been full of such stories. Herein if any drug was found to have a newly recognized effect or off-target effect, it was usually carried forward to take advantage of it [2]. Ashburn and Thor introduced the term — repurposing, which is the process to find the new use for existing drugs where drugs may or may not be part of public domain drugs comprised primarily of generic drugs [3]. This definition changed significantly with time, including active substances that either include failed drugs or drugs failed at the clinical level due to their profound toxicities and off-target effects. This widened definition excludes all the compounds that fall into the category of selective optimization of side activities (SOSA). In SOSA methodology, drugs withdrawn or failed drugs are chemically modified through chemical modification to be repurposed for a new indication [4]. The present chapter is put forth to expand the role of drug repurposing within the perspective of the scientific community working in academia and industry. Besides this, the chapter will also cover details on tools and techniques to identify drugs for repositioning and their application in identifying drugs for various diseases and disorders. The current review will also foresee the recent market analysis updates on the cost-effectiveness of drug discovery and development involving drug repurposing compared to traditional drug discovery, challenges involved with drug repurposing, and future perspectives.

# 2. BACKGROUND

One of the U.S. FDA reports showed that the number of new drugs approved by the FDA has declined since 1995. The report estimates that of the total approved drugs and vaccines, approximately 30% are repositioned drugs [5]. Some blockbuster drugs that have been discovered by repurposing methods include sildenafil, thalidomide, minoxidil, aspirin, methotrexate, and many more. Sildenafil was initially used as an antihypertensive drug, but Pfizer repurposes it to treat the erectile dysfunction-based condition. It is marketed as Viagra, which reveals great worldwide sales of approximately $2.05 billion. Thalidomide is yet another example that was marketed in 1957 for managing nausea in pregnant women. But due to skeletal defects in the newborn because of its teratogenic effect, it was discontinued from the market. However, thalidomide was then repurposed for erythema nodosum leprosum (ENL) and multiple myeloma and marketed successfully on the pharmaceutical drug market [6]. Drug repurposing, in general, is based on the fact that all the drugs approved or declined by regulatory agencies have already undergone thorough trials and safety assessments; thus, their repositioning is quick and does not require substantial funds comparatively to conduct extensive trials [7].

In contrast, traditionally, when a drug exhibits biological activity on numerous receptors, also called "polypharmacology," it was considered negative in search of a promiscuous drug candidate. However, polypharmacological currently presents a broader scope for identifying off-targets that may be utilized if the disease pathology is quite complex [8]. The system biology insertion into polypharmacological assessment has further recolonized the area of drug repurposing [6]. Repurposing drugs is often considered attractive since the process is less risky, more economical, and time-saving. Drug repurposing is essential and also a hot topic in modern drug technology as it boosts the economy as well in a short time. Some certain advantages reflected by drug repurposing involves cut in research and development cost and time saving. Generally, five long steps are involved in traditional drug discovery, these includes **i.** discovery of lead followed by preclinical studies; **ii.** review of safety; **iii.** clinical trials; **iv.** review by USFDA; **v.** post market surveillance and long-term safety assessment. However, drug repurposing involves four steps that are relatively very less in contrast to traditional discovery. The major steps include **i.** compound identification from the approved leads; **ii.** acquisition of lead compound(s); **iii.** validation of new target; and **iv.** FDA approval and market surveillance for safety parameters. Traditional *de novo* drug discovery takes a long time, from drug identification to the marketing of the particular drug, and it also takes high cost and high risk that creates less interest for an investor to invest in the pharmaceutical industry. Compared to this, the drug repositioning strategy requires lesser time and money to launch the drug in the market for the disease. In this case, the *in vitro* and *in vivo* (also do not require phase 1 clinical trials) screening, validation, and efficacy studies require lesser time and reduced cost, which grows the interest of the investor. In this process, repositioned compounds have gone through different safety and pharmacokinetics studies for drug development with zero error or leakage and 100% accuracy. It is disclosed that repositioning drugs save cost and accomplishes profits of around 40% from the market [9, 10]. It is estimated that repurposing requires 3-4 years to undergo significant clinical trials and an investment of around 1.6 billion dollars in contrast to 12 billion dollars on an average requirement for novel drug discovery [11]. Currently, drug repurposing has been practiced for the treatment of orphan, rare or neglected diseases where cost investment is very scarce, along with pandemics that require rapid discovery of putative drugs in a short span of time [12].

With many advantages, drug repurposing certainly also faces some significant hurdles. The important one includes the intellectual property considerations and availability of data and the compound [13]. It is possible to file a patent to protect the repurposed category drug in the pharmaceutical market. However, some Nations where the original drug was first patented may impose legal restrictions for obtaining a patent for its repurposed or second use. Also, many research groups continuously explore the secondary or multiple benefits of the drugs, so in that scenario, the literature may already be available in the public domain in the form of specialized literature or for off-label clinical use and hence may further restrict the patent obligations [6, 13]. Secondly, profitability is the primary factor on which major pharmaceutical companies focus. So, considering the original patent (obtained for first use), the data is protected for at least eight years in European Union and five years in the United States. If the second use has been detected during these years (8 or 5 years), the grant is further expanded by one year in European Union and by three years in the United States. Considering this short duration (1 and 3 years) provides a very narrow window of time to earn significant profits in lieu of the investment made. Hence, the acceleration for such discoveries is often faded by the pharmaceutical giants. Further, the availability of data and compound is also a setback to drug repositioning. The inaccessibility to secondary clinical trial data, disclosure of failed drugs, and selective collaborations between pharmaceutical drug discovery companies could pose a significant barrier to valuable data by all and hence may hamper the objective of drug repurposing. Further, the generic active pharmaceutical ingredients (API), if gone from the international market, may hinder the availability of that chemical to scientists from reliable vendors affecting the repurposing research tremendously [13 - 15]. Nevertheless, keeping the drawbacks aside, the quest to identify the old drugs for new use has raised significantly in recent years. The significant chunk for this breakthrough may be attributed to the Covid-19 pandemic, where the major reshuffling of the original drug candidates was done. A few of the reshuffled drugs also received emergency approval from the USFDA but were soon revoked because of the toxicities in Covid-19 patients. The primary drug(s) repurposed included hydroxyl chloroquine, tocilizumab, remdesivir, dexamethasone, ivermectin, *etc* [16]. Recently, the Drug Controller General of India has approved drug 2-DG medicine (2-Deoxy-D-Glucose) to be repurposed for adjunct therapy in Covid-19 treatment. 2-DG was developed as a joint venture of DRDO, India, in collaboration with Dr. Reddy's Laboratory. 2-DG is well known promising therapeutical effect against cancer, cardiovascular diseases, and Alzheimer's disease. It is observed that the level of proinflammatory cytokine IL-1$\beta$ is increased in people infected with SARS-CoV-2. The direct link between glucose metabolism and virus-induced cytokine storm has been established recently. An important by-product of glycolysis, *i.e.,* 3-phosphoglycerate has some role to play in the production of IL-1β. 2-DG was found to inhibit glycolysis which inhibits the induction of IL-1β. However, for its effects against SARS-CoV-2, 2-DG gets itself accumulated in the infected cells (host) selectively, owing to the cell's high energy requirement (glucose) for viral multiplication in the form of glucose. 2-DG acts as a pseudo substrate for glucose and cutoffs energy production and impairs the glycosylation process of the viral glycoprotein. This halts the virus progeny and consequently reduces the virulence inside the host cell by inhibiting the glycolysis process [17, 18].

## 3. LITERATURE TRENDS AND STATISTICS

Further, the popularity of drug repurposing may be analyzed from the data retrieved from the Scopus database on August 27, 2021. The data was searched using two keywords, 'Drug' AND 'Repurposing,' providing 11159 documents. The thorough analysis revealed (Fig. **1A**) that the first paper on drug repurposing came in 1965, with a significant boom coming after 2015. The year 2020 fetched 2600 publications, followed by 2227 publications in 2021 (till August 27, 2021). The publication types (Fig. **1B**) were mainly confined to Research articles (7084), Reviews (2631), Editorial (293), Notes (276), Conference papers (273), Book Chapters (233), *etc.* Considering the country-wise research scenario (Fig. **1C**), drug repurposing is focused primarily in United States (3831 publications), followed by China (1219 publications), United Kingdom (1213 publications) and India (1099 publications) . Moreover, the Scopus database also revealed a total of 19,821 patent results, with major accounting in the United States Patent & Trademark Office (16600), European Patent Office (1458), Japan Patent Office (1401), World Intellectual Property Organization (306), and the United Kingdom Intellectual Property Office (56).

## 4. TOOLS AND TECHNIQUES FOR DRUG REPURPOSING

Broadly talking, there are two effective strategies for drug repurposing. The first one is 'on target' drug repurposing, which involves the implementation of an existing pharmacological mechanism to the repurposed drug, and the second one is off-target drug repurposing that involves targeting the same drug-receptor but for different diseases [19]. An example of 'on target' drug repurposing is minoxidil, which was initially used for its vasodilator effect and antihypertensive properties. However, upon applying it to hair, it has also facilitated the blood vessel opening and nourishment to the follicles, and thus later, its application in hair growth was also realized. An example of off-target drug repurposing includes aspirin which was initially used for anti-inflammatory effects; however, its anticoagulant effect is also known to us. Herein aspirin involves a similar drug-receptor interaction but possesses a different mechanism in the treatment of inflammations and in preventing clot formation (inhibition of platelet aggregation).

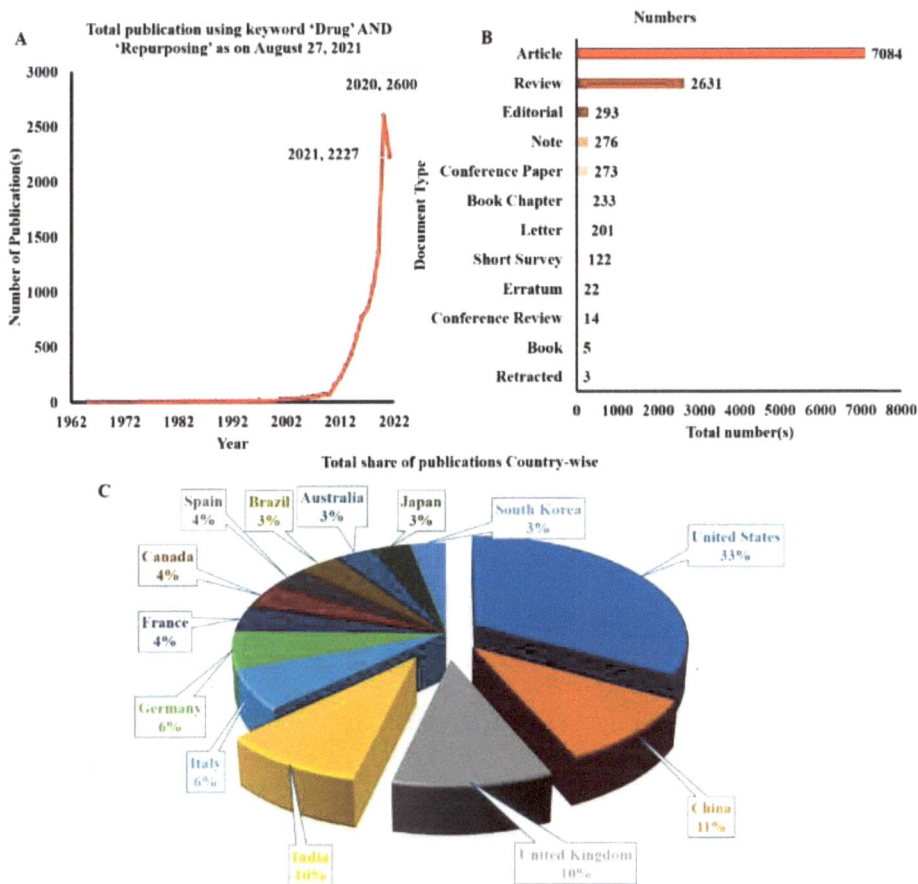

**Fig. (1).** Scopus search results (bar graphs and pie chart) were retrieved from the Scopus database using two keywords, 'Drug' AND 'Repurposing,' as of August 27, 2021. The data revealed (**A**) total publications in this area, (**B**) publication types, and (**C**) country-wise research scenario in current research for drug repositioning.

There are two major approaches of drug repurposing (Fig. **2**), including **i.** activity or profile based; **ii.** *in silico*-based approach, which is further divided into two sub-integrated methods, *i.e.,* network-based; and data-based drug repurposing [2]. The activity or profile-based repurposing includes experimental screening *via in vitro* and *in vivo* assays. However, this method is time-consuming but generally provides a lower probability of finding false hit(s). The second approach involves the computational technique that relies primarily on structural information of target proteins for high throughput screening of potential hits. Although this method is quick, it usually yields a high percentage of false hits during screening [20].

**Drug Repositioning**

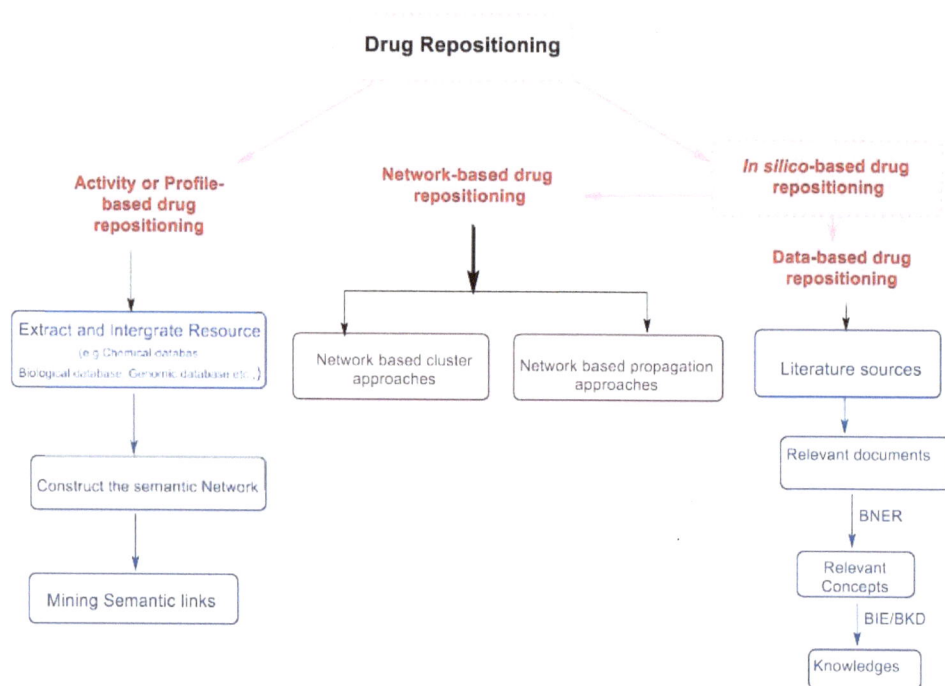

**Fig. (2).** A systematic diagram to showcase various approaches to achieve drug repurposing.

The major hurdle in repurposing involves identifying the off-patent molecules both from the approved and failed drug category. As per reports, the DrugBank database is enriched with 7800 drug candidates, among which the regulatory agencies have approved 2254. It is estimated that almost 80% of drug repositioning employs a target approach. This has been further boosted by the success of the Human Genome Project that offers approximately 6000 druggable targets to facilitate the repurposing ventures [9]. There are now several *in silico*-based drug repurposing strategies that may further be corroborated with activity or profile-based approaches to accelerate the repositioning of drug candidates. The crucial approaches include but may not be limited to network-based, semantics-based, or data-based drug repositioning.

Network-based approaches construct drug-disease networks that integrate numerous data sources considering gene expression, protein-protein interaction, and many more. Based on information from existing databases, interactions are extracted directly or indirectly *via* computational algorithms. There are two types of network-based approaches that are applied to explore existing core disease-associated genes. These are network-based cluster approaches and one network-based propagation approach. Network-based clustering approaches are used to identify biological entities from drug-disease, drug-drug, or drug-target relationships in a similar module of networks based on the same characteristics and topological structures to identify modules that could be used to discover novel drug-disease or drug-target relationships. The modules found by the approaches are also known as subnetworks. The drug Vismodegib, an inhibitor of the Hedgehog signalling pathway, was discovered to treat Gorlin syndrome. In contrast, iloperidone, an atypical antipsychotic used to treat schizophrenia, was discovered to be a novel potential hypertension medication. Another approach was network-based propagation, popularly used to find prospective candidate drugs. The workflow of these approaches was expanded to the genes sharing the neighbours in a Protein-Protein or gene-gene interaction network using a random walk propagation algorithm associated with a particular disease. These approaches can be classified into two groups based on how they propagate: local and global approaches. This approach identified a new indication for the drugs methotrexate, gabapentin, donepezil, risperidone, and cisplatin in Parkinson's disease, Crohn's disease, and anxiety-based diseases [21, 22].

Semantics-based approaches are commonly applied in data acquisition, image retrieval, and other related areas of drug development. Nowadays, these techniques used for the drug repositioning process consist of three phases. Firstly, to construct a semantic network built by extracting information from the medical database in order to extract biological entity relationships. After collecting the data from the preceding step, semantic networks construct based on current ontology networks. Furthermore, mining algorithms are established to forecast new semantic network relationships. Guillermo *et al.* proposed a hypothesis that similar drugs are interlinked with similar targets and similar outcomes, and immensely help in making drug-target relationships. A semantic network is constructed by drug-drug, drug-target, and target-target relationships. The findings show that the proposed approach made an accurate prediction about drug-target relationships [23]. Chen *et al.* constructed a semantic network based on drugs, targets, proteins, and diseases, including 290,000 nodes and 720,000 edges [24].

Further, there are many challenging tasks for the extraction of valuable and new biological entity correlations from existing literature. For this purpose, Text mining (TM) approaches have been extensively employed to overcome this challenge. This technique is rapidly being developed to mine new information from existing literature and uncovers the relationships between biological concepts or entities. The main workflow of the biological text mining pipeline consists of four phases: IR (information retrieval), BNER (biological name entity recognition), BIE (biological information extraction), BKD (biological knowledge discovery). In the first step, related documents are extracted from existing literature. After that, these associated documents must be filtered since they contain certain irrelevant concepts. In the next step, controlled vocabularies are used to identify crucial biological ideas in the BENR stage. In another two steps, BIE and BKD phases, relevant data is extracted to find and develop knowledge about the biological concept. Simultaneously, a potential correlation explored between knowledge from drug-disease and drug-target relation was detected. The most relevant example of drug repositioning in the clinical database is sildenafil. The drug was earlier diagnosed to treat pulmonary arterial hypertension, which was further repositioned to be used in erectile dysfunction, considering the side effects of the former. Many other examples were discovered *via* retrospective analysis, *e.g.,* aspirin in colorectal cancer and the drug raloxifene for breast cancer [7, 25]. Various databases required for *in silico*-based approach are compiled in Table **1**.

**Table 1. Databases employed for drug repurposing.**

| Data | Database Use |
|---|---|
| Drug chemical structure and activities | PubChem, CheEMBL, STITCH, |
| Structure of proteins | PDB, ProBis, PLIP |
| Clinical data | repoDB, repurposeDB |
| Structure of protein, transcriptional profile, and drug's activities | Open Targets, Drug Repurposing Hub, Drug Target Commons, |
| Drug-induced transcriptional response | Connectivity Map, LINCS |

## 5. CASE STUDIES OF BLOCKBUSTER DRUGS IDENTIFIED USING DRUG REPURPOSING

As discussed, drug repurposing is chiefly practiced to discover the treatment of orphan, rare, or neglected diseases because of the lack of investment in these diseases. Moreover, this approach is also reasonable in pandemics that require the rapid discovery of putative drugs in a short time. As per the estimate, approximately 90 percent of rare diseases do not have treatment; thus, drug repositioning looks pretty vital in such cases. Accidental discoveries have been the best example of drug repositioning and drug discovery [26 - 28]. The website http://drugrepur posing.info (last accessed on 29 August 2021) comprises 9040 drugs or drug-like candidates indicated for 475 biological purposes with 1016 molecular mechanisms with high correlation. Some important blockbuster repurposed drugs have been discussed herewith.

## 5.1. Aspirin

Aspirin is one of the most widely used drugs in the world. Acetylsalicylic acid (Aspirin), one of the oldest known drugs, was first launched in the market by Bayer in 1899 as an analgesic agent. This same drug was repurposed as an antiplatelet aggregation in low doses [29]. In 1971 Vane and co-workers came up with a landmark observation that aspirin blocked prostaglandin production by inhibiting cyclooxygenase (COX). It was the first time Dr. Lawrence observed that aspirin, originally administered for analgesic use for tonsillectomy patients, showcased increased bleeding as a side effect. It was further deciphered that aspirin

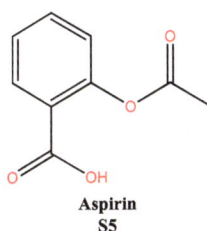

**Aspirin**
**S5**

inhibits the platelet aggregation *via* irreversible inhibition of the COX-1 enzyme utilised in the biosynthesis of prostaglandins analogue thromboxane [30, 31]. At low doses, *i.e.,* less than 300mg/day, aspirin binds selectively to COX-1 and exerts its antiplatelet aggregation effect, while at higher doses, it inhibits COX-2. This COX-1 enzyme is also involved in the synthesis of prostaglandins responsible for cytoprotection of the gastrointestinal tract [32]. It is further forecasted that aspirin may soon be repurposed for its action in oncology to treat several forms of malignant conditions. In colorectal cancer, aspirin controls cancer growth, and similar findings were also observed in many cancer types [33, 34].

## 5.2. Thalidomide

In 1962, WHO (world health organization) banned the use of thalidomide, an antiemetic drug that was used in early pregnancy state due to the degradation of transcription factor spalt-like family (SALL4) associated with the development. This leads to congenital disabilities associated with improper development of thumbs, ears or eyes and even conditions of congenital heart disease [35]. Thalidomide also inhibits the synthesis of proinflammatory cytokines, the major markers associated with the complications of leprosy. In 1998, thalidomide was repositioned as an orphan drug for the complication of leprosy [36]. The approval of this kind of drug with teratogenic toxicity is only possible for rare diseases. Like aspirin, thalidomide also possesses an antiangiogenic effect, a peculiar feature of drugs used to treat cancer. Due to its antiangiogenic, immunomodulatory, antiproliferative, and proapoptotic activities, thalidomide is now used as a first-line treatment for multiple myeloma, with the same precautions, *i.e.,* not to prescribe in the pregnancy stage [37].

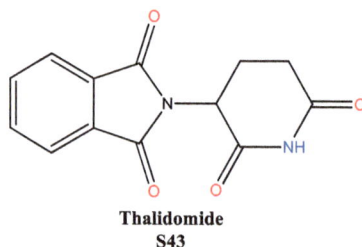

**Thalidomide**
**S43**

## 5.3. Sildenafil

Sildenafil is the world's most successful product of drug repurposing and the first drug that was repurposed before it reached to market. Initially, it was developed by Pfizer in 1990 for hypertension and angina-related cardiovascular diseases [38]. It produced vasodilation and inhibited the platelet aggregation by inhibiting PDE-5, a phosphodiesterase family enzyme having the ability to degrade cGMP, allowing vasoconstriction. During clinical trials conducted in the United Kingdom, an unexpected side effect has come into the picture in the form of penile erection. This side effect was the result of vasodilation which is produced due to the inhibition of PDE-5 that degrades the cGMP and ultimately leads to increased nitric oxide (NO) production [39]. In 1998 Pfizer utilized these physiological effects by launching sildenafil as _Viagra' to treat erectile dysfunction [40]. Pfizer continues to work on PDE-5 inhibitors, exploiting their vasodilatory effect. They found that one-fifth of the dose used in erectile dysfunction produces enough vasodilatory effect to treat pulmonary arterial hypertension [41]. In 2005, Pfizer got US FDA approval on the second sildenafil,

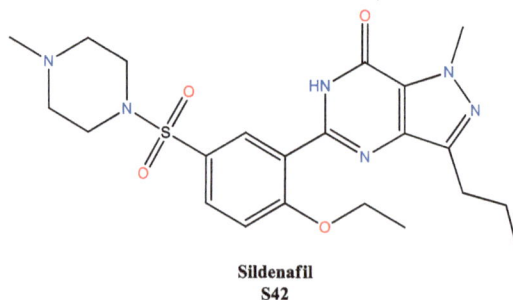

**Sildenafil**
**S42**

Revatio, for a rare disease, *i.e.,* pulmonary hypertension [42]. Sildenafil may soon again be repurposed for its effects against malignant disease. Enough evidence is now available showing its beneficial effect for cancer treatment, either alone or with other anticancer medicines. The nitric oxide (NO)/ PDE-5 dependent proapoptotic effect, along with activation of autophagy and modulation of the anti-tumor immunity of sildenafil, seems to be the primary mechanism for anti-cancer activity [43].

## 5.4. Amantadine

Initially, Amantadine was used to treat the Influenza A virus because of its prophylactic antiviral effect against Avian influenza. Later it was found that it can reduce Parkinson's disease, extrapyramidal syndromes, and akinesia. It got approved in 1969 [44]. However, this drug is now not recommended for the treatment of flu virus in the United States as it has been reported that these viruses have been resistant to amantadine for several years.

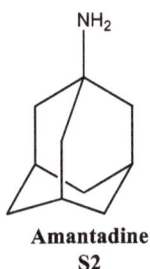

**Amantadine**
**S2**

## 5.5. Bupropion

Bupropion is another example of drug repurposing. Initially, it has been used in antidepressants. Lately, in clinical trials, participant helps to quit smoking, so it is used as a smoking remedy. The researcher found that Bupropion helps to alter chemical signals of the brain, diminishing the effect of removing nicotine. It got approved in 1997 [45].

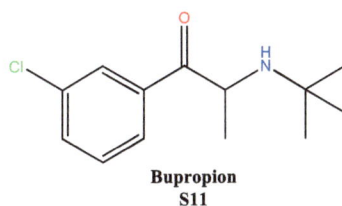

**Bupropion**
**S11**

## 5.6. Paromomycin

Paromomycin belongs to the category of aminoglycoside antibiotics employed as an inhibitor of protein synthesis in bacteria. It is repurposed for the treatment of visceral leishmaniasis and got approval in 2007 [46].

## 5.7. Finasteride

Finasteride, brand name Proscal, helps to shrink the enlarged prostate. Later in 1997, it was found to help treat male pattern baldness. It helps to inhibit the conversion of testosterone to dihydrotestosterone [47].

An exhaustive list of repurposed drugs and their original and repurposed use is compiled in Table **2** (adapted and revised from [7]). The relevant chemical structures are shown in Fig. (**3**).

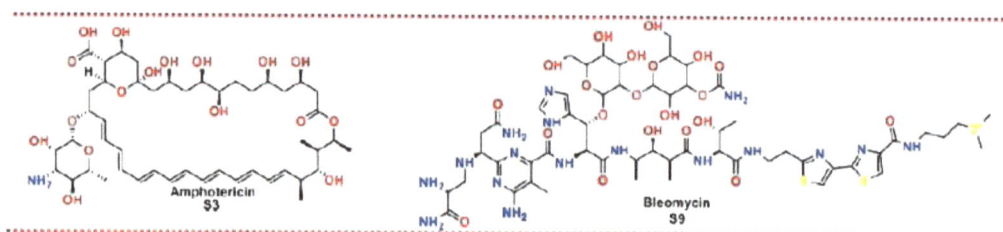

Fig. (**3**). Structure of Amphotericin and Bleomycin drug.

Table 2. List of reported repurposed drugs along with their original use of indication.

| Drug | Brand Name | Originally Discovered For | Repurposed Use | Chemical Structure |
|---|---|---|---|---|
| Allopurinol | Zyloprim | Cancer | Gout | Allopurinol S1 |
| Amantadine | Gocovri, | Influenza flu | Parkinson disorder | Amantadine S2 |

(Table 2) cont.....

| Drug | Brand Name | Originally Discovered For | Repurposed Use | Chemical Structure |
|------|-----------|--------------------------|----------------|--------------------|
| Amphotericin | Fungizone | Fungal infections caused by fungi | Anti-platelet | |
| Arsenic | Trisenox | Syphilis | Cancer (Leukemia) | |
| Aspirin | Aspir 81 | Inflammation, analgesia | Antiplatelet agent and colorectal cancer | |
| Atomoxetine | Strattera | Parkinson | Attention deficit | |
| Azathoprine | Azasan | Rheumatoid | Kidney transplant | |
| Bimatoprost | Lumigan | Glaucoma | Promoting eyelash | |

*(Table 2) cont.....*

| Drug | Brand Name | Originally Discovered For | Repurposed Use | Chemical Structure |
|------|------------|--------------------------|----------------|--------------------|
| Bleomycin | Bleocip | Cancer | Pleural effusion | Bleomycin S9 |
| Bromocriptine | Parlodel | Parkinson | Diabetes mellitus | Bromocriptine S10 |
| Bupropion | Aplenzin | Depression | Smoking cessation | Bupropion S11 |
| Celecoxib | Celebrex | Inflammation | Adenomatous | Celecoxib S12 |
| Colchicine | Colcrys | Gout | Recurrent pericarditis | Colchicine S13 |
| Colesevelam | Welchol | Hyperlipidemia | Diabetes mellitus | Colesevelam S14 |
| Cycloserine | Seromycin | Urinary tract | Tuberculosis | Cycloserine S15 |

(Table 2) cont.....

| Drug | Brand Name | Originally Discovered For | Repurposed Use | Chemical Structure |
|------|------------|--------------------------|----------------|--------------------|
| Cyclosporine | Gengraf | Rheumatoid | Transplant rejection | Cyclosporine S16 |
| Dapoxetine | Priligy | Analgesia and | Premature ejaculation | Dapoxetine S17 |
| Dapsone | Aczone | Leprosy | Malaria | Dapsone S18 |
| Disulfiram | Antabuse | Alcoholism | Melanoma | Disulfiram S19 |
| Doxepin | Silenor | Depressive | Antipruritic | Doxepin S20 |
| Duloxetine | Cymbatla | Depression | Stress urinary | Duloxetine S21 |
| Eflornithine | Vaniqa | Depression | Attention deficit | Eflornithine S22 |

*(Table 2) cont.....*

| Drug | Brand Name | Originally Discovered For | Repurposed Use | Chemical Structure |
|---|---|---|---|---|
| Everolimus | Afinitor | Renal Cancer | Renal transplant | Everolimus S23 |
| Fingolimod | Gilenya | Organ transplant rejection | Multiple sclerosis | Fingolimod S24 |
| Gabapentin | Gabarone | Seizures | Neuropathic pain | Gabapentin S25 |
| Gemcitabine | Infugem | Antiviral | Cancer | Gemcitabine S26 |
| Histrelin | Vantas | Prostate cancer | Precocious puberty | Histrelin S27 |
| Hydroxychloroquine | Plaquenil | Malaria | Covid-19 | |

(Table 2) cont.....

| Drug | Brand Name | Originally Discovered For | Repurposed Use | Chemical Structure |
|------|-----------|--------------------------|----------------|--------------------|
| Ketoconazole | Nizoral | Fungal | Cushing syndrome | |
| Lomitapide | Juxtapid | Hyperlipidemia | Familial | |
| Methotrexate | Trexall | Cancer | Rheumatoid arthritis | |
| Miltefosine | Impavido | Cancer | Visceral | |
| Minoxidil | Loniten | Hypertension | Alopecia | |
| Naltrexone | Vivitrol | Opioid | Alcohol withdrawal | |
| Naproxen | Anaprox | Inflammation, | Alzheimer disorder | |
| Nortriptyline | Pamelor | Depression | Neuropathic pain | |

*(Table 2) cont.....*

| Drug | Brand Name | Originally Discovered For | Repurposed Use | Chemical Structure |
|------|-----------|-------------------------|----------------|--------------------|
| Pemetrexed | Alimta | Mesothelioma | Lung cancer | Pemetrexed S37 |
| Propranolol | Inderal | Hypertension | Migraine control and | |
| Raloxifene | Evista | Osteoporosis, | Breast cancer | Raloxifene S39 |
| Retinoic acid | Aberela | Acne | Acute promyelocytic | |
| Rituximab | Rituxan | Various | Rheumatoid arthritis | Mab |
| Ropinirole | Requip | Parkinson's | Restless leg | |
| Sildenafil | Viagra | Angina | Erectile dysfunction, | Sildenafil S42 |
| Thalidomide | Thalomid | Morning | Leprosy, multiple | |
| Topiramate | Topamax | Epilepsy | Obesity | Topiramate S44 |

(Table 2) cont.....

| Drug | Brand Name | Originally Discovered For | Repurposed Use | Chemical Structure |
|------|-----------|--------------------------|----------------|--------------------|
| Zidovudine | Retrovir | Cancer | HIV/AIDS | |
| Zileuton | Zyflo | Asthma | Acne | |

## 6. DRUG REPURPOSING FROM AN ACADEMIC AND INDUSTRIAL EYE VIEW

The quest for translational research across the section of academia is rebalancing the methods and goals of drug discovery and bringing the traditional aspects of academia with the industry. The landscape and ambit of drug discovery are changing rapidly [28]. The academia and pharmaceutical industry should work in unison in order to have fruitful drug discovery and development. Drug repurposing is the cardinal example where both the important pillars of drug discovery and development are converging very well [2, 3]. It has been observed in the last decade that the baton of drug discovery projects has shifted from major pharmaceutical market players to hard-core academic setups. With the growing number of neglected and orphan diseases, orphan disease targets, and communicable diseases, it is strongly felt to have an efficient strategy for combating this, and thanks to drug repurposing, that came to the rescue [3]. There are several loopholes present in the *de novo* drug discovery process that has put the drug repurposing strategy into a central stage. Some notable hurdles of *de novo* drug discovery are already saturated chemical space, the innovation gap in the pharmaceutical industry, the higher attrition rate of newer scaffolds, the humongous cost involved in new drug development, the slow pace of drug discovery and growing concern for environmental concerns [48]. The repurposed drugs generate annual pharmaceutical revenue up to 25%, and over one-third of newly approved drugs recently are actually repurposed drugs [13]. Various government and non-for-profit organizations have sponsored various programs to promote drug repurposing. Some notable organizations which fund this initiative are NIH- National Center for Advancing Translational Sciences, Bill & Melinda Gates Foundation, and in India, CSIR (Council of Scientific and Industrial Research). Pharmaceutical companies have integrated a drug repurposing strategy in the life cycle management (LCM) of pharmaceutical products [49]. The below diagram Fig. (**4**) exhibits the interdisciplinary approach to drug repurposing. With the growing concern for environmental degradation, greener and more sustainable development approaches are largely being encouraged across various sectors. Pharmaceutical industries are now taking up and adopting the novel and greener approaches developed by academic setups for drug discovery and development [50, 51]. The drug repurposing strategy is relatively greener as compared to *de novo* drug discovery because it does not require the generation of a library of new chemical entities (NCE), which in turn would require lots of chemical reagents and solvents.

## 6.1. Integration of Pharmaceutical Industry and Clinical Studies

The drug discovery and development timeline is significantly shortened due to the availability of well-established safety data in preclinical models and known pharmacokinetic and manufacturing data. So, these drug candidates are often less likely to be failed on account of safety aspects unless severe drug-disease interactions are found [52, 53]. A plethora of gangbuster repurposed drugs, such as valproic acid, protease inhibitors, aspirin, hydroxy chloroquine, and propranolol, emerged based on previously standardized pharmacology and their off-level side effects [54, 55]. With the advent of computer aided drug design, *in-silico* studies and advanced proteomic data, drug repurposing has become systemic, robust, data driven and reliable [56]. The importance of drug repurposing could be understood with the astronomical surge in a number of publications over the years [19]. Fig. (**5**) depicts the advantages of the drug repurposing strategy. As the focus on translational and interdisciplinary research has grown in academia, the drug discovery process has also benefited from this. A fruitful collaboration between academia, small drug discovery start-ups and research laboratories could play a significant role in the drug-discovery process. As this would generate emphatic drug screening libraries, which could further accelerate the time required in search of suitable repurposing candidates.

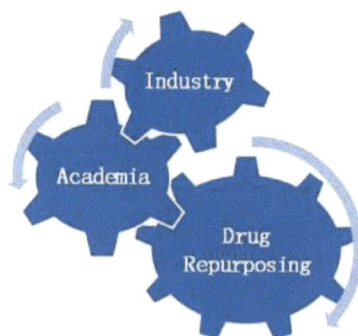

**Fig. (4).** Interplay of academia and industry in the drug repurposing strategy.

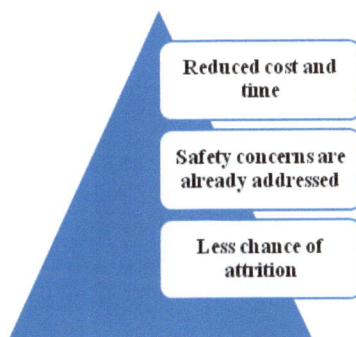

**Fig. (5).** Advantages of drug repurposing.

Drug repurposing involves several systemic steps and requires data from a variety of sources. It involves phenotypic screening, literature mining, and *in-silico* screening, and requires genomics data, clinical and pre-clinical data. Fig. (**6**) outlines the various steps involved in the drug repurposing study [57].

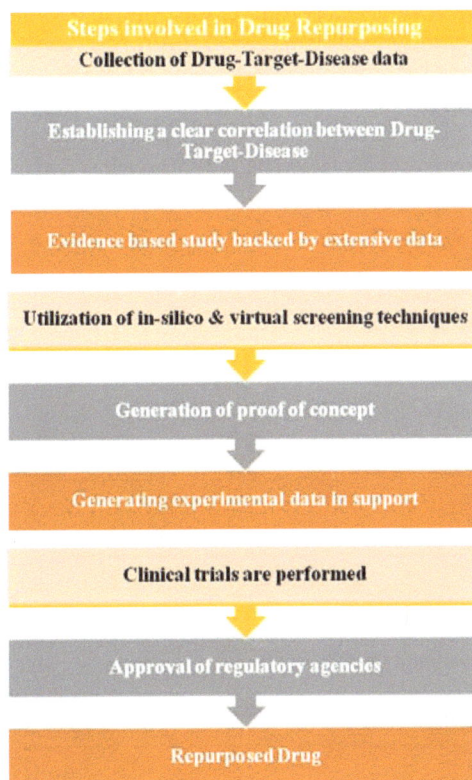

**Fig. (6).** Route map for drug repurposing.

The selection of a suitable approach for repurposing the drug is a crucial step in this process. The repurposing could be based on any of the three possible scenarios, such as a new target but old therapeutic indication, a new target as well as new therapeutic indication and an old target but new therapeutic indication [20]. After performing these steps properly, a suitable candidate for drug repurposing is achieved. Subsequently, the pharmaceutical industry will gear up for large-scale and emergency production of the drug. This reduces the time and launching cost required for a *de novo* drug discovery [15]. Recently the strategy of the old target but the new therapeutic indication was exploited for SARS-COV-2 treatment. The protease inhibitors and the RdRP inhibitors were two well-explored classes of drugs for the COVID-19 therapeutics. Viral protease inhibitors work by inhibiting protein translation and downstream proteolytic activities. Various protease inhibitors such as indinavir, lopinavir, sequinavir, and ritonavir were considered repurposing candidates against SARS-CoV-2 [16]. Fig. (7) depicts various protease inhibitors which were repurposed for COVID-19.

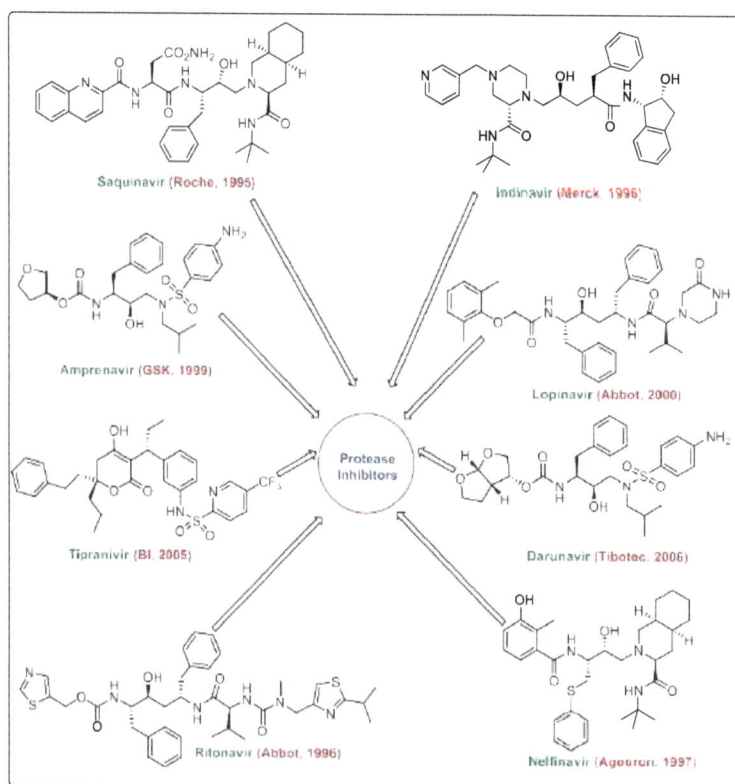

**Fig. (7).** Various protease inhibitors repurposed for SARS-COV-2.

Replication of the viral genome is mediated by a replication complex, including the RNA-dependent RNA polymerase (RdRp). RdRP inhibitors are a class of drugs that inhibits RNA-dependent RNA polymerase. Remdesivir is one such RdRP inhibitor repurposed for the Covid-19 pandemic, originally developed by Gilead Sciences in 2015 for HCV and has been explored for the treatment of the Ebola outbreak. Fig. (8) entails the mechanism of ramdesivir [58]. Remdesivir is a phosphoramidate prodrug that gets converted into an active NTP (nucleoside triphosphate) analog, which is called remdesivir triphosphate (RTP) [16].

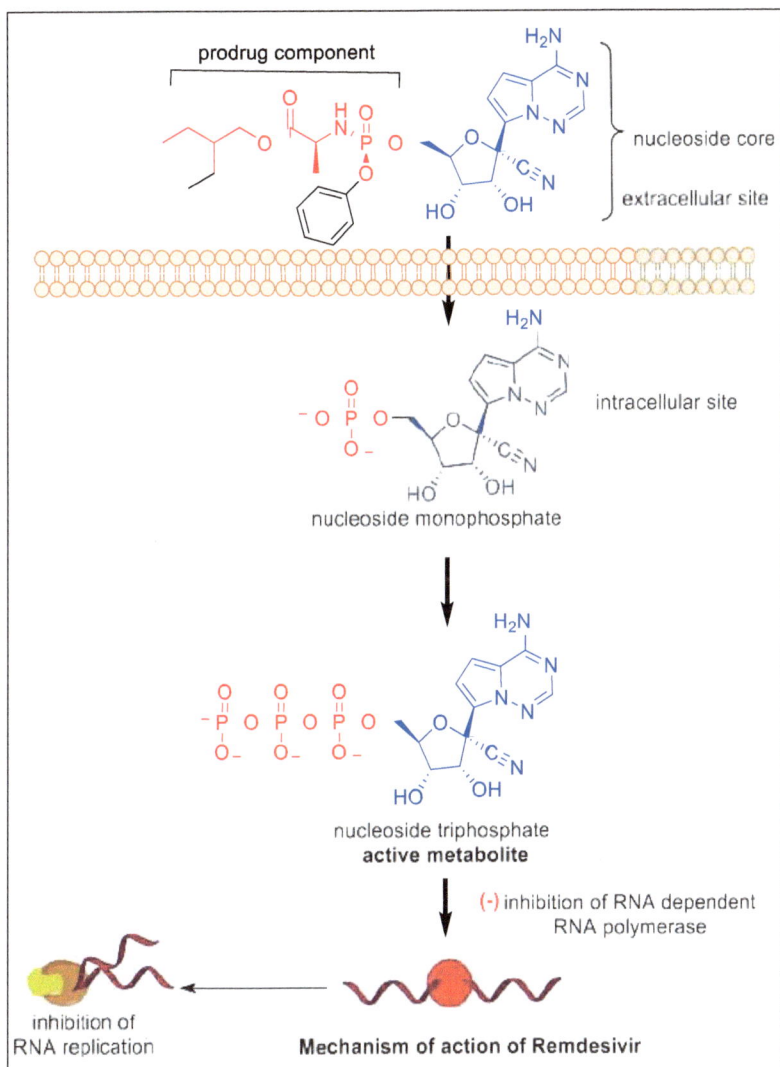

**Fig. (8).** Mechanism of action of Ramdesivir.

Similarly, for the same target but new indications scenario of the drug repurposing, tocilizumab was explored [59]. Tocilizumab is an immunosuppressive monoclonal antibody (mAb) drug originally developed by Hoffman-La-Roche and Chugai Pharmaceutical in 2003 for cytokine release syndrome in rheumatoid arthritis. However, treatment of moderately to severely active rheumatoid arthritis was approved by US FDA in 2010. It was the first biological therapy approved by the FDA for the treatment of systemic sclerosis-associated interstitial lung disease [60]. It acts by inhibiting the IL-6 receptor. It was found to antagonize both soluble and membrane bound IL-6 receptors generated by the pro-inflammatory cascade pathway in SARS-COV-2 infected patients [61].

The third scenario of drug repurposing is to find a new target and indication for an already known drug with well-established bioactivity and mechanism of action. This involves devising a completely new pharmacological or molecular target of a known drug. Drugs such as minoxidil, thalidomide, tamoxifen, celebrex, pentostatin, dapsone, rapamycin, and sildenafil are some of the drugs with known mechanisms of action successfully repurposed for a newer indication with novel molecular targets [20, 38, 52]. Hydroxychloroquine (HCQ) is one such drug repurposed for SARS-COV-2. Various mechanism of action is proposed for HCQ against COVID-19 infection, such as reducing immune cell activation in infected patients, inhibiting SARS-COV-2 virus entry into a human cell and inhibition of SARS-COV-2 virus fusion [62]. Another example includes the development of 2-DG, which acts as an antimetabolite for the natural glucose and cutoffs the energy source in host cells, thus affecting virus multiplication [17, 18].

## 6.2. Intellectual Coverage and Knowledge Transfer

The major drawback associated with drug repurposing is the lack of experts in the legal issues pertaining to this domain, as it is quite a novel field for both academia and industry. There is not much intellectual property protection mechanism for off-patent drugs [13]. The drug being repurposed for a new indication has already been exploited for various other indications and is well reported in the specialized literature. For off-patent drugs, a patent for the new indication can be obtained but could be challenged on the ground that it utilizes well-established strength and dosage form. So, its enforceability becomes a bone of contention among various pharmaceutical industries. Regulatory agencies across the world are often reluctant in recognizing the right of patentability and market protection for a repurposed drug. The best-case scenario envisioned was a situation where the drug being repurposed not only has a novel molecular mechanism for a newer indication but, at the same time, its formulation should also be unique. However, it should be kept in mind that derivatizing a known drug led to the creation of a new molecule itself and hence would not be considered a repurposed strategy. One more aspect related to the difficulty in implementing the patents for a repurposed drug (second indication) is a lack of coordination between various stakeholders involved in the supply chain of a medicine [63 - 65].

## 6.3. Regulatory Process Involved

Various regulatory agencies have their own laid-down procedures for granting market exclusivity right to a new chemical entity (NCE). European Union (EU) provides a data protection time period of 8 yrs during which no other generic company would be able to make use of the originator's data. EU also provides 2 years of market exclusivity to the originator. However, if the originator devised a new indication for the same drug during the 8 years period of exclusivity, one more year of protection would be given. It is evident that during the 2 years of market exclusivity to the originator, any generic company would not be able to market a product based on the data it collected. On the other hand, the United States (US) grants 5 years of market exclusivity to an NCE, which is extendable to 3 more years in case of finding a new indication. This extended period of exclusivity in the case of non-generic drugs constitutes an appropriate time to get an acceptable return on investment [66].

## 7. COST COMPARISON OF DRUG REPURPOSING VERSUS TRADITIONAL DRUG DEVELOPMENT

A medicinal chemist toolbox is now well equipped with advanced techniques such as bioinformatics/cheminformatics, *in-silico* studies, artificial intelligence, availability of biological and structural database, and structure-based drug design, which has further made drug repurposing strategy viable. The drug repurposing strategy has lots of benefits as compared to *de novo* drug discovery. One such biggest advantage is the cost involved. Table **3** compares a couple of parameters between drug repurposing strategies versus traditional drug development. Recent studies have estimated the cost involved in the development of a new drug to be somewhere around 2.6-2.8 billion US dollars [67]. On the contrary, a drug repurposing study requires only 1-1.6 billion US dollars [38, 68].

Table 3. Comparison of traditional drug discovery and drug repurposing strategy.

| S.No. | Parameters | *De novo* Drug Discovery | Drug Repurposing Strategy |
|-------|------------|--------------------------|---------------------------|
| 1. | Cost involved | To the tune of 2.8 billion USD | 1.6 billion USD |
| 2. | Time | Up to 12 years | 3 years |
| 3. | Duration of clinical trial | 6 years | 1-2 years |
| 4. | Success rate | 1 out of 10,000 (0.01%) | 3 out of 10 (30%) |

*(Table 3) cont.....*

| S.No. | Parameters | *De novo* Drug Discovery | Drug Repurposing Strategy |
|-------|------------|--------------------------|---------------------------|
| 5. | Regulatory requirements | Stringent | Somewhat relaxed |

## CONCLUSION

The drug repurposing strategy, despite being a promising strategy, has its own limitations and challenges. With the growing epidemics worldwide, given the high cost involved in traditional drug development and discovery of orphan diseases, it is high time to streamline drug repurposing and repositioning strategy. What is often considered as a 'valley of death' in the drug discovery fraternity, which is a lack of unison between basic and clinical sciences, is to be addressed. So, to avoid this, a more streamlined approach between various stakeholders involved in drug discovery and regulatory agencies is needed. Government incentives and industrial support to academia could do wonders in this area. A more robust technology transfer regime, better protection of intellectual property rights, collaborative industry-academia approach and better regulatory aspects would expedite the drug repurposing and repositioning.

## REFERENCES

[1]     Pushpakom, S.; Iorio, F.; Eyers, P.A.; Escott, K.J.; Hopper, S.; Wells, A.; Doig, A.; Guilliams, T.; Latimer, J.; McNamee, C.; Norris, A.; Sanseau, P.; Cavalla, D.; Pirmohamed, M. Drug repurposing: Progress, challenges and recommendations. *Nat. Rev. Drug Discov.,* **2019**, *18*(1), 41-58.
[http://dx.doi.org/10.1038/nrd.2018.168] [PMID: 30310233]

[2]     Xue, H.; Li, J.; Xie, H.; Wang, Y. Review of drug repositioning approaches and resources. *Int. J. Biol. Sci.,* **2018**, *14*(10), 1232-1244.
[http://dx.doi.org/10.7150/ijbs.24612] [PMID: 30123072]

[3]     Ashburn, T.T.; Thor, K.B. Drug repositioning: Identifying and developing new uses for existing drugs. *Nat. Rev. Drug Discov.,* **2004**, *3*(8), 673-683.
[http://dx.doi.org/10.1038/nrd1468] [PMID: 15286734]

[4]     Wermuth, C.G. Selective optimization of side activities: The SOSA approach. *Drug Discov. Today,* **2006**, *11*(3-4), 160-164.
[http://dx.doi.org/10.1016/S1359-6446(05)03686-X] [PMID: 16533714]

[5]     Aggarwal, S.; Verma, S.S.; Aggarwal, S.; Gupta, S.C. Drug repurposing for breast cancer therapy: Old weapon for new battle. *Semin Cancer Biol.,* **2021**, *68*, 8-20.

[6]     Jourdan, J.P.; Bureau, R.; Rochais, C.; Dallemagne, P. Drug repositioning: A brief overview. *J. Pharm. Pharmacol.,* **2020**, *72*(9), 1145-1151. Available From: https://doi.org/https://doi.org/10.1111/jphp.13273
[http://dx.doi.org/10.1111/jphp.13273] [PMID: 32301512]

[7]     Ko, Y. Computational drug repositioning: Current progress and challenges. *Appl. Sci.,* **2020**, *10*(15), 5076.
[http://dx.doi.org/10.3390/app10155076]

[8]     Liu, X.; Zhu, F.; Ma, X.H.; Shi, Z.; Yang, S.Y.; Wei, Y.Q.; Chen, Y.Z. Predicting targeted polypharmacology for drug repositioning and multi: Target drug discovery. *Curr. Med. Chem.,* **2013**, *20*(13), 1646-1661.
[http://dx.doi.org/10.2174/09298673311320130005] [PMID: 23410165]

[9]     Placchi, M.; Phillips, R. The benefits and pitfalls of repurposing drugs. **2018**. Available From: https//oliverdev. s3. Amaz. com/2018/11/07/21/59/08/240/Benefits

[10]    Elder, D.; Tindall, S. The many advantages of repurposing existing drugs. *Eur. Pharm. Rev.,* **2020**, *25*(3), 34-37.

[11]    Ojezele, M.O.; Mordi, J.; Adedapo, E.A. Drug repurposing: Cost effectiveness and impact on emerging and neglected diseases. *J. Camer. Aca. Sci.,* **2020**, *16*(1), 3-17.
[http://dx.doi.org/10.4314/jcas.v16i1.1]

[12]    Muthyala, R. Orphan/rare drug discovery through drug repositioning. *Drug Discov. Today Ther. Strateg.,* **2011**, *8*(3-4), 71-76.
[http://dx.doi.org/10.1016/j.ddstr.2011.10.003]

[13]    Talevi, A.; Bellera, C.L. Challenges and opportunities with drug repurposing: Finding strategies to find alternative uses of therapeutics. *Expert Opin. Drug Discov.,* **2020**, *15*(4), 397-401.
[http://dx.doi.org/10.1080/17460441.2020.1704729] [PMID: 31847616]

[14]    Agrawal, P. Advantages and challenges in drug re-profiling. *J Pharmacovigil S,* **2015**, *2*, 2.

[15]    Cha, Y.; Erez, T.; Reynolds, I.J.; Kumar, D.; Ross, J.; Koytiger, G.; Kusko, R.; Zeskind, B.; Risso, S.; Kagan, E.; Papapetropoulos, S.; Grossman, I.; Laifenfeld, D. Drug repurposing from the perspective of pharmaceutical companies. *Br. J. Pharmacol.,* **2018**, *175*(2), 168-180.
[http://dx.doi.org/10.1111/bph.13798] [PMID: 28369768]

[16]    Poduri, R.; Joshi, G.; Jagadeesh, G. Drugs targeting various stages of the SARS-CoV-2 life cycle: Exploring promising drugs for the treatment of Covid-19. *Cell. Signal.,* **2020**, *74*, 109721.
[http://dx.doi.org/10.1016/j.cellsig.2020.109721] [PMID: 32711111]

[17]    Mesri, E.A.; Lampidis, T.J. 2-Deoxy-d-glucose exploits increased glucose metabolism in cancer and viral-infected cells: Relevance to its use in India against SARS-CoV-2. *IUBMB Life,* **2021**, *73*(10), 1198-1204.
[http://dx.doi.org/10.1002/iub.2546] [PMID: 34418270]

[18]    Ardestani, A.; Azizi, Z. Targeting glucose metabolism for treatment of COVID-19. *Signal Transduct. Target. Ther.,* **2021**, *6*(1), 112.
[http://dx.doi.org/10.1038/s41392-021-00532-4] [PMID: 33677470]

[19]    Rudrapal, M.; Khairnar, J.S.; Jadhav, G.A. Drug repurposing (DR): An emerging approach in drug discovery. intechopen, **2020**.

[20]    Sahoo, B.M.; Ravi Kumar, B.V.V.; Sruti, J.; Mahapatra, M.K.; Banik, B.K.; Borah, P. Drug repurposing strategy (drs): Emerging approach to identify potential therapeutics for treatment of novel coronavirus infection. *Front. Mol. Biosci.,* **2021**, *8*, 628144.
[http://dx.doi.org/10.3389/fmolb.2021.628144] [PMID: 33718434]

[21]    Lotfi Shahreza, M.; Ghadiri, N.; Mousavi, S.R.; Varshosaz, J.; Green, J.R. A review of network-based approaches to drug repositioning. *Brief. Bioinform.,* **2018**, *19*(5), 878-892.
[http://dx.doi.org/10.1093/bib/bbx017] [PMID: 28334136]

[22]    Alaimo, S.; Pulvirenti, A. Network-based drug repositioning: Approaches, resources, and research directions. In: *Comput. Meth. Drug Rep*; Springer, **2019**; pp. 97-113.
[http://dx.doi.org/10.1007/978-1-4939-8955-3_6]

[23]    Palma, G.; Vidal, M.E.; Raschid, L. Drug-target interaction prediction using semantic similarity and edge partitioning. *Lect. Notes Comput. Sci.,* **2014**, *8796*, 131-146.
[http://dx.doi.org/10.1007/978-3-319-11964-9_9]

[24]    Chen, B.; Ding, Y.; Wild, D.J. Assessing drug target association using semantic linked data. *PLOS Comput. Biol.,* **2012**, *8*(7), e1002574.
[http://dx.doi.org/10.1371/journal.pcbi.1002574] [PMID: 22859915]

[25]    Tari, L. B.; Patel, J. H. Systematic drug repurposing through text mining. *Biomed. Lit. Min,* **2014**, 253-

267.

[26] Tanoli, Z.; Seemab, U.; Scherer, A.; Wennerberg, K.; Tang, J.; Vähä-Koskela, M. Exploration of databases and methods supporting drug repurposing: A comprehensive survey. *Brief. Bioinform.,* **2021,** *22*(2), 1656-1678.
[http://dx.doi.org/10.1093/bib/bbaa003] [PMID: 32055842]

[27] Issa, N.T.; Stathias, V.; Schürer, S.; Dakshanamurthy, S. Machine and deep learning approaches for cancer drug repurposing. In: *Seminars in cancer biology*; Elsevier, **2021**; 68, pp. 132-142.
[http://dx.doi.org/10.1016/j.semcancer.2019.12.011]

[28] Oprea, T.I.; Bauman, J.E.; Bologa, C.G.; Buranda, T.; Chigaev, A.; Edwards, B.S.; Jarvik, J.W.; Gresham, H.D.; Haynes, M.K.; Hjelle, B.; Hromas, R.; Hudson, L.; Mackenzie, D.A.; Muller, C.Y.; Reed, J.C.; Simons, P.C.; Smagley, Y.; Strouse, J.; Surviladze, Z.; Thompson, T.; Ursu, O.; Waller, A.; Wandinger-Ness, A.; Winter, S.S.; Wu, Y.; Young, S.M.; Larson, R.S.; Willman, C.; Sklar, L.A. Drug repurposing from an academic perspective. *Drug Discov. Today Ther. Strateg.,* **2011,** *8*(3-4), 61-69.
[http://dx.doi.org/10.1016/j.ddstr.2011.10.002] [PMID: 22368688]

[29] Bohuon, C.; Monneret, C. History of drug discovery. EDP sciences, **2012**.

[30] Vane, J.R. Inhibition of prostaglandin synthesis as a mechanism of action for aspirin-like drugs. *Nat. New Biol.,* **1971,** *231*(25), 232-235.
[http://dx.doi.org/10.1038/newbio231232a0] [PMID: 5284360]

[31] Vane, J.R.; Botting, R.M. The mechanism of action of aspirin. *Thromb. Res.,* **2003,** *110*(5-6), 255-258.
[http://dx.doi.org/10.1016/S0049-3848(03)00379-7] [PMID: 14592543]

[32] Cadavid, A.P. Aspirin: The mechanism of action revisited in the context of pregnancy complications. *Front. Immunol.,* **2017,** *8*, 261.
[http://dx.doi.org/10.3389/fimmu.2017.00261] [PMID: 28360907]

[33] Mills, E.J.; Wu, P.; Alberton, M.; Kanters, S.; Lanas, A.; Lester, R. Low-dose aspirin and cancer mortality: A meta-analysis of randomized trials. *Am. J. Med.,* **2012,** *125*(6), 560-567.
[http://dx.doi.org/10.1016/j.amjmed.2012.01.017] [PMID: 22513195]

[34] Rothwell, P.M.; Fowkes, F.G.R.; Belch, J.F.F.; Ogawa, H.; Warlow, C.P.; Meade, T.W. Effect of daily aspirin on long-term risk of death due to cancer: Analysis of individual patient data from randomised trials. *Lancet,* **2011,** *377*(9759), 31-41.
[http://dx.doi.org/10.1016/S0140-6736(10)62110-1] [PMID: 21144578]

[35] Donovan, K.A.; An, J.; Nowak, R.P.; Yuan, J.C.; Fink, E.C.; Berry, B.C.; Ebert, B.L.; Fischer, E.S. Thalidomide promotes degradation of SALL4, a transcription factor implicated in duane radial ray syndrome. *eLife,* **2018,** *7*, e38430.
[http://dx.doi.org/10.7554/eLife.38430] [PMID: 30067223]

[36] Raje, N.; Anderson, K. Thalidomide—a revival story. *N Engl J Med,* **1999,** *341*(21), 1606-1609.
[http://dx.doi.org/10.1056/NEJM199911183412110]

[37] Teo, S.; Stirling, D.; Zeldis, J. Thalidomide as a novel therapeutic agent: New uses for an old product. *Drug Discov. Today,* **2005,** *10*(2), 107-114.
[http://dx.doi.org/10.1016/S1359-6446(04)03307-0] [PMID: 15718159]

[38] Kauppi, D.M. Therapeutic drug repurposing, repositioning and rescue. *Drug Discov.,* **2015,** *16*, 16.

[39] Brazil, R. Repurposing viagra: The little blue pill'for all ills. *Pathophysiology,* **2018,** *14*, 20.

[40] Lexchin, J. Bigger and better: How pfizer redefined erectile dysfunction. *PLoS Med.,* **2006,** *3*(4), e132.
[http://dx.doi.org/10.1371/journal.pmed.0030132] [PMID: 16597172]

[41] Ghofrani, H.A.; Osterloh, I.H.; Grimminger, F. Sildenafil: From angina to erectile dysfunction to pulmonary hypertension and beyond. *Nat. Rev. Drug Discov.,* **2006,** *5*(8), 689-702.
[http://dx.doi.org/10.1038/nrd2030] [PMID: 16883306]

[42]   Dudley, J.; Berliocchi, L. Drug Repositioning: Approaches and applications for neurotherapeutics. CRC press, **2017**.
[http://dx.doi.org/10.4324/9781315373669]

[43]   Iratni, R.; Ayoub, M.A. Sildenafil in combination therapy against cancer: A literature review. *Curr. Med. Chem.*, **2021**, *28*(11), 2248-2259.
[http://dx.doi.org/10.2174/0929867327666200730165338] [PMID: 32744956]

[44]   Butterworth, R.F. Potential for the repurposing of adamantane antivirals for COVID-19. *Drugs R D.*, **2021**, *21*(3), 267-272.
[http://dx.doi.org/10.1007/s40268-021-00351-6] [PMID: 34152583]

[45]   Huecker, M. R.; Smiley, A.; Saadabadi, A. Bupropion StatPearls: Treasure Island, **2017**.

[46]   Vallières, C.; Singh, N.; Alexander, C.; Avery, S.V. Repurposing nonantifungal approved drugs for synergistic targeting of fungal pathogens. *ACS Infect. Dis.*, **2020**, *6*(11), 2950-2958.
[http://dx.doi.org/10.1021/acsinfecdis.0c00405] [PMID: 33141557]

[47]   Chavez-Dozal, A.A.; Lown, L.; Jahng, M.; Walraven, C.J.; Lee, S.A. *In vitro* analysis of finasteride activity against *Candida albicans* urinary biofilm formation and filamentation. *Antimicrob. Agents Chemother.*, **2014**, *58*(10), 5855-5862.
[http://dx.doi.org/10.1128/AAC.03137-14] [PMID: 25049253]

[48]   Mouchlis, V.D.; Afantitis, A.; Serra, A.; Fratello, M.; Papadiamantis, A.G.; Aidinis, V.; Lynch, I.; Greco, D.; Melagraki, G. Advances in *de novo* drug design: From conventional to machine learning methods. *Int. J. Mol. Sci.*, **2021**, *22*(4), 1676.
[http://dx.doi.org/10.3390/ijms22041676] [PMID: 33562347]

[49]   Global Drug Repurposing Service Providers Market - A Look at Repurposed Drugs in the Fight Against COVID-19, 2020. Available From: https://www.prnewswire.com/news-releases/2020-glob-l-drug- repurposing-service-providers-market---a-look-at-repurposed-drugs-in-the-fight-against-covid-19-301130140.html

[50]   Anastas, P.; Eghbali, N. Green chemistry: Principles and practice. *Chem. Soc. Rev.*, **2010**, *39*(1), 301-312.
[http://dx.doi.org/10.1039/B918763B] [PMID: 20023854]

[51]   Jadhavar, P.S.; Kumar, D.; Purohit, P.; Pipaliya, B.V.; Kumar, A.; Bhagat, S.; Chakraborti, A.K. Sustainable approaches towards the synthesis of quinoxalines. In: *Green Chemistry: Synthesis of Bioactive Heterocycles*; Springer, **2014**; pp. 37-67.
[http://dx.doi.org/10.1007/978-81-322-1850-0_2]

[52]   Schcolnik-Cabrera, A.; Juárez-López, D.; Duenas-Gonzalez, A. Perspectives on drug repurposing. *Curr. Med. Chem.*, **2021**, *28*(11), 2085-2099.
[http://dx.doi.org/10.2174/0929867327666200831141337] [PMID: 32867630]

[53]   Baker, N.C.; Ekins, S.; Williams, A.J.; Tropsha, A. A bibliometric review of drug repurposing. *Drug Discov. Today*, **2018**, *23*(3), 661-672.
[http://dx.doi.org/10.1016/j.drudis.2018.01.018] [PMID: 29330123]

[54]   Talevi, A. Drug repositioning: Current approaches and their implications in the precision medicine era. *Expert Rev. Precis. Med. Drug Dev.*, **2018**, *3*(1), 49-61.
[http://dx.doi.org/10.1080/23808993.2018.1424535]

[55]   DeMonaco, H.J.; Ali, A.; Hippel, E. The major role of clinicians in the discovery of off-label drug therapies. *Pharmacotherapy*, **2006**, *26*(3), 323-332.
[http://dx.doi.org/10.1592/phco.26.3.323] [PMID: 16503712]

[56]   Gns, H.S.; Gr, S.; Murahari, M.; Krishnamurthy, M. An update on drug repurposing: Re-written saga of the drug's fate. *Biomed. Pharmacother.*, **2019**, *110*, 700-716.
[http://dx.doi.org/10.1016/j.biopha.2018.11.127] [PMID: 30553197]

[57]    Corsello, S.M.; Bittker, J.A.; Liu, Z.; Gould, J.; McCarren, P.; Hirschman, J.E.; Johnston, S.E.; Vrcic, A.; Wong, B.; Khan, M.; Asiedu, J.; Narayan, R.; Mader, C.C.; Subramanian, A.; Golub, T.R. The drug repurposing hub: A next-generation drug library and information resource. *Nat. Med.,* **2017,** *23*(4), 405-408.
[http://dx.doi.org/10.1038/nm.4306] [PMID: 28388612]

[58]    Tian, L.; Qiang, T.; Liang, C.; Ren, X.; Jia, M.; Zhang, J.; Li, J.; Wan, M.; YuWen, X.; Li, H.; Cao, W.; Liu, H. RNA-dependent RNA polymerase *(RdRp)* inhibitors: The current landscape and repurposing for the COVID-19 pandemic. *Eur. J. Med. Chem.,* **2021,** *213*, 113201.
[http://dx.doi.org/10.1016/j.ejmech.2021.113201] [PMID: 33524687]

[59]    Denton, C. P.; Khanna, D. Rational repurposing of tocilizumab for treatment of lung fibrosis in systemic sclerosis. *Lancet Rheumatol.,* **2021,** *3*(5), e321-e323.
[http://dx.doi.org/10.1016/S2665-9913(21)00111-9]

[60]    Actemra fda approval history Available From: https://www.drugs.com/history/actemra.html (accessed on Aug 30 2021).

[61]    Samaee, H.; Mohsenzadegan, M.; Ala, S.; Maroufi, S.S.; Moradimajd, P. Tocilizumab for treatment patients with COVID-19: Recommended medication for novel disease. *Int. Immunopharmacol.,* **2020,** *89*(Pt A), 107018.
[http://dx.doi.org/10.1016/j.intimp.2020.107018] [PMID: 33045577]

[62]    Joshi, G.; Thakur, S.; Mayank, ; Poduri, R. Exploring insights of hydroxychloroquine, a controversial drug in Covid-19: An update. *Food Chem. Toxicol.,* **2021,** *151*, 112106.
[http://dx.doi.org/10.1016/j.fct.2021.112106] [PMID: 33722600]

[63]    Fetro, C.; Scherman, D. Drug repurposing in rare diseases: Myths and reality. *Therapie,* **2020,** *75*(2), 157-160.
[http://dx.doi.org/10.1016/j.therap.2020.02.006] [PMID: 32241561]

[64]    Smith, R.B. Repositioned drugs: Integrating intellectual property and regulatory strategies. *Drug Discov. Today Ther. Strateg.,* **2011,** *8*(3-4), 131-137.
[http://dx.doi.org/10.1016/j.ddstr.2011.06.008]

[65]    Halabi, S.F. The drug repurposing ecosystem: Intellectual property incentives, market exclusivity, and the future of new medicines. *Yale JL Tech.,* **2018,** *20*, 1.

[66]    Breckenridge, A.; Jacob, R. Overcoming the legal and regulatory barriers to drug repurposing. *Nat. Rev. Drug Discov.,* **2019,** *18*(1), 1-2.
[http://dx.doi.org/10.1038/nrd.2018.92] [PMID: 29880920]

[67]    Wouters, O.J.; McKee, M.; Luyten, J. Estimated research and development investment needed to bring a new medicine to market, 2009-2018. *JAMA,* **2020,** *323*(9), 844-853.
[http://dx.doi.org/10.1001/jama.2020.1166] [PMID: 32125404]

[68]    DiMasi, J.A.; Grabowski, H.G.; Hansen, R.W. Innovation in the pharmaceutical industry: New estimates of R&D costs. *J. Health Econ.,* **2016,** *47*, 20-33.
[http://dx.doi.org/10.1016/j.jhealeco.2016.01.012] [PMID: 26928437]

**CHAPTER 3**

# Pharmaceutical Potential of Pyrimidines as Antiviral Agents

**Dina Nath Singh**[1,*] and **Nisha Verma**[1]

[1] *K.S. Saket PG College, Dr. Ram Manohar Lohia Avadh University, Ayodhya-224001, India*

**Abstract:** Antiviral drugs are a class of medicines particularly used for the treatment of viral infections. Drugs that combat viral infections are called antiviral drugs. Viruses are among the major pathogenic agents that cause a number of serious diseases in humans, animals and plants. Viruses cause many diseases in humans, from self-resolving diseases to acute fatal diseases. The strategies for the development of antiviral drugs are generally focused on two different approaches, *i.e.*, targeting the viruses themselves or the host cell factors. Antiviral drugs that directly target viruses include the inhibitors of virus attachment, inhibitors of virus entry, uncoating inhibitors, polymerase inhibitors, protease inhibitors, nucleotide reverse transcriptase, inhibitors of nucleoside and the inhibitors of integrase. The inhibitors of protease (ritonavir, atazanavir and darunavir), viral DNA polymerase (acyclovir, tenofovir, valganciclovir and valacyclovir) and integrase (raltegravir) are listed among the top 200 drugs by sales during the2010. Still, there are no effective antiviral drugs available for many viral infections. There is a couple of drugs for herpes viruses, many for influenza and some new antiviral drugs for treating hepatitis C infection and HIV. This chapter gives an overview of the pyrimidines and hetero annulated pyrimidines that have been reported to be active against viral infections; identification of novel pyrimidine leads may be used in the designing of new potent, selective and less toxic novel therapeutic agents having promising antiviral activity. An effort has been made to compile all the possible information regarding antiviral pyrimidines and bring them together to make easy availability of the existing literature on the subject. The objective of this chapter is to provide the structural and antiviral activity information as well as methods being used for the screening of the antiviral activity and antiviral potential $IC_{50}/ED_{50}/CC_{50}$ values of the reported active pyrimidines are briefly discussed.

**Keywords:** Antiviral drugs, Antiviral pyrimidines, Inhibitory actions, Mechanisms of action.

---

\* **Corresponding author Dina Nath Singh**: K.S. Saket PG College, Dr. Ram Manohar Lohia Avadh University, Ayodhya-224001, India; Tel: +919415188503; E-mail: dnsinghsaket@yahoo.com

**Ashok Kumar Jha & Ravi S. Singh (Eds.)**

# 1. INTRODUCTION

The treatment of specific viral diseases requires specific antiviral drugs, *e.g.*, antibiotics for bacteria. In contrast to the complex structure of protozoa, fungi, and helminths, in viruses, the nucleic acid, protein coating and viral enzymes, including the coating of lipids, simply constitute the viral structural framework. Moreover, for replication, viruses utilize all the machinery of the cell and are hence treated as typically obligate intracellular pathogens. Under such conditions, it is a very difficult task for scientists to design and synthesize potential antiviral agents, which are only selectively toxic against viruses [1], as viruses are very tiny agents either made up of DNA or RNA and are also causal organisms of various diseases in animals and plants. Hence, in order to combat humans and viruses, different strategies are needed to adopt against each other. Antiviral drugs inhibit the growth of the viral pathogen, unlike the action of most antibiotics drugs which kill the targeted pathogens. Therefore, it is very difficult to search such drug targets that would only interfere with the virus without affecting the host's cell. Furthermore, due to continuous changing in the viral strains, the development of effective antiviral drugs and vaccines is a very complicated task [2].

The discovery and approval of idoxuridine in June 1963 as an effective antiviral agent opened a new area of discovery of antiviral drugs. Since then, a large number of antiviral drugs have been discovered for treating the virus disease in humans, and many others are also in clinical trials [3].

The process of discovery and development of an antiviral drug is very tedious and consists of a number of stages which include identification of the target, biological screening, generation of lead molecules and lead optimization, studies at the clinical level, registration of the drug, *etc* [4]. Continuous research on the discovery of potential antiviral agents is an urgent need in order to control the millions of human fatalities due to viral infections worldwide over the course of human civilization.

## 1.1. DNA Virus

The herpes viruses, papilloma viruses, poxviruses and adenoviruses and other DNA viruses generally have double standard DNA, leaving single-digit DNA that enters the cell centre and develops new viruses.

## 1.2. RNA Virus

The measles, influenza, colds, mumps, polio, meningitis, retroviruses (T-cell leukaemia, AIDS), arenaviruses and other RNA viruses are single descriptors.

RNA does not enter the cell centre. DNA copy of the viral RNA is formed by using the viral RNA, this process is organized by the host genome followed by retroviruses.

## 1.3. Steps of Viral Infections

The initial stage of viral infection is the entry of the viral DNA in the host cell and then releasing of new viruses after the replication (which includes a viral attachment, invasion, uncoating, replication, assembly and release) of that DNA. Hence, the first stage of viral infection is the attachment and penetration in which the virus attaches to a host cell, followed by injecting its genetic material into the host cell. Then incorporation of the viral genetic material (RNA or DNA) itself into the genetic material of the host cell and inducing it to replicate the viral genome, this step comprises uncoating, replication, assembly and release. Thus newly created viruses are released from the host cell either by breaking the cell, budding off through the cell membrane or by waiting for cell death [5, 6].

## 1.4. Inhibitory Action of Antiviral Agents

Two modes of inhibitory action due to antiviral drugs include targeting viral function and targeting cellular function that the virus needs. Generally, nucleic acid polymerases are divided into three categories *viz.* DNA dependent DNA polymerase, RNA dependent RNA polymerase and DNA dependent RNA polymerase. Due to the high mutability of the viruses and newly developed drug resistant viruses, the developments of vaccines and synthetic effective chemotherapy agents against influenza virus (flu) are of limited use [7, 8]. Designing and synthesis of potential antiflu drugs are based on the use of several potential molecular targets, *viz.* M2 proteins [9], endonuclease [10], hemagglutin [11] and neuraminidase [12], as revealed by various viral replicative cycles. A few drugs, namely rimantadine and amantadine, are only currently available for the treatment of Influenza, which provide limited protection as they have activity limitations and work as M2 inhibitors against influenza A by blocking the ion channel of the M2 protein [13]. Zanamivir and oseltamivir are potential neuraminidase (NA) inhibitors that displayed significant antiviral activity when taken intranasally, but poor NA if given systematically. However, the poor bioavailability of these drugs is a major concern as it is rapidly eliminated through renal excretion [14]. The orally active antiviral drug, namely oseltamivir, has side effects of nausea and vomiting. However, a recent report revealed that drug resistant strain of influenza A was developed in 20% of children when treated with oseltamivir [15, 16] and partially drug-resistant H5N1 strain 1 to oseltamivir was also recently reported [17, 18]. Thus the emergence of drug resistant strain of influenza needs to search for new and effective drugs against this mutant viral species. Worldwide, 175 million people [19, 20] infected with hepatitis C virus (HCV) remains one of the main public health problems. For treating HCV, the currently available drug is the combination of pegylated IFNα-2b and ribavirin [21], but this treatment is not responded to 20% of patients infected with HCV having genotype 2 or 3 and 50% with HCV having genotype 1 [22 - 24]. Therefore, a new treatment option based on more potent and specific inhibitors of HCV replication is currently needed in order to improve the recent antiviral treatment strategies. Patients suffering from chronic viral hepatitis B (HBV) were treated with (α-IFN, Intron A), but this drug has a limitation as less than one and half of the chronic hepatitis B viral patients fulfilling treatment eligibility due to its expensiveness and serious side effects [25 - 27]. Enzyme NS5b RNA dependent RNA polymerase is proved to be a prominent therapeutic target for the development of new anti-HCV agents [28, 29]. Infections with coxsackie viruses, and in particular with CVB3, are the most common cause of viral myocarditis. Moreover, these viruses are found to be responsible for the development of some other symptoms like pancreatitis, meningitis as well as encephalitis [30]. There is recently no approved antiviral therapy for treating picornaviral infections either in men or animals. Numerous compounds have been reported in the past as selective inhibitors of enteroviruses [31]. For example, pleconaril entered clinical trials but was not approved by FDA for the treatment of common cold symptoms in HRV-infected patients [32]. Murine subtype of parainfluenza is known as Sendai virus (SV) [33, 34]. Viruses PIVs causing upper and lower respiratory tract infections are recognized as significant human pathogens, however there is no licensed antiviral therapy till today for treating the PIV infections. A broad-spectrum antiviral agent namely ribavirin is found to be effective against PIV in cell culture and effectively treated the lower respiratory tract disease in immunocompromised hosts [35]. However, its efficacy of ribavirin is still debatable [36]. Furthermore, the potential environmental release of ribavirin has caused major concerned in hospital personals and was also proved to be a potential teratogenicity in the rodent model [37]. At present, there is no effective mono therapy against respiratory viruses, particularly for para influenza viruses. Non-nucleoside reverse transcriptase inhibitors (NNRTIs) of HIV-1 RT are currently considered as a potential anti HIV therapy due to their diversity and specificity in targeting this enzyme [38]. But NNRTIs of HIV-1 RT suffer efficacy related issues due to the emergence of mutant viral strains [39, 40]. Therefore, it is genuine to search for new chemical entities having broad-spectrum activity against mutant RT enzymes with minimal cytotoxicity. Few cyclic and acyclic fused pyrimidine nucleosides were reported in the literature as promising anti-herpetic drugs with selective activity against herpes simplex virus (HSV-1 and HSV-2)and varicella zoster virus (VZV) [41, 42]. However, there is still an urgent need to prepare more active cyclic and acyclic pyrimidine nucleoside, having lesser side effects in comparison to the existing drugs.

## 2. CURRENT STATUS OF ANTIVIRAL AGENTS IN CLINICAL USE

### 2.1. Iodo-2'- deoxyuridine (IDU)

The IDU (5-Iodo-2'- deoxyuridine) is the first anti HSV drug [43] to be licensed for clinical use [44]. The discovery of (E)-5-(2-bromovinyl)-2'-deoxyuridine (BVDU) as a promising and selective anti-HSV agent, as it has selectivity to specific phosphorylation by the virus-encoded TK [45], has become the lead for the development of a new class of antiviral agents. The diversity of acyclic nucleoside phosphonates such as adefovir, cidofovir and tenofovir [46 - 48] was found to be an entirely new class of antiviral agents. The antiviral drug trifluridine (TFT) was found to be reported as an effective anti-HSV agent [49]. The amantadine was reported to be the first antiviral drug against influenza [50] and ribavirin has also been proven as a broadspectrum antiviral drug [51]. 9-(2-Hydroxyethoxymethyl) guanine, namely acyclovir, is considered the basis of 2'-deoxiguanosin and exhibited antiviral effects after manipulating on acyclovir triphosphate and became the first specific antiviral agent as acyclovir is activated by a specific virus-induced enzyme, thymidine kinase (TK) [52]. Specificity of the acyclic guanosine analogue (acyclovir) against herpes viruses encoding for a specific viral TK (*i.e.*, HSV) has led to the synthesis of (S)-9-(2, 3-dihydroxypropyl)adenine [(S)-DHPA], which act as a broad-spectrum antiviral agent [53, 54]. Acyclovir displayed less inhibitory effect against VZV than DVBU, but unlike to acyclovir, BVDU has inhibitory potential against HSV-1, which is much more than HSV-2. Moreover, new DVBU analogue having promising activity against VZV has also been synthesized [55].

dihydroxypropyl)adenine

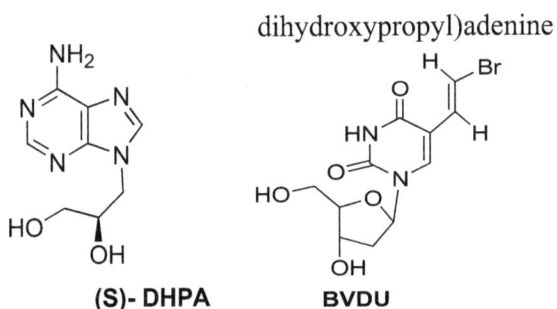

**(S)- DHPA**    **BVDU**

### 2.2. Valaciclovir

Valaciclovir (amino acid esters of acyclovir) was ultimately selected as the anti-HSV drug due to its better oral absorption profile as compared to acyclovir [56], and it has now become the standard drug being used orally against HSV infections. By following the acyclovir, a large number of acyclic guanosine analogues were synthesized and well documented as effective drugs against HSV. Among acyclic guanosine analogues, ganciclovir was the most prominent. Ganciclovir monophosphate replaces Ganciclovir. The oral prodrug of ganciclovir is valganciclovir and famciclovir is the prodrug of penciclovir. Antiviral drug cidofovir [(S)-1-(3-hydroxy-2-phosphonylmethoxypropyl) cytosine] has been approved for the treatment of cytomegalovirus (CMV) retinitis in patients suffering from AIDS [57]. For the treatment of cytomegalovirus, ganciclovir is found to be superior to acyclovir [58, 59].

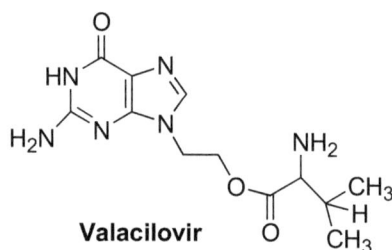

**Valacilovir**

## 2.3. Penciclovir

The antiviral activity of penciclovir is similar to acyclovir, and its *in vitro* inhibitory effect against herpes simplex 1 and 2 types and VZV infection is similar to acyclovir [60]. The penciclovir has now only been claimed as a topical plan for treating cold sores, and intravenous form was utilized for the treatment of mucocutaneous herpes in immuno-debilitated patients.

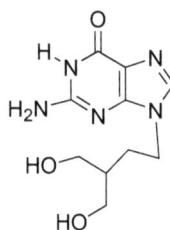

**Penciclovir**

## 2.4. Famciclovir

It is the prodrug of penciclovir and is converted into penciclovir by deacetylating in the digestive tract, blood and liver. It is also effective against the shingles virus & genital herpes virus [61].

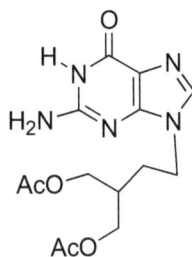

**Famciclovir**

## 2.5. Foscarnet

It is a trisodium phosphonoformate and a typical inorganic pyrophosphate. It is given intravenously. The clinical result of foscarnet is similar to ganciclovir against cytomegalovirus and has shown a better response than vidarabine for the treatment of the patients suffering from acyclovir resistant HSV [62].

## 2.6. Ribavirin

Ribavirin has shown broad spectrum antiviral activity. *In vitro*, it has a wide range of activity against RNA infections. The clinical suitability of this drug has been demonstrated detailed by administrating orally and intravenously against dengue as well as against hepatitis C when given orally by mixing ribavirin with interferon [63].

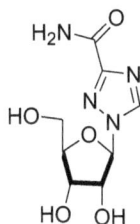

**Ribavirin**

## 2.7. Lamivudine

It was initially synthesized as an antiretroviral drug and basically a pyrimidine nucleoside. Lamivudine is prescribed as a reverse transcriptase inhibitor (NRTI), and in combination with some other drugs, it is found to be effective for the treatment of HIV-1 and monotherapy of the hepatitis B virus [64].

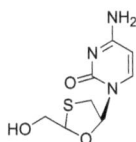

**Lamivudine (3TC)**

## 2.8. Amantadine and Rimantadine

Both drugs, namely amantadine and rimantadine, suppress influenza viral replication by blocking the M2 protein virus particle channel. Amantadine has a higher oral bioavailability as compared to rimantadine antiviral drug and these drugs are also found to be effective in the treatment of influenza infection [65].

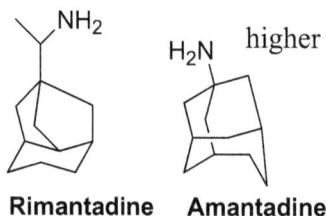

**Rimantadine**     **Amantadine**

## 2.9. Interferon alpha

It is a glycoprotein and found to be effective against diseases caused by varieties of viral infections such as HSV, hepatitis B and C virus and Kaposi's sarcoma. It is not suitable when given orally but behaves as a good drug candidate when administered either by subcutaneous infusion or intramuscular. Interferon alpha is produced in microbes by recombinant deoxyribose nucleic acid strategy [66]. Acyclic nucleoside phosphonates with (S)-HPMPA have also shown inhibitory activity against retrovirus infections and DNA virus [40].

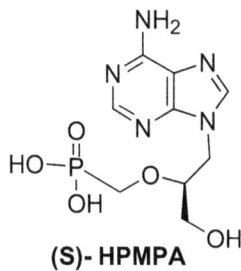

**(S)- HPMPA**

## 2.10. Adefovir

Adefovir's prodrug PMEA has been approved against the hepatitis B viral infection (HBV), and TDF, an oral prodrug of tenofovir, was found to be effective and approved against HIV infections [46.47]. An antiviral drug, cidofovir, and its cyclic analogue, were found to have potential activity against DNA virus infections [48]. Drugs HEPT and TIBO were introduced as specific antiviral agents against HIV-1 [67, 68], leading to the discovery of many promising reverse transcriptase inhibitors as anti HIV drugs belonging to the class of non-nucleoside. Furthermore, anti HIV activity is also encountered in some bicyclams [69, 70]. Cidofovir, by its promising efficacy value, is also used as an off-level drug against other DNA viruses' infections such as HSV and VZV resistant toacyclovir [71 - 74].

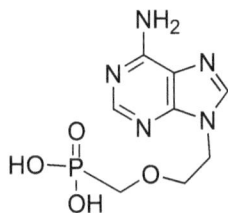

**Adifovir**
**(PMEA)**

## 2.11. Remdesivir

It is a novel antiviral prodrug of an ATP analog that inhibits the RNA dependent RNA polymerase and declines the viral genome's replication, thereby checking its production. Its pharmacological effect is broadly studied in MERS and SARS coronavirus infections [75, 76] and used against Ebola virus and Marburg viral infections.

## 2.12. Nitazoxanide

It is a broad spectrum antiviral agent which declines viral replication by interfering with the host regulated pathways and has been used for the treating of SARS corona virus and MERS Corona virus-2 infections. It upregulates the host mechanisms thereby is intrusive with the viral infections and hence viruses target to bypass the host cellular defenses [77]. This drug acts against influenza viruses at post translational stage and also blocks viral emagglutinin [78].

## 3. PYRIMIDINES AS ANTIVIRAL AGENTS

Pyrimidine derivatives play a very significant role in viral chemotherapy, as a wide range of antiviral activities have been shown to be associated with the pyrimidines. Despite a gradual increase in a large number of antiviral agents, patients still have no choice except to compromise with the side effects and the lack of the inhibitory effect of compounds against the virus resistant to existing classes of antiviral drugs, hence, there is a need to develop new antiviral agents, which may be highly potent and most effective, capable of producing a curative effect and causing least side effects and effective against those viral infections that are not responded by current antiviral drugs. The drug development programme is a very fascinating exercise and aims at the development of new lead, when the lead molecule is synthesized; it is further subjected to the synthesis of homologs and analogs. Thus lead generation and lead optimization are the two important aspects for chemists in the design of new compounds of biological significance.

## 3.1. Thio-arabinosylpyrimidine Nucleosides

A series of 2'- deoxy - 2'fluoro -4'- thio-arabinosylpyrimidine nucleosides have been synthesized and subjected to anti HSV-1 and anti HSV-2 activity evaluation *in vitro* [79]. The antiviral profile of the tested compounds showed that only β-anomers of 5-ethyluracil, 5-iodouracil, 5-chloroethyluracil, and 5-iodocytosine derivatives are potent and selective against HSV-1 and HSV-2 except for 5-fuorouracil derivative, 1-(2-deoxy-2-fuoro-4-thio-β-D-arabino-pentofur- anosyl)-5-fuorouracil **(1)** ($ED_{50}$ HSV-1 >27µg/mL, HSV-II >27 µg/mL and 5-hydroxyethyluracil derivative, 1-(2-deoxy-2-fuoro-4-thio-β-D-arabino- pento-furanosyl)-5-(2-hydroxyethyl)uracil) **(2)** ($ED_{50}$ HSV-I 27 µg/mL, HSV-II >27 µg/mL). Of these three analogues, (1-(2-deoxy-2-fuoro-4-thio-β-D-arabino-pentofur-anosyl)-5-ethyluracil **(3)**, 1-(2-deoxy-2-fuoro-4-thio-β-D-arabino-pentofur-anosyl)-5-iodouracil **(4)** and 1-(2-deoxy-2-fuoro-4-thio-β-D-arabino-pentofur-anosyl)-5-fuorocytosine **(5)**, the antiviral profile of the 5-ethyluracil derivative **3** ($ED_{50}$ HSV-1 0.012 µg/mL, HSV-II 0.11 µg/mL) is noteworthy. While 5-iodouracil derivative **4** ($ED_{50}$ HSV-1 0.037 µg/mL, HSV-II 0.32 µg/mL) and 5-iodocytosine derivative **5** showed weak cytotoxicity. The 5-ethyluracil derivative **3** did not show any cytotoxicity up to 100 µg/mL. None of the α-anomers of pyrimidine derivatives showed any antiviral activities. Acyclovir ($ED_{50}$ HSV-I 0.32 µg/mL, HSV-II 0.32 µg/mL) served as a standard control [80].

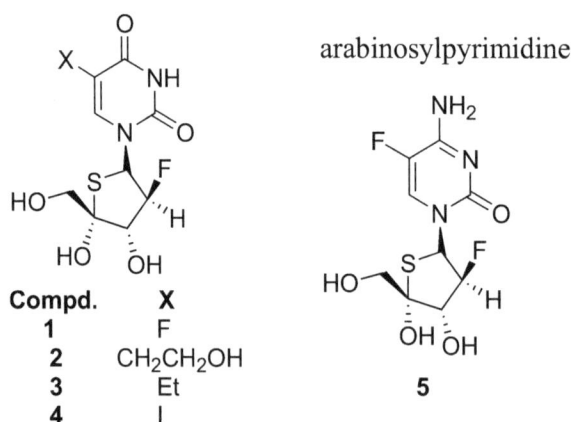

| Compd. | X |
|--------|-----------|
| 1 | F |
| 2 | CH₂CH₂OH |
| 3 | Et |
| 4 | I |

## 3.2. Acyclic Pyrimidine Nucleosides

Novel classes of 5-substituted acyclic pyrimidine nucleosides, 1-[(2-hydroxyethoxy)methyl]-5-(1-azidovinyl)uracil (**6**), 1-[(2-hydroxy-1-(hydroxy methyl)ethoxy)methyl]-5-(1-azidovinyl)uracil (**7**), and 1-[4-hydroxy-3-(hydroxymethyl)-1-butyl]-5-(1-azidovinyl)uracil (**8**) have been prepared and *in vitro* screening was also done. Compounds **6-8** displayed promising and selective anti-HBV activity against DHBV infected primary duck hepatocytes [81] with $EC_{50}$ 0.01-0.1 $\mu$g/mL. Among them, compound **8** was the most active anti-DHBV agent and displayed activity with an $EC_{50}$ value of 0.01-0.05 $\mu$g/mL comparable to standard compound (-)-$\beta$-L-2',3'-dideoxy-3'-thiacytidine (3-TC) ($EC_{50}$) 0.01-0.05 $\mu$g/mL. All newly synthesized compounds did not show any detectable toxicity against a panel of 60 human cancer cell lines [82].

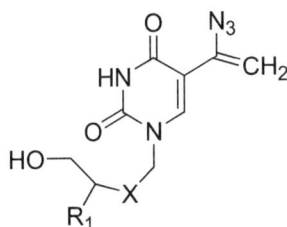

| Compd. | X | $R_1$ |
|--------|------|------------|
| 6 | O | H |
| 7 | O | $CH_2OH$ |
| 8 | $CH_2$ | $CH_2OH$ |

## 3.3. Lyxofuranosyl Pyrimidines

Compounds, lyxofuranosyl, 2'-fluoroxylofuranosyl, 3'-fluoroarabinofuranosyl, and 2'-fluoro-2',3'-didehydro-2',3'-dideoxyribose pyrimidine nucleoside analogues have been synthesized and screened for their antiviral activities against hepatitis B virus [83, 84]. Among them, compounds 1-(2-deoxy-$\beta$-D-lyxofuranosyl)thymine (**9**), 1-(2-deoxy-$\beta$-D-lyxofuranosyl)-5-trifluoromethylur acil (**10**), 1-(2-deoxy-2-fluoro-$\beta$-D-xylofuranosyl) uracil (**11**), 1-(2-deoxy-2-fluoro-$\beta$-D-xylofuranosyl) thymine (**12**), 2',3'- dideoxy-2',3'-didehydro-2'-fluorothymidine (**13**), and 2',3'-dideoxy-2',3'-didehydro-2'-fluoro-5-ethyl uridine (**14**) have exhibited promising anti-HBV activity against DHBV in primary duck hepatocytes with $EC_{50}$ values of 4.1, 3.3, 40.6, 3.8, 0.2, and 39.0 $\mu$M, respectively. Compounds **9, 10, 11, 12, 13**, and **14** ($EC_{50}$= 41.3, 33.7, 19.2, 2.0, 4.1, and 39.0 $\mu$M, respectively) exhibited significant activity against wild-type human HBV in 2.2.15 cells. Intriguingly, **10, 12, 13**, and **14** retained sensitivity against lamivudine-resistant HBV containing a single mutation (M204I). Compound **13** was found to be the most effective inhibitor of drug-resistant HBV with an $EC_{50}$ of 4.1 $\mu$M as 50% inhibition was not reported in the case of reference drug lamivudine at 44 $\mu$M concentration against drug-resistant strain. Tested compounds did not exhibit cytotoxicity to host cells at the tested concentrations [85].

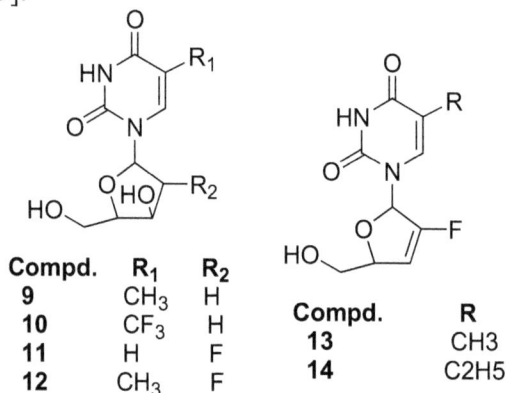

| Compd. | R₁ | R₂ |
|--------|-----|-----|
| 9 | CH₃ | H |
| 10 | CF₃ | H |
| 11 | H | F |
| 12 | CH₃ | F |

| Compd. | R |
|--------|------|
| 13 | CH3 |
| 14 | C2H5 |

## 3.4. 2'-Deoxyuridine Analogues

2'-deoxyuridine analogues have been prepared and screened for their antiviral potential. The HCV subgenomic replicon system has been used to assess the inhibitory activity of the compounds [86]. Among the compounds tested, 2'-deoxyuridine analogues, 5-iodoethynyl-2'- deoxyuridine (15), 5-(1-chloro-2-iodo)-2'-deoxyuridine (16) and 5-(1-bromo-2-iodo)vinyl-2'-deoxyuridine (17) have shown the significant selectivity index 3.2, 2.7 and 14.8, respectively on hepatitis C viral replication. It is worth noting that ribavirin in the same system had an SI < 1. The synthesized uridine derivatives 18, 19 and 20 have shown significant inhibition having $EC_{50}$ of 58, 162 and 75 µM, respectively, against replicon of hepatitis C virus, with a $CC_{50}$> 200 µM for 19 and 20. The selectivity index against HCV, for 18, 19 and 20, was also comparable to 3.2, 1.5 and 2.8, respectively [87].

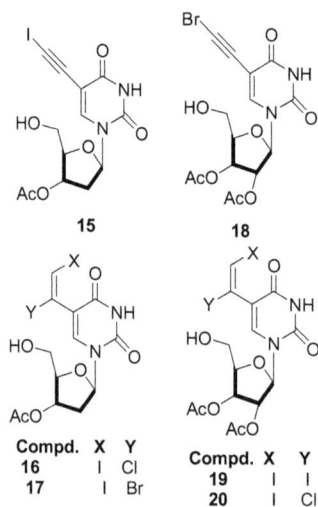

15

18

| Compd. | X | Y |
|--------|---|----|
| 16 | I | Cl |
| 17 | I | Br |

| Compd. | X | Y |
|--------|---|----|
| 19 | I | I |
| 20 | I | Cl |

## 3.5. 1-H- pyrimidine-2,4-diones

6-arylvinyl analogues of human immuno deficiency viral drugs (Emivirine and SJ-3366) were synthesized and screened for their antiviral potential against HIV-1 [88, 89]. Among them, compounds 1-ethoxymethyl, 1-(2-propynyloxymethyl), and 1-(2-methyl-3-phenylallyloxymethyl) substituted 6-[1-(3,5-dimethylphenyl) vinyl]-5-ethyl-1H-pyrimidine-2,4-dione **(21, 22,** and **23)** displayed promising activities against HIV-1 wild type ($CC_{50}$ 0.035 µM, $IC_{50}$>100 µM for **21**, $CC_{50}$ 0.03 µM, $IC_{50}$ 36 µM for **24**, $CC_{50}$ 0.03 µM, $IC_{50}$ 5 µM for **25**, $CC_{50}$ 0.03 µM, $IC_{50}$>100 µM for **22**, $CC_{50}$ 0.03 µM, $IC_{50}$ 31 µM for **23**) in the range of Efavirenz ($IC_{50}$, 0.01 µM, $CC_{50}$>100 µM), Emivirine ($IC_{50}$ 0.02 µM, $CC_{50}$>100 µM) and moderate activities against Y181C and Y181C+K103N mutant strains were also observed. These five most active compounds towards the wild type HIV-1 were also screened against HIV-1 strains with Y181C and Y181C+K103N mutations. Both strains are typically resistant to NNRTIs, Emivirine, Nevirapine, and Delavirdine and for the latter, also Efavirenz. Compounds **24** and **25** were inactive at the higher concentration, while **21** ($IC_{50}$, 17 µM against Y181C, $IC_{50}$, 29 µM against Y181C+K103N), **22** ($IC_{50}$, 17 µM against Y181C, $IC_{50}$, 23 µM against Y181C+K103N) and **23** ($IC_{50}$, 7 µM against Y181C, $IC_{50}$, 100 µM against Y181C+K103N) showed marginally higher activity against the Y181C single mutated strain than Emivirine ($IC_{50}$, 44 µM against Y181C and $IC_{50}$, >100 µM against Y181C+K103N). Compounds **21** and **22** were also found to be active against the double mutated strain Y181C+K103N [90].

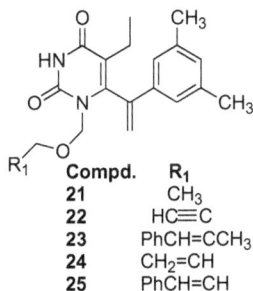

| Compd. | $R_1$ |
|--------|-------|
| 21 | $CH_3$ |
| 22 | $HC\equiv C$ |
| 23 | $PhCH=CCH_3$ |
| 24 | $CH_2=CH$ |
| 25 | $PhCH=CH$ |

## 3.6. Pyrimidin-4(3H)-ones

A series of novel 2-(phenylaminocarbonylmethylthio)-6-(2,6 dichlorobenzyl)-pyrimidin-4(3H)-ones were prepared and screened for their anti-HIV potential in MT-4 cells [91]. Most of screened new7 compounds displayed moderate to significant activities against wild-type HIV-1 with an $EC_{50}$ ranging from 4.48 µM to 0.18 µM. Among them, 2- [(4-bromophenylamino)carbonylmethylthio]-6-(2, 6-dichlorobenzyl)-5-methylpyrimidin-4(3H)-one **26** was reported most promising compound ($EC_{50}$ = 0.18 ± 0.06 µM, $CC_{50}$>243.56 µM, SI >1326) [92].

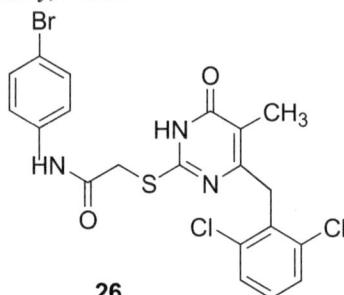

**26**

## 3.7. Pyrimidinyl-1,3-thiazolidin-4-ones

A series of 2-(2,6-dihalophenyl)-3-(substituted pyrimidinyl)-1,3-thiazolidin-4-ones have been designed on the prediction of QSAR studies. The synthesized pyrimidinyl-1,3-thiazolidin-4-ones were screened against HIV and were found to be prominent HIV-1 reverse transcriptase inhibitors [93 - 95]. Among the compounds tested, compounds **27** and **28** were found to be highly active in inhibiting HIV-1 replication in MT-4 and in CEM cells with selectivity indexes of >10,000 with $EC_{50}$ having a range of 22–28 nM [96].

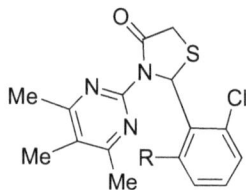

| Compd. | R |
|--------|---|
| 27 | Cl |
| 28 | F |

## 3.8. S-alkylated Pyrimidin-4(3*H*)-ones

A series of *S*-alkylated dihydro alkoxy benzyl oxo pyrimidine (*S*-DABO) analogues having naphthyl methyl substitution at C-6 and a β-carbonyl group on the *C*-2 side chain were synthesized and evaluated for their anti-HIV activities in MT-4 cells [97, 98]. Among the compounds tested, compound 5-isopropyl -2-[(4'- methoxy phenyl carbony-methyl) thio] -6- (1-naphthylmethyl)pyrimidin -4(3*H*)-one **(29)** was found to be most active against HIV-1 and also against the double mutated strain of HIV(Y181C and K103N) in the micro molar range with $IC_{50}$ 0.030 ± 0.002μM, $CC_{50}$ ≥203 μM and SI was found to be ≥6766 against HIV-1 in MT-4 cells [99].

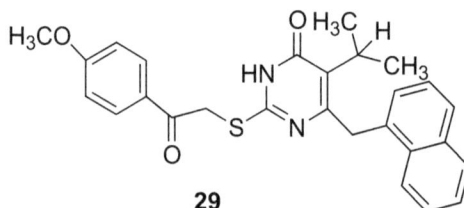

**29**

## 3.9. [2-(Phosphonomethoxy) Ethoxy] Pyrimidines

The 5-cyano and 5-formyl 2,4-diamino-6-[2-(phosphonomethoxy) ethoxy] pyrimidines **(30 and 31)** and the bis phosphonic acid **32** have been screened against several DNA and retroviruses for their inhibitory activity. The screening result revealed that compounds **30** and **31** have an inhibitory effect against HIV at 0.0027–0.011 µmol/mL and also against MSV at 0.0095–0.021 µmol/mL. The antiviral potency of the tested compounds was found to be comparable to 5-unsubstituted 2,4-diamino-6-[2-(phosphonomethoxy)-ethoxy]pyrimidine [100, 101] against HIV, but was inferior to the inhibitory values against MSV. The observed inhibitory values for compounds **30** and **31** were also comparable to standard reference drugs such as adefovir and tenofovir. No appreciable cytotoxicity for these compounds was reported against E6SM, HEL, or CEM cell growth, and did not alter microscopically visible cell morphology [102].

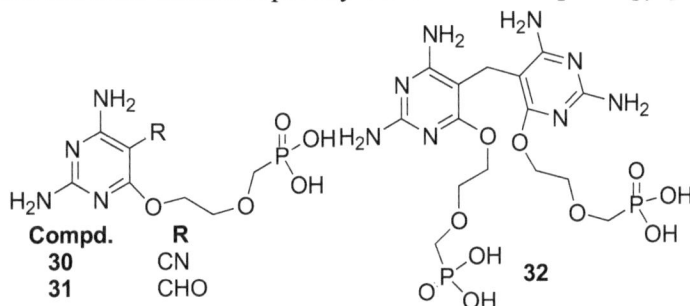

| Compd. | R |
|--------|------|
| 30 | CN |
| 31 | CHO |

## 3.10. 4-(3*H*)-Pyrimidinones, and Uridines

4-(3*H*)-Pyrimidinone and Uridines were prepared and screened for their antiviral activity against para influenza 1 (Sendai) Virus [103]. Among them, only compounds 1,3-dimethyl-6-(2'-phenyl -2'-oxiranylmethyl)uracil **(33)** and 1,3-dimethyl-6-(2'methyl-2'-tetrahydrofurylmethyl)uracil **34** were found to display prominent anti-parainfluenza 1 (Sendai) viral activity. Active compounds **33** ($EC_{50}$ 0.18 µM, $CC_{50}$ 3.7µM) and **34** ($EC_{50}$ 1.11, $CC_{50}$ 1380µM) were found as potent and selective inhibitors of para influenza 1 (Sendai) virus. Finally, **34** was identified by a selectivity index of about 200, as the magnitude of antiviral activity 1 order higher than the most active compound **33** [104].

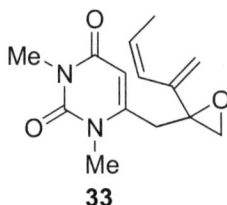

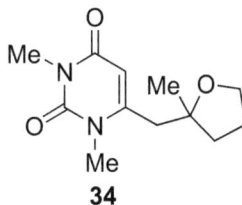

### 3.11. 5-(1-Azido-2-haloethyl) Uracils

Novel acyclic nucleoside analogues of 5-(1-Azido-2-haloethyl) uracils were prepared and screened for their antiviral activities in culture against HSV-1, strains KOS and E-377, HSV-2, strain MS, VZV, strain Ellen and HCMV, strain (AD-169) infected human foreskin fibroblast (HFF) or Vero cells [105, 106]. Among them, only compound **35** exhibited the most potent activity against VZV ($EC_{50}$ 2.4 $\mu$M), comparable to acyclovir ($EC_{50}$ 2.6 $\mu$M). Interestingly, acyclic derivatives of 5-(1-azido-2-haloethyl) uracil were also identified, having inhibitory potential to HCMV. Compound 1-[4-hydroxy-3-(hydroxymethyl1)-1-butyl]-5-(1-azido-2-chloro ethyl) uracil (**36**) was also an effective antiviral agent in the *in vitro* assays against HCMV ($EC_{50}$ 3.1 $\mu$M) and DHBV ($EC_{50}$ 0.31-1.55 $\mu$M). No tested compounds displayed any detectable toxicity to several stationary and proliferating host cells [107].

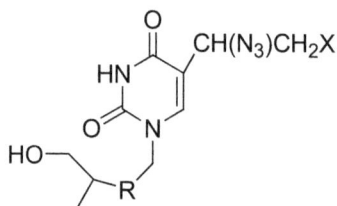

| Compd. | R | R$_1$ | X |
|--------|-----|--------|-----|
| 35 | O | CH$_2$OH | I |
| 36 | CH$_2$ | CH$_2$OH | Cl |

### 3.12. 6-[2-(Phosphonomethoxy)alkoxy]pyrimidines

6-[2-(Phosphonomethoxy)alkoxy]pyrimidines were synthesized and their antiviral screening profile revealed that only compounds 2,4-diamino-6-[2 (phosphono methoxy)ethoxy]pyrimidine (**37**) and 2-amino-4-hydroxy-6-[2 (phosphono methoxy)ethoxy]-pyrimidine (**38**) were found to be potent against two wild type VZV and two TK-deficient VZV strains [108 - 110].

Compounds **37** & **38** exhibited an inhibitory effect against herpes simplex virus type 1 (HSV-1), HSV-2, and the thymidine kinase (TK)-deficient TK-/HSV-1 strain [111], having $EC_{50}$ between 6.5 and 24 $\mu$g/mL and more active against the above mentioned wild type viral strains ($EC_{50}$: 0.6-2.5 $\mu$g/mL), and not active at subtoxic concentrations against cytomegalovirus (CMV). Compound **37** was inactive against adenovirus type 2 and type 3 infections in HEL cells. Compounds **37** and **38** were also exquisitely inhibitory to MSV in C3H/3T3 cell cultures ($EC_{50}$: 0.04-0.08 $\mu$g/mL). Compound **37** was found to be very effective ($EC_{50}$: 0.4-0.8 $\mu$g/mL) against HIV-1 and HIV-2 in CEM cell cultures. In contrast, **38** was not inhibitory at 0.8 $\mu$g/mL, which is at a concentration close to its toxicity threshold [112].

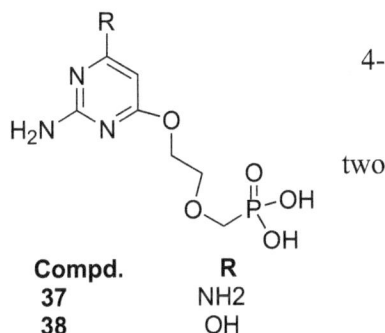

| Compd. | R |
|--------|------|
| 37 | NH2 |
| 38 | OH |

### 3.13. (*Z*)- and (*E*)-[2-Fluoro-2- (hydroxymethyl) cyclopropylidene]methyl-pyrimidines

(*Z*)- and (*E*)-[2-Fluoro-2- (hydroxymethyl) cyclopropylidene]methyl-pyrimidines, a new class of methylene cyclopropane analogues of nucleosides, have been synthesized and screened againstHSV-1 and VZV [113, 114]. Among them, only thymine *Z*-isomer *Z*)-1-{[(2-fluoro-2-hydroxymethyl)cyclopropylidene]-methyl} thymine (**39**) was found to be more effective against HSV-1 in BSC-1 cells (ELISA, $EC_{50}$ 2.5 $\mu$M) and inactive against HSV-1 or HSV-2 in Vero or HFF cells. Cytosine and thymine *Z*-isomers **39** and (*Z*)-1-{[(2-fluoro-2-hydroxy methyl)cyclopropylidene]-methyl}cytosine (**40**) were active against varicella zoster virus (VZV) in HFF culture in the submicromolar range with $EC_{50}$ 0.62 $\mu$M [115].

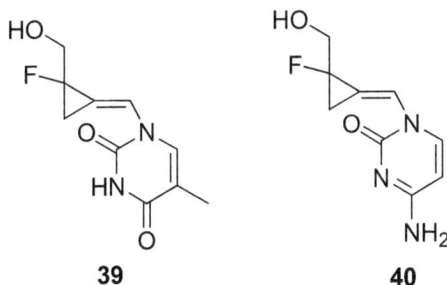

**39**                    **40**

### 3.14. Pyrimidines Carbonucleosides

The antiviral activity of the synthesized pyrimidines carbo nucleosides has been evaluated by the plaque-reduction method against cytomegalovirus (CMV) in PEU cells and HSV-1 and HSV-2, in Vero cells [116, 117]. Among the carbonucleosides, compounds **41** (CMV, HSV-1 and HSV-2, $EC_{50}$ =10.0 $\mu$M) **42** (CMV and HSV-2,$EC_{50}$ = 0.97 $\mu$M ;HSV-1,$EC_{50}$ =10.0 $\mu$M) and **43** (CMV $EC_{50}$ =10.0 $\mu$M, HSV-1 and HSV-2 $EC_{50}$ =0.97$\mu$M) were found to exhibit good efficacy against three virus species tested, while no cytotoxicity was observed for any of the compounds [118].

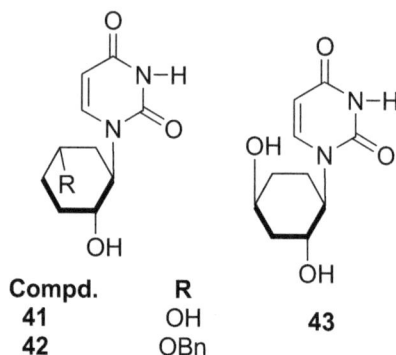

| Compd. | R |
|--------|-----|
| 41 | OH |
| 42 | OBn |

43

## 3.15. Suitably Substituted Pyrimidines

Pyrimidines derivatives **44-48** were prepared and screened for their antiviral potentials. Among the compounds screened, 5-bromo-6-dibromomethyl-substituted pyrimidine **44** was found to have moderate inhibitory potential against TK+VZV (EC$_{50}$ 8.8 $\mu$M) and TK-VZV (EC$_{50}$ 10.5 $\mu$M). Compound **45** displayed slight activity and not highly specific activity against TK+-VZV (EC$_{50}$ 8.1 $\mu$M) and TK-VZV (EC$_{50}$ 7.4 $\mu$M). Compound **46** was marginal active against the CMV AD-169 strain (EC$_{50}$ 45 $\mu$M), CMV Davis strain (EC$_{50}$ 20 $\mu$M), TK+VZV (EC$_{50}$ 80 $\mu$M), and TK-VZV (EC$_{50}$ 45 $\mu$M). Moreover, C-6 fluoro phenyl alkenyl pyrimidine **47** showed moderate activity against Coxsackie B4 virus (EC$_{50}$ 24 $\mu$M) and CMV Davis strain (EC$_{50}$ 38 $\mu$M). Comparisons of the potency of the tested compounds to standard reference revealed that 5-bromo-6-dibromomet-yl-substituted pyrimidine **44** was 3-fold more potent against TK-VZV than acyclovir and 16-fold more potent than brivudin. Besides, compound **44** was 16-fold more active against TK-VZV than acyclovir and 84-fold more active than brivudin and 2-fold less active than acyclovir. Against TK+-VZV, compound **47** was found to be 6-fold more potent against Coxsackie B4 virus than ribavirin. Furthermore, fluorophenyl alkylated pyrimidine derivatives **46** and **47** showed no cytotoxic effect. Compounds **44-48** were also screened for their cytostatic activities. Among the screened compounds, the 5-bromo-6-dibromomet-yl-substituted pyrimidine derivative **44** was found to exhibit the most significant cytotoxic activity against the malignant tumor cells. Generally, fluoroalkyl pyrimidine derivatives showed more prominent cytostatic effects compared to the fluorophenyl pyrimidine series. Hence, **45** and **48,** against all tested tumor cell lines, showed remarkable inhibitory activity. Therefore, from the fluoro alkylated pyrimidine series, compound **45** emerged as the most interesting leading compound with cytostatic and antiviral activities that could be used in future lead optimization [119].

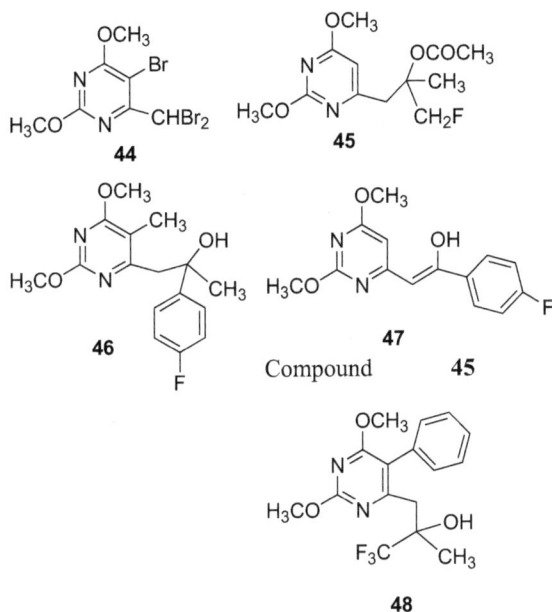

**44**   **45**

**46**   **47**

Compound **45**

**48**

## 3.16. 2-Deoxy-1, 5-anhydro-D-mannitol Nucleosides with Pyrimidine Base Moiety

Compounds 2-deoxy-1, 5-anhydro-D-mannitol nucleosides containing a pyrimidine base moiety **49** and **50** have been synthesized and displayed antiviral activity against HSV-1 and CMV. Compound **49** displayed MIC values of 7.0 µg/ml against HSV-1 and compound **50** exhibited MIC values of 10.0 µg/ml against cytomegalovirus. The minimum cytotoxic concentration required to cause a microscopically detectable alteration of normal cell morphology was > 400 µg/ml. The concentration required to reduce cell growth by 50% was 30 µg/ml. Acyclovir (HSV-1, MIC: 0.004 µg/ml) and ganciclovir (CMV, MIC: 1.0 µg/ml) were used as standard drugs in the same assay [120].

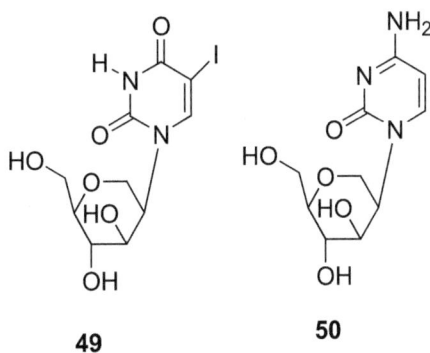

**49**   **50**

### 3.17. 5-Ethyl and E-5- (2-bromovinyl) Uracil-(benzoyloxymethyl) Pyrrolidine

5-Ethyluracil-(benzoyloxymethyl) pyrrolidine **51** was tested in a broad antiviral assay such as HSV-1 and -2, varicella zoster virus (VZV), human cytomegalovirus (HCMV), HIV-1 and -2, vaccinia virus and vesicular stomatitis virus [121, 122]. Antiviral screening result revealed that compound **51** was only found to be a specific inhibitor of vaccinia virus (IC$_{50}$ 40 µM, toxic at ≥ 201µM) with comparable activity to BVDU (IC$_{50}$ 12 µM, toxic at ≥ 1200 µM) and the conversion of the ethyl side chain of **51** to an E-5-(2-bromovinyl) functionality as in **52**, which resulted in a compound with no activity and increased toxicity (69 µM) [123].

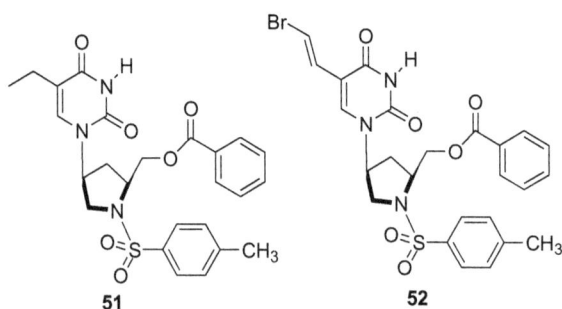

**51**                     **52**

### 3.18. Dihydroxypyrimidine Carboxylates

Patients suffering from hepatitis C virus (HCV) are a serious concerned world health problem, and hence in order to overcome this situation, novel therapies are in urgent demand [124 - 126]. The polymerase of the hepatitis C virus is responsible for the replication of viral RNA. Compound dihydroxy pyrimidine carboxylate, 2- phenyl-5,6-dihydroxypyrimidine-4-carboxylic acid **53** (IC$_{50}$ 30 *µ*M), has been synthesized as a novel, reversible inhibitor of the HCV NS5B polymerase [127, 128]. A series of 5,6-dihydroxy-2-(2-thienyl)pyrimidine- 4-carboxylic acids were further developed among the tested compound. Only 2-[3-({[(2-chlorobenzyl)amino]carbonyl}amino)-2-thienyl]-5,6-dihydro-xypyrimidine -4-carboxylic acid **(54)** (EC$_{50}$ 9.3 *µ*M, IC$_{50}$ 0.15 *µ*M) exhibited activity in the cell-based HCV replication assay [129].

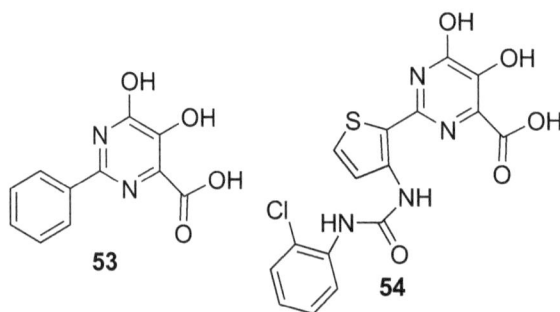

**53**                     **54**

## 3.19. 2', 3'-Dideoxynucleoside Analogs

Several analogs of 3' -fluoro (or chloro) and 2',3'-difluoro 2',3'-dideoxynucleoside were prepared and subjected to *in vitro* antiviral activities evaluation against duck hepatitis B virus, human HBV, and HCV [130, 131]. Among the tested compounds, only compounds 5-hydroxymethyl-3'-fluoro-2-,3'-dideoxyuridine **(55)**, 5-iodo-3'-fluoro-2',3'-dideoxyuridine **(55)** and 1-(3-chloro-2,3-dideoxy-β-D-erythro-pentofuranosyl)-5-fluorouracil **(57)** displayed inhibition up to 30-40% at 20µM against HCV. Ribavirin showed 50% inhibition at 20µM and served as a standard reference. Compound 5-Iodo derivative **(56)** showed most inhibition against HCV, and it exhibited a reduction in cellular RNA levels in Huh-7 cells. Compounds, **55**, **56** and **57** exhibited the best anti-DHBV activity with $EC_{50}$ values of 1, 5 and 10 µg/mL, respectively. 5-hydroxymethyl-30-fluoro-20,30-dideoxyuridine **(55)** and 1-(3-chloro-2,3- dideoxy-β-D-erythro-pentofuranosyl)-5-fluorouracil **(57)** showed the most inhibition without cytotoxicity against both viruses [132].

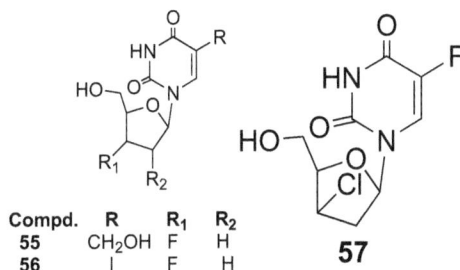

| Compd. | R | $R_1$ | $R_2$ |
|--------|-------|-------|-------|
| 55 | CH₂OH | F | H |
| 56 | I | F | H |

**57**

## 3.20. Acyclic Pyrimidine Nucleosides

Prepared acyclic pyrimidine nucleosides (5-chloro-1- [(2-hydroxy-1-(hydroxy methyl) ethoxy) methyl]-uracil **(58)**, 5-(2-bromovnyl)-1-[(2-hydroxy-1-(hydroxy methyl)ethoxy)-methyl]uracil **(59)** and 5-bromo-6-methyl-1-[(2-hydroxy-1-(hydroxymethyl)ethoxy)-methyl]uracil **(60)**) were screened *in vitro* against duck hepatitis B virus (DHBV) and exhibited most significant activity having $EC_{50}$ value of 4-20, 3-15, and 16.2-32.4 µM, respectively [133, 134]. Anti-DHBV activity shown by compounds **58** and **59** was found to be comparable to ganciclovir ($EC_{50}$) 4 $\mu$M [135]. Cell-based DNA replication assays were used to measure the antiviral potency of **58** and **60** against lamivudine-resistant HBV. The screening result showed that compounds **58** and **60** retained activity as compared to the wild-type HBV. The potential of anti-HBV activity of compound **60** was slightly decreased against double-mutant HBV, but **58** & **60** were still sensitive to lamivudine-resistant single as well as double mutant HBV strains [136].

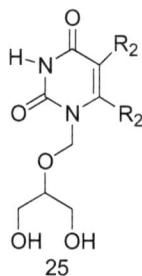

| Compd. | R₁ | R₂ |
|--------|----|----|
| 58 | H | Cl |
| 59 | H | HC=CHBr |
| 60 | CH₃ | Br |

### 3.21. 5-Fluorocytosine Analogous and (R)-oxaselenolane Nucleosides

Cytosine, 5-fluorocytosine analogous and (R)-oxaselenolane nucleosides were prepared and subjected to *in vitro* Anti-HIV and Anti-HBV activity evaluations. Cytosine and 5-fluorocytosine analogs (61 and 62) had shown promising anti-HIV activity having $EC_{50}$ values of 0.88 and 0.51 $\mu$M, respectively. Against anti-HBV, both compounds have $EC_{50}$ value of 1.2 $\mu$M with no toxicities up to 100 $\mu$M in various cell lines (PBM, CEM, and Vero). 3TC (Lamivudine) was used as a standard drug exhibiting activity at $EC_{50}$, 0.07 and 0.0089 $\mu$M against HIV and HBV, respectively. Interestingly, the $\alpha$-isomer (63) also displayed moderate antiviral activity against HIV, having no toxicities up to 100 $\mu$M in PBM, CEM, and Vero cells [137]. Compound 5-fluoro derivative 62 was found to be more potent as compared to the cytosine analogue 61 against HIV-1 [138 - 141].

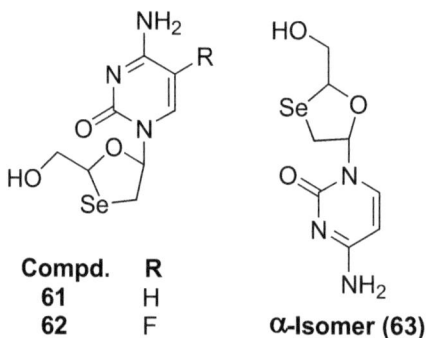

| Compd. | R |
|--------|---|
| 61 | H |
| 62 | F |

α-Isomer (63)

### 3.22. 2', 3'-β-L-Dideoxy-5-azacytidine

A new class of compound, L-nucleoside, 2',3'-dideoxy-β-L-5-azacytidine (64), was prepared and *in vitro* evaluated against HIV-1, HBV, HSV-1, HSV-2, L1210, P388, S-180, and CCRF-CEM cells [142]. Compound 64 has shown potent anti-HBV activity at approximately the same level as 2',3'-dideoxy-β-D-cytidine (ddC) with $ED_{50}$ values of 1.5 and 1.0 $\mu$M, respectively. Therefore, compound 64 was found to exhibit a selective inhibitor of HBV with no cytotoxicity [142] against L1210, P388, S-180, and CEM cells having $EC_{50}$ 100 μM. On the contrary, D-enantiomer of **64** was found to be inactive against HBV [143].

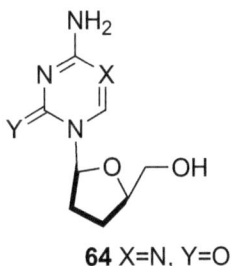

**64** X=N, Y=O

### 3.23. 5-, 6-, or 5,6-Substituted Acyclic Pyrimidine Nucleosides

A group of 5-substituted, 6-substituted or 5, 6-substituted acyclic pyrimidine nucleosides with a 1-[(2-hydroxyethoxy)methyl] moiety were prepared and screened for their antiviral potential. Among tested compounds, 5-bromo (**65**), 5-chloro (**66**), 5-amino (**67**), and 5-trifluoromethyl (**68**) analogues were found to be active and displayed 50% inhibition of DHBV replication at 3.7-18.5, 0.4-2.2, 5.0, and 3.9-39.3 μM, respectively. Moreover, compounds belong to the series of 6-substituted and 5,6- disubstituted, 6-methyl (**69**), 6-carbomethoxy (**70**), 5-iodo-6-methyl (**71**), and 5-nitro-6-methyl (**72**) derivatives, which showed approximately equiactive anti-DHBV activity ($EC_{50}$ 20.4-40.9 μM). Antiviral drugs, abacavir and lamivudine (3-TC), served as standard drugs in this assay.

In the DHBV studies, among the analogues, compound **66** ($EC_{50}$ 0.4-2.2 μM) was identified as the most active lead, but it was 10-times less potent as compared to the standard drug 3-TC ($EC_{50}$, 0.04-0.2 μM). 5-bromo derivative **65** was found to exhibit approximately 9-fold less activity ($EC_{50}$, 3.7-18.5 μM) than **66** confirmed by the SAR study. In contrast, compound **73** having 5-iodo substituent was found to exhibit less inhibitory potential to DHBV replication having an $EC_{50}$ value of 32 μM as compared to either **65** or **66**. SAR studies revealed that for this series of compounds, halogen substituent at 5-position is essential for anti-DHBV activity. The activity of a group of 5-, 6-, or 5, 6-substituted acyclic pyrimidine nucleosides against wild-type HBV was also examined against human hepatitis B virus in 2.2.15 cells. In 2.2.15 cells screening, among the tested group of compounds, 5-, 6-, or 5, 6-substituted acyclic pyrimidine nucleosides, compound **66** was found to be most active having $EC_{50}$ value of 4.5-45.4 μM as compared to standard reference 3-TC ($EC_{50}$) 2.1- 4.4 μM). In the cell-based DNA replication assays against lamivudine resistant HBV, the antiviral activity in the B1 cell line with single-mutant HBV of 5-, 6-, or 5, 6- analogues, only compounds **65**, **66** and

**68** were found to have notably inhibitory with $EC_{50}$ values of 18.5-37.7, 4 .5-45.4, and 39.3 μM respectively. Moreover, the D88 cell line against lamivudine-resistant HBV with double mutations compounds **65** and **66** also exhibited better response having $EC_{50}$ values of 3.7-45.4 μM as compared to the standard reference drug abacavir ($EC_{50,}$ 3.4-16.9 μM) used in this screening [144].

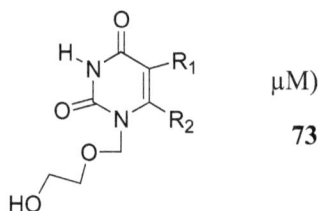

| Compd. | R$_1$ | R$_2$ |
|--------|-------|-------|
| 65 | Br | H |
| 66 | Cl | H |
| 67 | NH$_2$ | H |
| 68 | CF3 | H |
| 69 | H | CH$_3$ |
| 70 | H | COOCH$_3$ |
| 71 | I | CH$_3$ |
| 72 | NO$_2$ | CH$_3$ |
| 73 | I | H |

### 3.24. 2-Alkylamino-6- substituted-3,4-dihydro-5-alkylpyrimidin-4(3H)-ones

Compounds belonging to DABOs family *viz.* 2-Alkylamino-6-[1-(2,6 difluorophenyl)alkyl]-3,4-dihydro-5 alkylpyrimidin-4(3H)-ones [145] having different side chains like alkyl and aryl amino at C-2 position of pyrimidine ring [146] were synthesized and screened for their anti HIV1 and cytotoxic activity in MT-4 cells taking nevirapine and emivirine as reference drugs [($IC_{50,}$ 0.04 μM against HIV-1 rRT for Emivirine) and ($IC_{50,}$ 0.035 μM against HIV-1 rRT for 2-cyclopentylamino -6- [1-(2,6-difluorophenyl) ethyl]- 3,4 - dihydro-5-methylpyrimidin- 4(3H)-one) **74**]. Compound **74** also exhibited $EC_{50}$ 0.16 μM against Y181C HIV-1 mutant variant with the fold resistance value Y181C/Wt IIIB 5.3, which was found to be lower as compared to its counterpart **75**, which showed an inhibitory effect with $EC_{50}$ 0.2 μM against Y181C/Wt IIIB 13. Furthermore, no cytotoxicity was observed for MT-4 cells at doses as high as 200μM ($IC_{50} \geq 200$ μM) for compounds 6-(2,6-difluoro phenylmethyl)-3,4-dihydro-2-(2-methoxyethyl) aminopyrimidin-4(3H)-one **(76)**, 6-(2,6-difluoro phenylmethyl)-3,4-dihydro-2-(2-cyclohexyl) aminopyrimidin-4(3H)-one **(77)** and 6-(2,6-difluorophenylmethyl)-3,4-dihydro-5-methyl-2-(2-isopropyl)aminopyrimidin-4(3H)-one **(78)** [147].

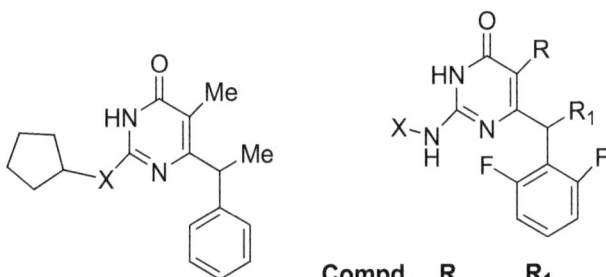

| Compd. | X |
|--------|---|
| 74 | NH |
| 75 | S |

| Compd. | R | R$_1$ | X |
|--------|---|-------|---|
| 76 | H | H | CH$_3$O C$_2$H$_5$ |
| 77 | H | H | Cyclohexyl |
| 78 | Me | H | isoPropyl |

## 3.25. Pyrimidine- 2,4-dione

Compound 6-(3,5-dimethylbenzyl)-5-ethyl-1-(4-iodobenzyl-oxymethyl)- 1H-pyrimidine- 2,4-dione (**79**) was synthesized and evaluated against antiviral activity, screening profile revealed that compound **79** exhibited potent activity against HIV-1 virus with wild type and mutated virus having EC$_{50}$ and CC$_{50}$ 0.007µM and CC$_{50}$ 19µM, respectively [148].

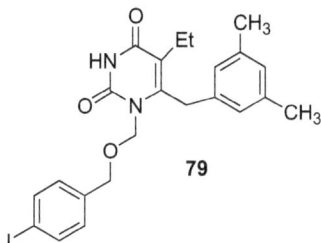

**79**

## 3.26. 2-Arylcarbonylmethylthio-6-arylmethylpyrimidin-4(3H)-ones

A novel series of compounds, namely, 2-arylcarbonylmethylthio-6-arylmethylpyrimidin-4(3H)-ones were prepared and screened *in vitro* for anti-HIV activities in MT-4 cells [149]. Most of these synthesized compounds showed an EC$_{50}$ range from 8.97 µM to 0.010 µM having moderate to potent activities against wild-type HIV-1. Among them, compound 6-(3,5-dimethylbenzyl)-5-ethyl – 2-(phenylcarbonylmethylthio)pyrimidin-4(3H)-one (**80**) was identified as the most significant compound having EC$_{50}$ = 0.010 µM, SI > 31,800 associated with moderate activity against the HIV-1 double mutant RT strain K103N + Y181C [150].

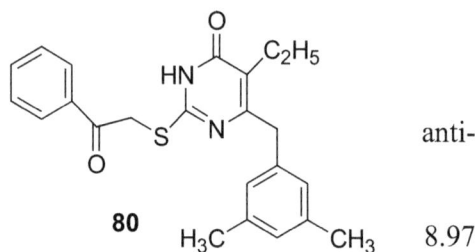

**80**     anti- 8.97

### 3.27. (5-Ethyl-4,6-dimethylpyrimidin-2-yl) Thiazolidin-4-one

A series of novel thiazolidin-4-ones were prepared and screened *in vitro* as HIV-1 reverse transcriptase inhibitors [151]. The screening results showed that some of the newly synthesized compounds, 2-(2,6-dichlorophenyl)-3-(5-ethyl-4,6-dimethylpyrimidin-2-yl)thiazolidin-4-one **(81)** and 2-(2-chloro-6-fluorophenyl)-3-(5-ethyl-4,6-dimethylpyrimidin-2-yl)thiazolidin-4-one **(82)**, in which ethyl group is present at 5-position on N-3 pyrimidine ring, were found to be best ones having $IC_{50}$ value of 0.26 μM and 0.23 μM, respectively [152].

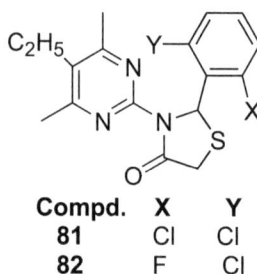

| Compd. | X | Y |
|--------|---|---|
| 81 | Cl | Cl |
| 82 | F | Cl |

### 3.28. N-1-Alkylated-5-Aminoaryalkylsubstituted-6-Methyluracils

N-1-alkylated-5-aminoaryalkylsubstituted-6-methyluracils have been synthesized and evaluated as potent inhibitors of HIV-1 RT [153].Among the synthesized compounds, the most active compounds against HIV-1 RT were 1-(ethoxymethyl)-5-[(2,4,5-trichloro-phenylamino)-methyl]-6-methyluracil **(83)** [($IC_{50}$ 0.82 μM)], 1-(benzyloxymethyl)-5-[(methyl-phenylamino)-methyl]- 6-methyluracil **(84)** [($IC_{50}$ 3.49 μM)] and 1-(benzyloxymethyl)-5-(cyclohexylaminomethyl)-6-methyluracil **(85)** [($IC_{50}$ 5.09 μM)]. Compounds **83-85** were found to be more active than nevirapine ($IC_{50}$ 10.60 μM) at concentrations 2- to 13-fold compared to nevirapine. Nevirapine was used as a reference compound here; $IC_{50}$ for nevirapine was 10.60 μM [154].

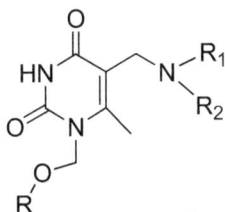

| Compd. | R | R$_1$ | R$_2$ |
|--------|---|-------|-------|
| 83 | C$_2$H$_5$ | H | 2,4,5-trichlorophenyl |
| 84 | C$_6$H$_5$CH$_2$ | CH$_3$ | C$_6$H$_5$ |
| 85 | C$_6$H$_5$CH$_2$ | H | Cyclohexyl |

## 3.29. N, N-disubstitutedaminopyrimidin-4(3*H*)-ones

A new DABOs series such as F2-*N,N*-DABOs having an *N,N*-disubstituted amino group or a cyclic amine at the pyrimidine-C2 position [155], as well as a small alkyl group or a hydrogen atom at C5 or at the benzylic position and also the suitable 2,6-difluorobenzyl moiety at the C6 position were prepared and screened against both wt and mutant HIV-1 strains [156, 157]. Among the compounds screened, compounds, 6-[1-(2,6-difluorophenyl)ethyl]-3,4-dihydro-2-n-propyl methyl aminopyrimidin-4(3*H*)-one **(86)**, 6-[1-(2,6-difluorophenyl)ethyl]-3,4-dihydro-2-dimethylamino-5-methylpyrimidin-4(3*H*)-one **(87)**, 6-[1-(2-6-difluorophenyl)ethyl]-3,4-dihydro-2-ethylmethylamino-5-methylpyrimidin-4(3*H*)-one **(88)**, 6-[1-(2,6-difluorophenyl)ethyl]-3,4-dihydro-2-isopropylmethyl amino-5-methylpyrimidin-4(3*H*)-one **(89)** and 6-[1-(2,6 difluorophenyl)ethyl]-3,4-dihydro-2-n-propylmethylamino-5-methylpyrimidin-4(3*H*)-one **(90)** were found to be potent in cellular assays. The most of the prepared F2-*N,N* DABOs were proved to be highly active against both wt and mutant HIV-1 strains, at the sub micromolar to nanomolar range. Compounds **86, 87, 88, 89 and 90** showed sub nanomolar potency against wt HIV-1 having EC$_{50}$ value of (0.0006, 0.0003, 0.0003, 0.0005 and 0.0007 µM), respectivelty. More interestingly, against the Y181C mutant strain, compound **89** having EC$_{50}$ 0.0007 µM & compound **90** having EC$_{50}$ 0.0006 µM were observed to be more potent than *NH*-DABOs and *S*-DABOs. Compounds efavirenz and nevirapine were taken as reference drugs [158].

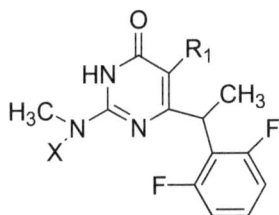

| Compd. | R$_1$ | X |
|--------|-------|---|
| 86 | H | n-Pr |
| 87 | Me | Me |
| 88 | Me | Et |
| 89 | Me | i-Pr |
| 90 | Me | n-Pr |

## 3.30. Substituted 5,6-dihydroxypyrimidine-4-carboxamide

A class of *N*-benzyl-5,6-dihydroxypyrimidine-4 carboxamides was prepared and screened for their anti HIV1activity [159]. Among the compounds screened, compound 2-[1-(dimethylamino)-1-methylethyl]-*N*-(4-fluorobenzyl)-5,6-dihydro xypyrimidine-4-carboxamide **91** was found to be more active with a CIC95 of 78 nM in the cell-based assay in the presence of serum proteins [160 - 162].

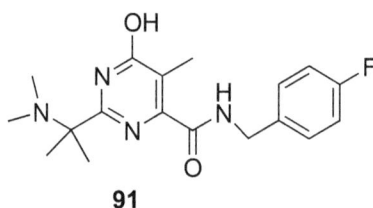

**91**

## 3.31. 4'-*C*-Substituted Nucleosides

4'-*C*-Ethynyl-*β*-D-*arabino*- and 4'-*C*-ethynyl-2'-deoxy- *β* -D-*ribo*-pentofuranosyl pyrimidine nucleosides were prepared and subjected to *in vitro* anti-HIV activity screening. Among these, compounds, 4'-*C*-ethynyl nucleosides, [(1-(4-*C*-ethynyl-*β*-D-*arabino*-pentofuranosyl)cytosine **(92)**, 1-(2-deoxy-4-*C*-ethynyl- *β*-D-*ribo*-pentofuranosyl)-5-methylcytosine **(93)**, 1-(2-deoxy-4-*C*-ethynyl-*β*-D-*ribo*-pentofuranosyl)-cytosine **(94)**, and 1-(2-deoxy-4-*C*-ethynyl- *β* -D-*ribo*-pentofuranosyl)-5-fluorocytosine **(95)**] were found to be significantly active having $EC_{50}$ value 0.0048 *μ*M for compounds **92** and **94**, and compounds **93** and **95** having $EC_{50}$ value 0.011 and 0.030*μ*M, respectively. These compounds also displayed potent antiviral activity against a wild-type clinical HIV-1 strain (HIV-1104 pre) and a multi-dideoxynucleoside-resistant infectious molecular clone (HIV-1MDR) with comparable $EC_{50}$ values. Compound **95** was least toxic (SI: >3333) and potent against all HIV strains tested [163].

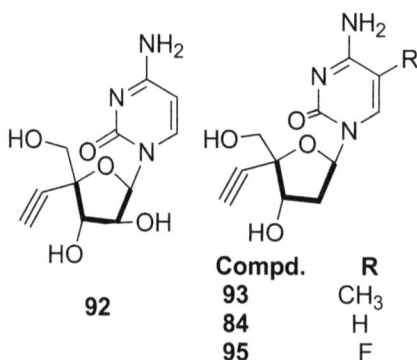

| Compd. | R |
| --- | --- |
| 93 | CH$_3$ |
| 84 | H |
| 95 | F |

**92**

### 3.32. β-L-2',3'-Didehydro-2',3'-dideoxy-2'-fluoro-4'-thionucleosides

β-L-2',3'-Didehydro-2',3'-dideoxy-2'-fluoro-4'-thionucleosides (*β*-L-2'-F-4'-S-d4Ns) were prepared and antiviral activity of the prepared compounds was evaluated against HIV-1 and compound AZT was taken as a reference drug [164]. Among these nucleosides, two pyridines, the cytosine(+)-1-[(1*S*,4*R*)-2,3-dideoxy-2,3-didehydro-2-fluoro-4-thio-*β*-L-ribofuranosyl]cytosine **(96)** and (+)-1-[(1*S*, 4*R*)-2,3-dideoxy-2,3-didehydro-2-fluoro-4-thio-*β*-L-ribofuranosyl]-5-fluorocyto sine **(97)** showed most potent anti-HIV activities (EC$_{50}$) 0.12 and 0.15 $\mu$M, respectively and no significant cytotoxicity up to 100 $\mu$M in CEM, human PBM, and Vero cells. Compound 96 was found to exhibit cross-resistance to a 3TC-resistant variant [165].

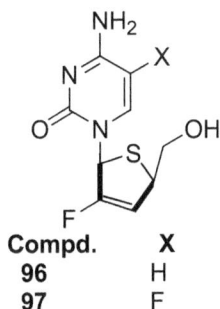

| Compd. | X |
|--------|---|
| **96** | H |
| **97** | F |

### 3.33. 5-Substituted-2,4-diamino-6-[2-(phosphonomethoxy) Ethoxy]pyrimidines

5-Substituted-2,4-diamino-6-[2-(phosphonomethoxy)ethoxy]pyrimidines were synthesized and evaluated against HIV-1, HIV-2 and moloney murine sarcoma virus [166, 167]. Among the compounds synthesized, the most active compounds were 5-methyl derivative 2,4-diamino-5-methyl-6-[2-(phosphonomethoxy) ethoxy]-pyrimidine **(98)**, 2,4-diamino-5-bromo-6-[2 (phosphonomethoxy) ethoxy]-pyrimidine **(99)** and 2,4-diamino-5-chloro-6-[2 (phosphonomethoxy) ethoxy]-pyrimidine **(100)** with EC$_{50}$ value ranging from 0.00016 to 0.007 $\mu$mol/mL, respectively. Compound **98** was also found to be very effective against HIV-1 and HIV-2 in CEM cell cultures with EC$_{50}$ value 0.00023-0.00043 $\mu$mol/mL. Compound **99** and **100** were also active, though less efficient, against these viruses at EC$_{50}$ values of 0.0031-0.0095 $\mu$mol/mL & these values were comparable to that of adefovir and tenofovir [168].

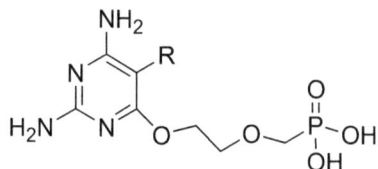

| Compd. | R |
|--------|-----|
| 98 | CH₃ |
| 99 | Br |
| 100 | Cl |

### 3.34. D- & L-Cyclopentenyl Nucleosides

D- and L-Cyclopentenyl nucleosides were synthesized and screened for their antiviral activity against RNA viruses such as HIV and West Nile virus. Among the prepared compounds, only D-(-) nucleosides exhibited significant activity. D-(-)-nucleosides, cytosine, CPE-C) [169] analogues, (1'$R$,2'$S$,3'$R$)-1-[2-3-dihydroxy-4-hydroxymethyl-4-cyclopenten-1-yl]cytosine (**101**) exhibited potent antiviral activity having $EC_{50}$ 0.06 $\mu$M but showed significant cytotoxicity in PBM, CEM, and Vero cells. 5-Fluorocytosin analogue, (1'$R$,2'$S$,3'$R$)-1-[2-3-dihydroxy-4-hydroxymethyl-4-cyclopenten-1-yl]-5-fluorocytosine (**102**) displayed moderately potent antiviral activity ($EC_{50}$ 5.34 $\mu$M) in PBM, CEM, and Vero cells with significant cytotoxicity. Also, cytosine (**101**) and 5-fluorocytosine (**102**) analogues have shown most potent anti-West Nile virus activity ($EC_{50}$ 0.2-3.0 and 15-20 $\mu$M, respectively). The synthesized nucleosides were also evaluated against West Nile virus *in vitro* (Table **1**). D-Cytosine (**101**) and D--fluorocytosine (**102**) analogues exhibited the most potent antiviral activity having $EC_{50}$ 0.2-3.0 and 15-20 $\mu$M, respectively [170].

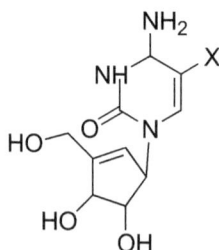

| Compd. | X |
|--------|---|
| 101 | H |
| 102 | F |

## 3.35. 2-(2,6-dihalophenyl)-3-(substituted pyrimidinyl)-1,3-thiazolidin-4-ones

A series of 2-(2,6-dihalophenyl)-3-(substituted pyrimidinyl)-1,3-thiazolidin-4-ones were prepared and screened as HIV-1 reverse transcriptase inhibitors *in vitro* anti-HIV assay [171]. The screening results showed that only compounds 2-(2,--dichlorophenyl)-3-(4,5,6-trimethylpyrimidin-2-yl)thiazolidin-4-one **(103)** and 2-(2-chloro-6-fluorophenyl)-3-(4,5,6-trimethylpyrimidin-2-yl)thiazolidin-4-one **(104)** have been proved highly potent and selective anti-HIV- 1 agents, with $EC_{50}$ value ranging of 22–28 nM and selectivity indexes of P10,000 in MT-4 as well as in CEM cells. Hence, in MT-4 cells, compounds **103** and **104** were more than 10-fold active and in CEM cells, activity was 50-fold more active than TBZ1 [172].

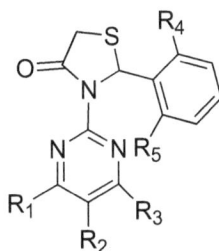

| Compd. | $R_1$ | $R_2$ | $R_3$ | $R_4$ | $R_5$ |
|--------|-------|-------|-------|-------|-------|
| **103** | Me | Me | Me | Cl | Cl |
| **104** | Me | Me | Me | Cl | F |

## 3.36. N-1 Alkyl Substituted Pyrimidines

A series of N-1 alkyl substituted pyrimidines were prepared and screened for their antiviral activities among the synthesized N-1 alkyl substituted pyrimidines, 1-[(2-hydroxy-1-(hydroxymethyl)ethoxy)methyl]-5-vinyluracil **(105)** ($EC_{50}$ 0.3–1.0 μg/ml), a 5-vinyl derivative with a (2-hydroxy-1-(hydroxymethyl) ethoxy)-methyl moiety, which emerged as the most active compound. The analogue, 1-[4-hydroxy-3 (hydroxymethyl)-1-butyl]-5-vinyluracil **(106)** containing a 4-hydroxy-3-(hydroxymethyl)-1-butyl chain was found to be approximately 3-fold less potent ($EC_{50}$ 1.0–3.0 μg/ml) than **105** [173]. In contrast, 1-[(2-hydroxyethoxy)methyl]-5-vinyluracil **(107),** a 5-vinyl pyrimidine, with 2-hydroxyethoxy methyl substituents, was weakly inhibitory to DHBV replication ($EC_{50}$>10 μg/ml). The anti-DHBV activity displayed by **105** was compared with the standard drug *ganciclovir* (GCV), $EC_{50}$ 1.5 μg/ml, *penciclovir* (PCV), $EC_{50}$0.3 μg/ml), and pyrimidine, *lamivudine,* ($EC_{50}$ 0.01–0.05 μg/ml) as measured in the DHBV infected primary duck hepatocyte cultures. In contrast, all of the compounds described were devoid of activity against TK$^+$ HSV-1 and TK$^-$ HSV-1. *Famciclovir*, a prodrug of PCV, was investigated in order to increase oral bioavailability and was shown highly potent as an anti-HBV agent in clinical studies [174, 175].

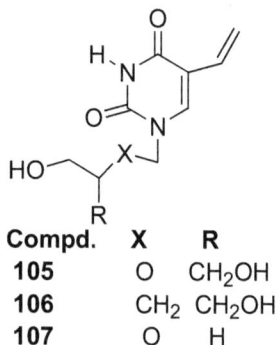

| Compd. | X | R |
|--------|-----|--------|
| 105 | O | $CH_2OH$ |
| 106 | $CH_2$ | $CH_2OH$ |
| 107 | O | H |

## 3.37. 2-(Phosphonomethoxy) Alkyl Derivatives of Pyrimidine Based Acyclic Nucleosides

2-(Phosphonomethoxy) alkyl derivatives of purine and pyrimidine based acyclic nucleoside phosphonates (ANPs) possess significant antiviral and cytostatic activity [176, 177]. Among ANPs, particularly 9-[2-(phosphonomethoxy)ethyl]adenine (PMEA, adefovir and [(R)-2-phosphonomethoxypropyl]adenine ((R)- PMPA, tenofovir is a commercially available drug active against DNA viruses and retroviruses [178 - 183]. 5-unsubstituted 2, 4-diamino-6-[2 (phosphonomethoxy)- ethoxy]pyrimidine (**108**) has antiviral activity against HIV ($EC_{50}$, 0.0016-0.0031 µmol/ml; MSV ($EC_{50}$, 0.00015 µmol/ml). Compounds **109** and **110** are the 5-cyano and 5-formyl derivatives, respectively, and have been synthesized and displayed inhibitory effect against HIV ($EC_{50}$,0.0027–0.011 µmol/ml), and against MSV ($EC_{50}$,0.0095–0.021 µmol/ml), these antiviral (HIV) potencies were comparable with those found for **108** but inferior values were found for MSV. The antiviral HIV and MSV activity exhibited by compounds **109** and **110** were also comparable to those recorded for adefovir HIV ($EC_{50}$, 0.0033- 0.0066 µmol/ml), MSV ($EC_{50}$, 0.0022 µmol/ml), tenofovir HIV ($EC_{50}$, 0.0012- 0.0014 µmol/ml), and MSV ($EC_{50}$, 0.0046 µmol/ml). Adefovir (PMEA) and tenofovir [(R)- PMPA] were used as reference drugs for the antiviral activity evaluation assays. Furthermore, 5-methyl 2, 4-diamino-6-[2 (phosphonomethoxy)-ethoxy]pyrimidine (**111**) displayed greater HIV and MSV activity (HIV $EC_{50}$, 0.00023- 0.00023,; MSV $EC_{50}$, 0.00016 µmol/ml) than that of **109** and **110**. Thus SAR study revealed that the suitable variation of the group at position 5 may provide the lead molecule as AntiHIV and AntiMSV agents [184].

| Compd. | R |
|--------|-----|
| 108 | H |
| 109 | CN |
| 110 | CHO |
| 111 | CH₃ |

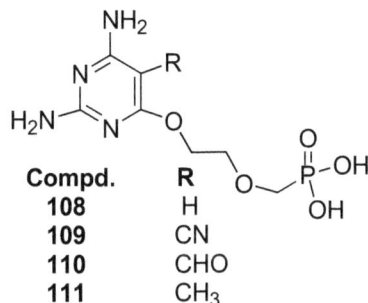

## 3.38. (-)-β-D-(2R,4R)-dioxolane-thymine-5'-O-aliphatic Acid Esters and Amino Acid Esters

A series of (-)-β-D-(2R,4R)-dioxolane-thymine-5'-O-aliphatic acid esters and its amino acid esters were synthesized as prodrugs of DOT [185, 186]. Synthesized compounds were screened against anti-HIV *viz.* HIV-1LAI in human peripheral PBM cells and cytotoxicity in PBM, CEM and Vero cells [187, 188]. Among the synthesized compounds, dioxolane thymine-5'-O-valeric ester (**112**), dioxolane thymine-5'-O-octanotic ester (**113**) and dioxolane thymine-5'-O-dodecanoic ester (**114**) showed improved anti-HIV potency *in vitro* without an increase in cytotoxicity in comparison to the parent drug (EC$_{50}$, 0.4, 0.6, 0.8 μM and EC$_{50,}$ 2.5, 4.3, 3.2 μM for compounds **112**, **113** and **114**, respectively). Cytotoxicity IC$_{50}$ of most active compounds **112-114** (5'-O-aliphatic acid esters) displayed the same IC$_{50}$ value, which was >100 μM in PBM, CEM and Vero cells except for compound **112** having IC$_{50,}$ 49 μM in Vero cells. Parent drug, DOT, displayed EC$_{50}$ 0.68 μM and EC$_{90}$ 4.0 μM against HIV-1LAI, and cytotoxicity IC$_{50}$ was >100 μM in the same assay at the concentration of the cell tested [189].

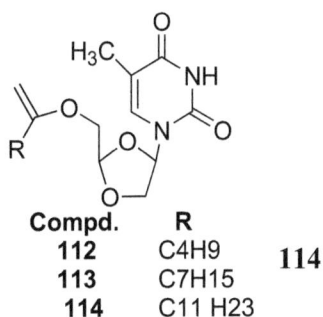

| Compd. | R |
|--------|--------|
| 112 | C4H9 |
| 113 | C7H15 |
| 114 | C11 H23 |

114

### 3.39. 2',3'-Dideoxy-3'-thiacytidin-5'-yl O-alkyl Carbonates

*In vitro*, screening of lamivudine prodrugs against anti-HIV activity in primary PBMCs infected with HIV [190] and the activities were compared with those of 3TC as a standard drug. Among the compounds screened, 2',3'-dideoxy- 3'-thiacytidin-5'-yl O-butyl (**3TC-Buta,115**), 2',3'-dideoxy-3'-thiacytidin-5'-yl O-pentyl (**3TC-Penta,116**), and 2',3'-dideoxy-3'-thiacytidin-5'-yl O-hexyl (**3TC-Hexa,117**) proved to be promising as candidates. Compound 2',3'-dideoxy--'-thiacytidin-5'-yl O-pentyl carbonate (**116,3TC-Penta**) has SI 20784 ± 4535 equivalent to that of 3TC. It should be noted that this compound showed a potent $IC_{50}$ (0.065 μM, 3 times lower than the parent drug) but also a higher toxicity ($CCID_{50}$ = 1286 μM). Compound 3TC-**Buta115** ($IC_{50}$ 0.200 ± 0.001μM) was found to be equipotent to lamivudine concerning its $IC_{50,}$ giving, as a result, relevant SI 22,500, and **3TC-Hexa 117** ($IC_{50}$ 0.250 ± 0.001μM, SI 3428 ± 1002) has 10-fold lower SI than that of 3TC (($IC_{50}$ 0.200 ± 0.060μM, SI 20000±4535) [191].

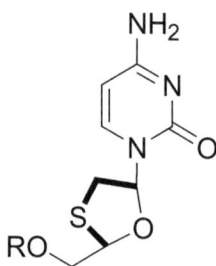

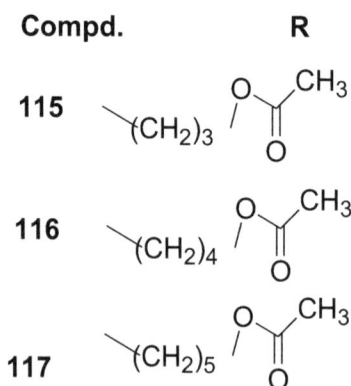

### 3.40. Pyrimidine–pyrazolones

Two pyrimidine–pyrazolone derivatives **118** and **119** were prepared and displayed antiviral activities *in vitro* that exceeded the activity of cidofovir against cowpox virus (CV) and vaccinia virus (VV). For pyrimidinylidene monopyrazolone **118**, $EC_{50}$, as defined by the CPE assay [192], was CV; $EC_{50,}$ 0.3 µM, VV; $EC_{50,}$ 1.7 µM and for compound **119**, CV; $EC_{50}$ 1.8 µM, VV; $EC_{50}$ 20 µM. The effective concentration to reduce viral cytopathogenicity (CPE) by 50% ($ED_{50}$) for cidofovir against CV and VV was 7.1 µM, and 3.2 µM, respectively. Compounds **118** and **119** were somewhat more active against CV than against VV and provided strong leads to novel orthopoxvirus antivirals. The CV is often considered to be a closer model to the smallpox variola virus than VV [193].

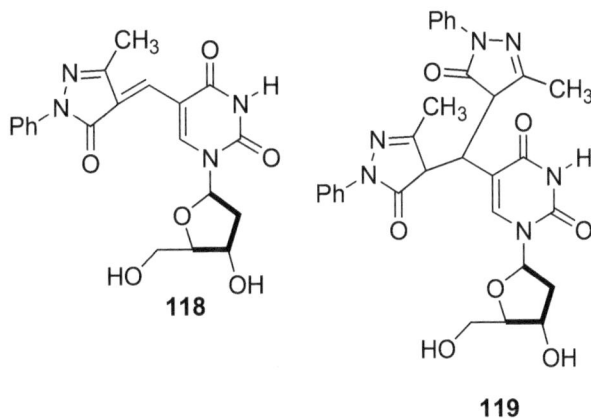

**118**

**119**

## 3.41. N-1 (1, 5-anhydro-2, 3- dideoxy-D-arabino-hexitolyl) -5-Substituted Pyrimidines

5-Substituted pyrimidines, 5-iodouracil **(120)**, 5-ethyluracil **(121)** and 5-trifluoromethyl analogue **(122)**, bearing a 1,5-anhydro-2,3- dideoxy-D-arabino-hexitol moiety at N- 1, were demonstrated to show potent anti-HSV-I activity by the conformational studies of the viral thymidine kinase (TK) [194 - 196]. Among the compounds with the highest selectivity index, it was observed that these compounds are not active in the absence of viral TK, which points to the importance of intracellular phosphorylation as a biological activation process [197].

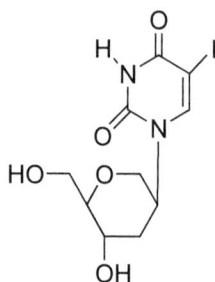

| Compd. | R |
|--------|-----|
| **120** | I |
| **121** | CH$_2$CH$_3$ |
| **122** | CF$_3$ |

## 3.42. C-3' Modified Ribose Nucleosides

C-3' modified ribose nucleosides were prepared and screened *in vitro* against the antiviral activity such as influenza virus, both A and B viral strains. Among the synthesized nucleosides, only compound **123** displayed potent influenza virus activity. Compound 172 showed EC$_{50}$ 18 µg/mL against Flu A (H5N1, Vietnam/1203/2004H) and EC$_{50}$ 7.7 µg/mL against Flu B (Florida4/2006) and inhibitory activity (IC$_{50}$ > 100 µg/mL) of influenza virus infection of MDCK cells [198].

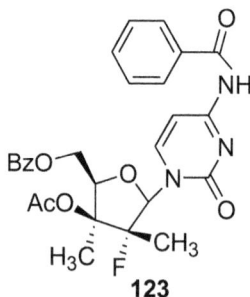

**123**

## 3.43. 5-Hydroxy-5, 6-dihydro-6-substituted Uracils

5-Hydroxy-5, 6-dihydro-6-substituted uracil derivatives were synthesized. Among the compounds screened, only compound **124** was found to be a strong inhibitor of Sendai virus (SV) production measured by decreased haemagglutinin titre (HAU). Sendai virus is an enveloped RNA virus with six major structural proteins with haemagglutinin-neuroaminidase (HN). Compound **124** induced reduction of haemagglutinating activity in the supernatants of infected cells indicates a decreased release of mature viral particles. The concentrations of compound **124** lower than 1 mg/ml had no effect on haemagglutinin production. At higher concentrations, the inhibitions were dose-dependent 10 mg/ml was able to give a 50% inhibition and reached maximum values (87.5% inhibition) at 100 mg/ml and this dose was not toxic for the cell, as confirmed by microscopic examination of the monolayers and by vital dye exclusion. Compound **124** has the ability to slightly inhibit the HIV-I virus at a concentration of 100 mg/ml and **124** was also able to inhibit HSV-1 replication by 98%, without any toxic effect on uninfected cells at high concentrations, but in this case, a cytotoxic effect was observed [199].

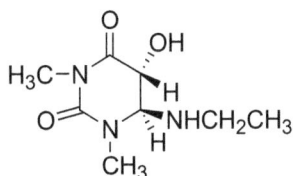

**124**

## 4. HETEROANNULATED PYRIMIDINES AS ANTIVIRAL AGENTS

### 4.1. Pyrazolo [3,4-d] Pyrimidines

Novel pyrazolo [3,4-d] pyrimidine derivatives and acyclic S-nucleosides of pyrazolo[3,4-d]pyrimidines were prepared and screened for antiviral activity. Among the tested, some pyrazolo [3,4-d] pyrimidines exhibited promising antiviral activity in the Plaque infectivity assay [200]. The reported activity is either due to virucidal effect or virus adsorption or effect on virus replication for both HAV and HSV-1 at concentrations of 10 $\mu g/10^5$ and 20 $\mu g/10^5$ cells. Among the tested compounds, only pyrazolo[3,4-d] pyrimidines 1-(5, 6-dihydronaphtho [1',2':4,5] thieno [2,3-d] pyrimidin-11-yl)-1H- pyrazolo [3,4-d] pyrimidine-4 (3H)-one **(125)**, 1-(5, 6-dihydro naphtho[1',2':4,5] thieno [2,3-d]pyrimidin-11-yl) -1H-pyrazolo [3,4-d] pyrimidine-4(3H)- thione **(126)**, acyclic S-nucleosides of pyrazolo[3,4-d]pyrimidine derivatives, 4-(2-methoxyethylsulfanyl)-1-(5,6-dihydro naphtho[1',2':4,5]thieno [2,3d]pyrimidin-11-yl)-1H-pyrazolo[3,4-d]pyrimidine **(127)**, 4-(dimethoxyethylsulfanyl) -1-(5,6 dihydronaphtho [1',2':4,5]thieno[2,3-d] pyrimidin-11-yl)-1H-pyrazolo[3,4-d] pyrimidine **(128)**, 4-(2-hydroxyethyl sulfanyl)-1-(5,6-dihydronaphtho[1',2' :4,5]thieno[2,3-d]pyrimidin-11-yl)-1H-pyra zolo[3,4-d]pyrimidine **(129)** and 4-(hydroxyethox yethylsulfanyl)-1-(5,6-dihyro-naphtho[1',2':4,5]thieno[2,3-d]pyrimidin-11-yl)-1H-pyrazolo[3,4-d] pyrimidine **(130)** displayed the highest anti-HAV activity having concentration of 10 $\mu g/10^5$ cells, as compared to amantadine and acyclovir used as a reference drugs. Furthermore, the fused pyrazolopyrimidine derivatives also revealed higher anti-HSV-1 activity than S-acyclic nucleoside derivatives, **128–130** at a concentration of 20 $\mu g/10^5$ cells. In the same assay, **125** and **126** also exhibited promising anti-HAV activity at a concentration of 10 $\mu g/10^5$ cells [201].

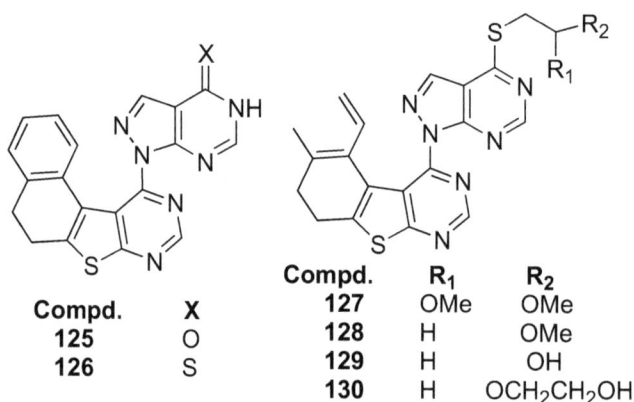

| Compd. | X |
|--------|---|
| 125 | O |
| 126 | S |

| Compd. | R₁ | R₂ |
|--------|-----|-----|
| 127 | OMe | OMe |
| 128 | H | OMe |
| 129 | H | OH |
| 130 | H | OCH₂CH₂OH |

## 4.2. Bicyclic Furanopyrimidine Deoxy Nucleosides

Novel bicyclic furanopyrimidine deoxy nucleosides were synthesized and screened for their inhibitory potential, and tested nucleosides proved to be potent inhibitors against two strains of thymidine kinase competent (TK⁺) VZV and two strains of thymidine kinase deficient virus (TK⁻) [202 - 205]. Among the compounds screened, compounds **131, 132 and 133** showed a potent and selective TK dependent anti-VZV activity, with EC$_{50}$ values [0.02 μM/VZV(OKA), 0.03 μM/ VZV(YS) for **131**, 0.01 μM/VZV(OKA), 0.02 μM/ VZV(YS) for **132** and 0.05 μM/VZV(OKA), 0.03 μM/ VZV(YS) for **133**]. The CC$_{50}$ was observed >200 μM for both compounds. Compounds **131** and **132** exhibited the same EC$_{50}$ value at >5 μM against both strains of HCMV with an MCC value at 20 μM. The chlorobutyl compound **133** is a particularly promising lead compound, with 9.7–30 μM activity against both strains of HCMV and cytotoxicity at 200 μM. Particularly, compound **133** is very interesting as it has poor cytotoxicity [206].

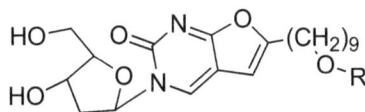

Compd.     R
131        $C_4H_9$
132        $C_5H_{11}$
133        $(CH_2)_4Cl$

## 4.3. 2,3-Dihydrofuro[2,3-*d*] Pyrimidin-2-ones

Discovery of the potent anti-varicella zoster virus action of lipophilic alkyl furanopyrimidine 2'-deoxynucleosides [207, 208] encouraged the synthesis of 2',3'-dideoxy sugar analogues, which are devoid of anti-VZV activity but are potent and selective inhibitors of HCMV. The synthesized dideoxy alkyl furano pyrmidines 3-[2',3'-dideoxy-ribo-$\beta$-D-furanosyl]-6-octyl-2,3- dihydrofuro[2,3-*d*] pyrimidin-2-one **(134)**, 3-[2',3'-dideoxy-ribo- $\beta$ -D-furanosyl]-6-nony--2,3-dihydrofuro[2,3-*d*]pyrimidin-2-one **(135)**, 3-[2',3'-dideoxy-ribo- $\beta$ -- -furanosyl]-6-decyl-2,3-dihydrofuro[2,3-*d*]pyrimidin-2-one **(136)**, 3-[2',3- -dideoxy-ribo- $\beta$ -D-furanosyl]-6-undecyl-2,3-dihydrofuro[2,3-*d*]pyrimidin-2-one **(137)** and 3-[2',3'-dideoxy-ribo- $\beta$ -D-furanosyl]-6-dodecyl-2,3- dihydrofuro[2,3-*d*]pyrimidin-2-one **(138)** were found to exhibit potent antiviral activity with $EC_{50HMCV}$ 2.5, 1.2, 2.6, 1.4 and 3.7 µm for **134, 135, 136, 137,** and **138,** respectively and $EC_{50AD\ 169}$ 3.0, 1.3, 3.2, 1.2 and 5.0 for **134, 135, 136, 137,** and **138,** respectively at ca. 1-5 $\mu$M and in excess of 200 $\mu$M with cytotoxicity. This is comparable to reference drugs for CMV, ganciclovir, less potent than cidofovir and more potent than foscarnet. Thus 2',3'-dideoxy sugar analogues proved to be new leads for the discovery of new drugs of this class, having improved therapies for HCMV [209].

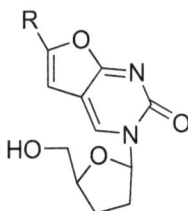

Compd.     R
134        $C_8H_{17}$
135        $C_9H_{19}$
136        $C_{10}H_{21}$
137        $C_{11}H_{23}$
138        $C_{12}H_{25}$

## 4.4. 6-(Alkyn-1-yl)furo[2,3-*d*]pyrimidin-2(3*H*)-one Nucleosides

6-(Alkyn-1-yl)furo[2,3-*d*]pyrimidin-2(3*H*)-one nucleosides were synthesized and screened against VZV in human embryonic lung (HEL) cells [207, 210, 211]. Among the synthesized compounds, the 2'-deoxy series exhibited the most potent anti- VZV activity, which was highest for 6-(octyn-1-yl) **139** and 6-(decyn-1-yl) **140** derivatives. The $EC_{50}$ values for 3-(2-deoxy-$\beta$-D-*erythro*-pentofuranosyl)-6-(octyn-1-yl)furo- [2,3-*d*]pyrimidin-2(3*H*)-one **139** were1.5 $\mu$M with a TK+ strain and ~25$\mu$M with two TK- strains. The anti-VZV activity of **140** was equal to that of acyclovir. Compound, 3-(2 –deoxy -$\beta$- D- *erythro* - pentofuranosyl) -6-(decyn-1-yl)furo-2,3-*d*] pyrimidin-2(3*H*)-one (**140** had $EC_{50}$ values7.4$\mu$M/7.6 $\mu$M with AD169/ Davis comparable to those of ganciclovir (GCV), ($EC_{50}$ value(5.1$\mu$M/ 8.7 $\mu$M with AD169/ Davis), and the 6-(octyn-1-yl) homologue **139** $EC_{50}$ (21$\mu$M/19 $\mu$M with AD169/ Davis) also showed activity against HCMV in HEL cells [212].

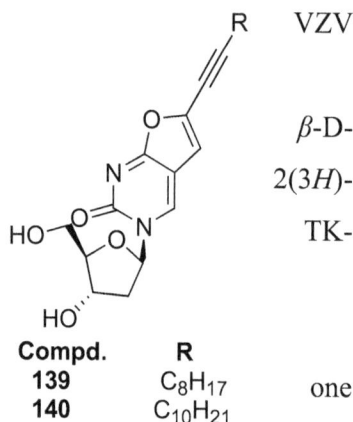

| Compd. | R |  |
|--------|------|------|
| **139** | $C_8H_{17}$ | one |
| **140** | $C_{10}H_{21}$ |  |

## 4.5. Imidazo [1,2-c] Pyrimidine-5-one

A series of novel base-modified imidazo[1,2-c]pyrimidine nucleosides were synthesized; among them, only 2-aminomethyl-6-(2,3,5-tri-O-tert-butyl dimethylsilyl-$\beta$-D-ribofuranosyl)-5-oxo-5,6-dihydro-imidazo[1,2-c] pyrimidine-5-one (**141**) displayed activity, at a cytotoxic concentration ($CC_{50}$ 9.6 $\mu$M, MCC 20 M), having $EC_{50}$ 7.3 $\mu$M (AD-169 strain) and 8.9 $\mu$M (Davis strain) against cytomegalovirus. The ganciclovir served as a reference drug, and displayed MCC values at 5.1 and 4.7 M against AD-169 and Davis strains, respectively [213].

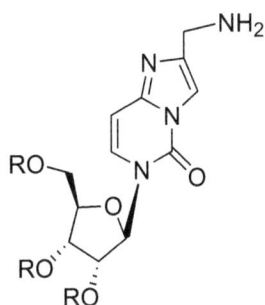

**141**    **R=** $(CH_3)_2Si\ C(CH_3)_3$

## 4.6. Furo [2,3-d]pyrimidin-2-ones

A series of novel acyclic nucleosides in the 5-alkynyl and 6-alkylfuro [2,3-d]pyrimidine were prepared and screened against HSV and HIV activity. The antiviral [214] and cytotoxicity assays against PBM, CEM and VERO cells [215] were performed by adopting the procedure given in the literature [214, 215]. Compounds 3-N-(2-hydroxy-ethoxymethyl)-6-pentyl-2,3-dihydrofuro[2,3-d]pyrimidin-2-one **(142)** and 3-[4-hydroxy-3-(hydroxymethyl)-2-butenyl]-6-(4-pentylphenyl)furo[2,3-d]pyrimidin-2(3H)-one **(143)** showed $EC_{50}$ of 2.7 and 4.9 µM, respectively, against HIV-1 and against HSV compounds **142** and **143** displayed $EC_{50}$ 6.3 and 4.8 µM, respectively [216].

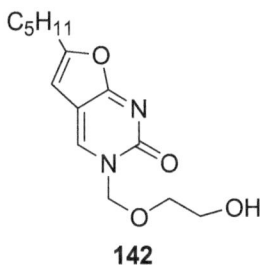

**142**

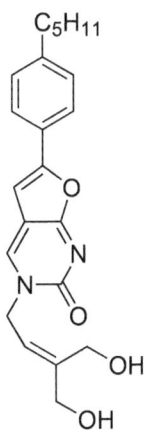

**143**

## 4.7. 2,3-Thieno[2,3-d]pyrimidin-2-one Nucleosides

A new class of anti VZV nucleosides 2,3-dihydrofuro[2,3-d]pyrimidin-2-one nucleoside **(144)** and some of its thieno analogues in which oxygen at 7 position is substituted by sulfur **145-149** [202, 207] were prepared and screened as inhibitors for VZV in human embryonic lung (HEL) cells. The activity of newly synthesized nucleosides **145-149** is compared to lead compound **144** and acyclovir (ACV) was taken as a standard reference. Among the thieno analogues, antiviral activity against VZV of compound **147** having $EC_{50}$ 0.005±0.003 µM) was found to be superior to the **144** VZV ($EC_{50}$ 0.008µM) and acyclovir ACV; ($EC_{50}$ 1.5±0.6µM). Short chain compounds **145** and **146** were not cytotoxic at the highest tested concentration (50–200 µM) and longer chain analogues **147-149** showed toxicity at 5 to 50 µM [217].

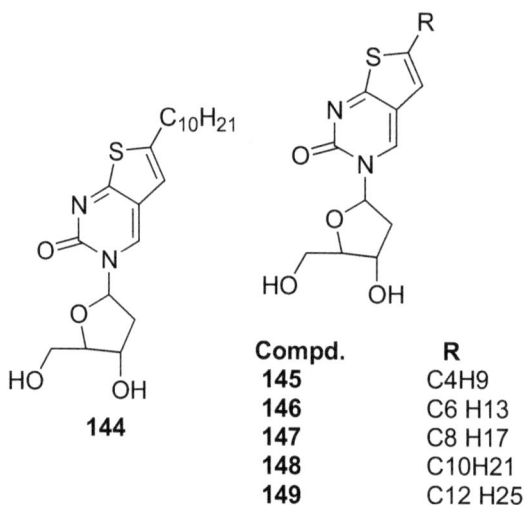

| Compd. | R |
|--------|------|
| 145 | C4H9 |
| 146 | C6 H13 |
| 147 | C8 H17 |
| 148 | C10H21 |
| 149 | C12 H25 |

## 4.8. 6-(Alkyl-heteroaryl)furo[2,3-*d*]pyrimidin-2(3*H*)-one Nucleosides

6-(Alkyl-heteroaryl)furo[2,3-*d*]pyrimidin-2(3*H*)-one nucleosides were synthesized and screened against VZV and HHCMV in Human Embryonic Lung Cell Cultures, which showed that the most potent compound among the tested was decyl derivative **150**. Compound **150** having $EC_{50}$ 0.066-0.094 *µ*M was found to be ~10-times more inhibitory to VZV in comparison to the decenyl derivative **151** ($EC_{50}$0.72-1.2 *µ*M) as well as also more potent as compared to decynyl analogue **152** ($EC_{50}$ 2.7 *µ*M) [218].

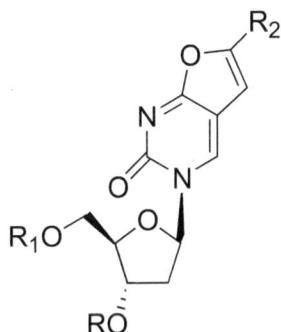

| Compd. | R | $R_1$ | $R_2$ |
|---|---|---|---|
| 150 | OH | OH | $HC{=}CHC_8H_{17}$ |
| 151 | H | H | $C_{10}H_{21}$ |
| 152 | OAc | OAc | $C{\equiv}CC_8H_{17}$ |

## 4.9. Alkenyl Substituted Aryl Bicyclic Furano Pyrimidines

Novel aryl bicyclic furano pyrimidines having alkenyl substitution were synthesized and screened *in vitro* against Varicella Zoster Virus (VZV), which showed inhibition of VZV TK-catalysed [$^3$H] thymidinephosphorylation [202, 219] by test compounds, revealing that compound **153** was more inhibitory ($IC_{50}$: 0.33 μM) than **154** and **155** ($IC_{50}$: 2.7–3.2 μM), whereas the para derivative in the C5-series **156** was more inhibitory ($IC_{50}$: 2.6 μM) than **157** and **158** ($IC_{50}$: 160–416 μM) [220].

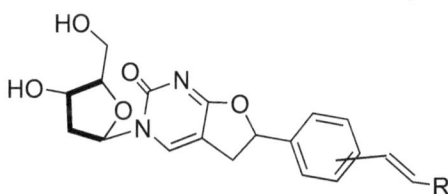

| Compd. | | R | Compd. | | R |
|---|---|---|---|---|---|
| 153 | ortho | R= $CH_3$ | 156 | para | R = n-Pr |
| 154 | meta | R = $CH_3$ | 157 | ortho | R= n-Pr |
| 155 | para | R = $CH_3$ | 158 | meta | R = n-Pr |

## 4.10. Pyrrolo[2,3-d]pyrimidine

A novel series of pyrrolo[2,3-d]pyrimidine compounds were synthesized and screened against influenza virus. Among them, one derivative, 4-(3-piperidinyl benzylamino)-2-methyl-7H-pyrrolo[2,3-d]pyrimidine **(159)** showed promising activity against both A ($IC_{50}$ 2.3μm) and B ($IC_{50}$ 5.1 μm) strains. The compound had activity comparable to amantadine ($IC_{50}$1.25 μm) [221], the drug currently used for influenza A infections. However, administered by the oral route to mice

[222], **159** had no antiviral effect. Since one of the reasons for this difference may have been extensive metabolism by the oral route [223].

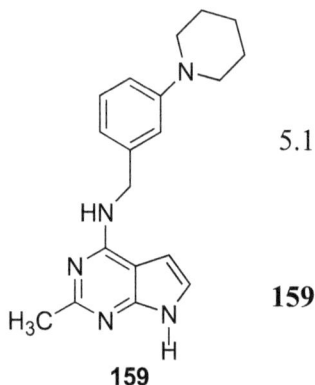

5.1

**159**

**159**

## 4.11. Pyrazolo[3,4-d]pyrimidines

Compound **160** was synthesized and exhibited significant activity against human enterovirus 68 (IC$_{50}$ 0.18 µM), human enterovirus 71 (IC$_{50}$ 0.35–0.52 µM), echovirus 9 (IC$_{50}$ 0.30 µM), and coxsackie viruses A and B (IC$_{50}$ 0.05–0.94 µM). Compound **160** was reported to be highly active against most of the serotypes of enteroviruses, in sub-micromolar range concentration and also exhibited a very low cytotoxic effect on the uninfected rhabdomyosarcoma (RD) host cells (IC$_{50}$>25 µM). Other compounds of pyrazolo[3,4-d]pyrimidines were also prepared and screened in a plaque reduction assay [224], which showed very specific for human enteroviruses. The pyrazolo[3,4-d]pyrimidines with a thiophene substituent **161-165** exhibited high activity against coxsackievirus B3 (IC$_{50}$ 0.063–0.089 µM) and were moderately active against enterovirus 71 (IC$_{50}$ =0.32–0.65 µM). No cytotoxic effect was observed toward RD (rhabdomyosarcoma) cell lines (CC$_{50}$>25µM) [225].

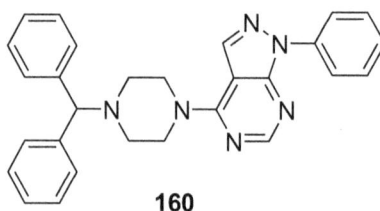

**160**

## 4.12. Pyrazolo[1,5-a]-pyrimidines

A class of novel 2-amino-3-nitro-7-hydroxypyrazolo[1,5-a]-pyrimidine derivatives **(166-171)** was prepared and found to be a potent inhibitor of coxsackie virus B3 (CVB3). The 50% inhibitory concentration and therapeutic index (TI) exhibited by compounds are **166** ($IC_{50}$, 3.94 µg/ml, TI ($CC_{50}$:$IC_{50}$), >25.9), **167** ($IC_{50}$, 29.60 µg/ml, TI ($CC_{50}$:$IC_{50}$), >3.4), **168** ($IC_{50}$, 20.35 µg/ml, TI ($CC_{50}$:$IC_{50}$), >3.2), **169** ($IC_{50}$, 50.29 µg/ml, TI ($CC_{50}$:$IC_{50}$), >2.0), **170** ($IC_{50}$, 5.81 µg/ml, TI ($CC_{50}$:$IC_{50}$), >17.2) and **171** ($IC_{50}$, 17.53 µg/ml, TI ($CC_{50}$:$IC_{50}$), >3.8) against coxsackie virus B3 in HeLa cells [226].

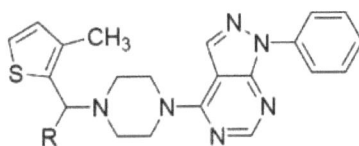

| Compd. | R |
|---|---|
| 161 | Ph |
| 162 | 2-CH₃Ph |
| 163 | 2-BrPh |
| 164 | 2-pyridyl |
| 165 | 2,5-dimethyl-3-isoxazolyl |

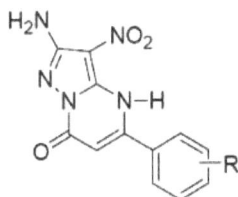

| Compd. | R |
|---|---|
| 166 | 2,4-Cl-5-NO₂ |
| 167 | H |
| 168 | 2-F |
| 169 | 4-F |

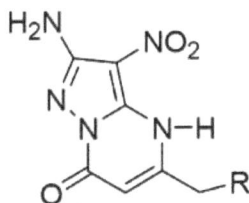

| Compd. | R |
|---|---|
| 170 | NHNH-C₆H₄-F-4 |
| 171 | NHNH-C₆H₄-OCH₃-4 |

## 4.13. Hybrid Diarylbenzopyrimidine Analogues (DABPs)

A series of novel of hybrid diarylbenzopyrimidine analogues (DABPs) were synthesized and screened against HIV in MT-4 cell cultures [227]. Most of the synthesized DABPs exhibited significant anti wild-type HIV-1 activity and also against mutant viruses. Particularly, compound 4-(2-(4-cyanophenylamino)quinazolin-4-yloxy)-3,5 -dimethylbenzonitrile **172** displayed most significant activity against wild-type HIV-1 having $EC_{50}$ 1.8 nM and selectivity index up to 111,954. Compound **172** also showed excellent potency against L100I, K103N, Y188L, and K103N + Y181C mutant strains with $EC_{50}$ values 18, 3.6, 36, and 60 nM, respectively, and is more active than efavirenz. Therefore, compound **172** can serve as the basis for further modification in searching for more effective candidates for improved anti-HIV-1 chemotherapy. Some other compounds, 4-(4-(mesityloxy)quinazolin- 2-ylamino)benzonitrile **(173)**, 4-(2-(4-cyanophenylamino)quinazolin-4-yloxy)-3, 5-dimethoxybenzonitrile **(174)**, 3-chloro-4-(2-(4-cyanophenylamino) quinazolin-4-yloxy)-5-methoxy-benzonitrile **(175)**, 3-chloro-4-(2-(4-cyanophenylamino)quinazolin-4-yloxy)-5-ethoxybenzonitrile **(176)**, 4-(2-(4-cyanophenylamino)quinazolin-4-yloxy)-3,5-diethoxybenzonitrile **(177)** and 4-(6-Chloro-2-(4-cyanophenylamino)quinazolin-4-yloxy)-3,5-dimethylbenzonitrile **(178)** also showed high anti-HIV-1 potency ($EC_{50}$ = 11, 8.7, 4.7, 7.5, 16, and 8.5 nM, respectively) and excellent selectivity indices (SI = 3215, 22,005, 46,947, 2969, 6771, and 13,832, respectively) [228].

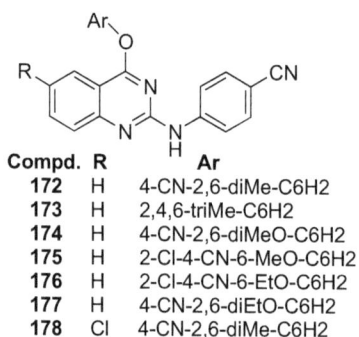

| Compd. | R | Ar |
|--------|---|-----|
| 172 | H | 4-CN-2,6-diMe-C6H2 |
| 173 | H | 2,4,6-triMe-C6H2 |
| 174 | H | 4-CN-2,6-diMeO-C6H2 |
| 175 | H | 2-Cl-4-CN-6-MeO-C6H2 |
| 176 | H | 2-Cl-4-CN-6-EtO-C6H2 |
| 177 | H | 4-CN-2,6-diEtO-C6H2 |
| 178 | Cl | 4-CN-2,6-diMe-C6H2 |

## 4.14. Bicyclo Furano Pyrimidines

Bicyclo furano pyrimidine derivatives **(179-182)** were synthesized and found to be highly effective, having significant selectivity against VZV. The effective concentrations of compounds **179**, **180**, **181** and **182** needed to inhibit VZV-induced cytopathicity by 50% ($EC_{50}$) were found to be 0.0001, 0.28, 0.005 and 1.0 μM, respectively against VZV TK$^+$YS, and minimum concentrations of compounds **179**, **180**, **181** and **182** required to induce a microscopically visible alteration of cell morphology (MCC) were found to have values of >20, >50, >200 and >200 μM, respectively [229].

| Compd. | X |
|--------|-----|
| 179 | O |
| 180 | $CH_2$ |

**182**

compounds **179, 180, 181**

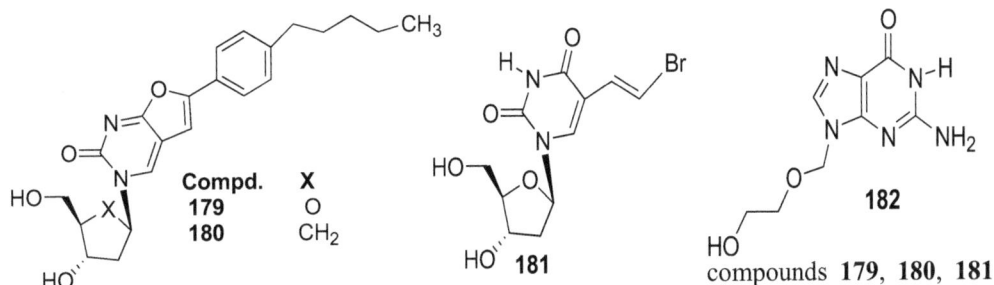

## 4.15. Unsaturated Nucleosides

A series of L-β-3'-cyano-2', 3'-unsaturated nucleosides were prepared and screened *in vitro* against HIV-1 in human PBM cells. Among the compounds tested, only **183** (EC$_{50}$ 21.7 mM), **184** (EC$_{50}$ 38.0 μM), **185** (EC$_{50}$ 67.4 μM), and **186** (EC$_{50}$ 74.8 μM) exhibited modest anti-HIV activity. Only the guanosine analogue displayed cytotoxicity (IC$_{50}$ 46.7 μM) [230].

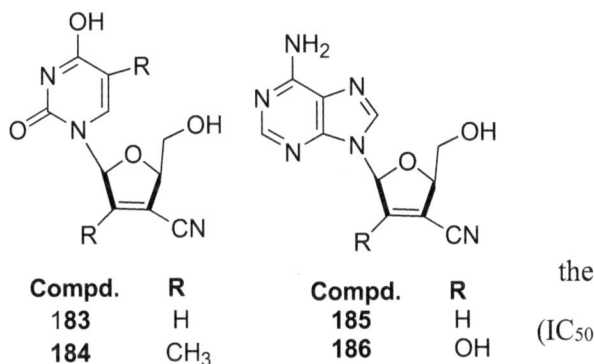

| Compd. | R |
|--------|------|
| 183 | H |
| 184 | $CH_3$ |

| Compd. | R |
|--------|------|
| 185 | H |
| 186 | OH |

the

(IC$_{50}$

## 4.16. Acyl (thio)urea and 2H-1,2,4-thiadiazolo [2,3-a] pyrimidine derivatives

Substituted acyl (thio) urea and *2H*- 1, 2, 4-thiadiazolo [2,3-a] pyrimidines were synthesized and evaluated their antiviral activity against both of their cell cultures and enzymatic activity against influenza (H1N1) virus. Compounds **187** and **188** displayed significant activity having IC$_{50}$ 0.08 and 0.09 μm, respectively. Compounds **187** and **188** were proved to be a novel class of highly potent and selective inhibitors of influenza virus. In the same assay, zanamivir was taken as a reference drug, having IC$_{50}$ 0.05 μm for the cell culture inhibitory activity [231].

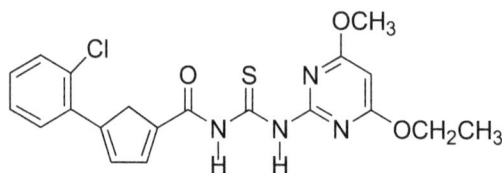

**187**

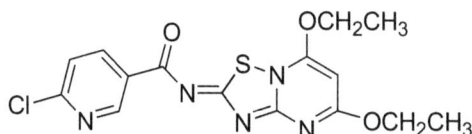

**188**

## 4.17. Substituted Thiopyrimidine and Thiazolopyrimidine Derivatives

Substituted thiopyrimidine and thiazolopyrimidine derivatives were prepared and evaluated against HSV-1 by the plaque reduction assay; a concentration of 2 and 5 mg/mL was used in the initial screening. Among the compounds tested, 2-(2, 4-dioxopentan-3-ylthio)-1,6-dihydro-4-(1,2,3,4-tetrahydronaphthalen-6-yl)-6- (3,4-dimethoxy phenyl) pyrimidin-5(4H)-one **(189)** and 5-(3,4- Dimethoxyphenyl)-2-methyl-7-(5, 6, 7, 8-tetrahydronaphthalen-2-yl)-2H-thiazolo-[3,2-a]pyrimidine-3,6(5H,7H)- dione **(190)** showed virucidal activity against HSV-1. Compounds **189** and **190** exhibited 90% inhibition and were found to be highly significant. The antiviral activity of compounds **189** and **190**  was also compared to the standard drug acyclovir and the result confirmed that the activity of **189** and **190** gave high % inhibition at low concentrations. A study on the mechanism of action of compounds **189** and **190** showed their virucidal activity against HSV-1. The chemical configuration of these compounds contains heterocyclic moieties, which may alter virus epitopes that inhibit virus attachment [232].

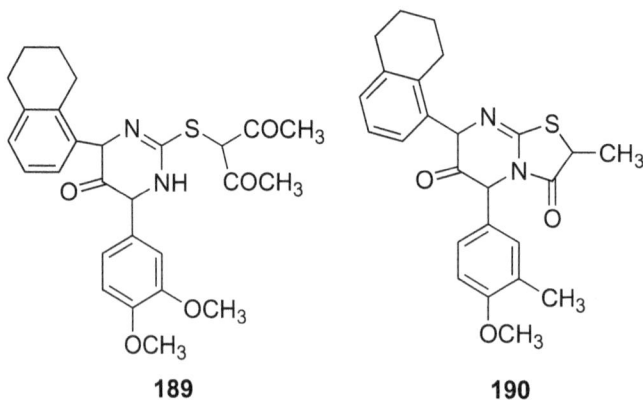

**189**                                          **190**

# CONCLUSION

One hundred ninety chemically defined synthetic pyrimidines have been reported in the literature. Some of them displayed potent antiviral activity and provided the structural basis for lead generation and lead optimization, in order to achieve potent clinical agents in the future. Pyrimidines continue to be an important source of molecular diversity and compounds with unique pharmacological activity. The aim of this chapter is to achieve this goal by the examination of the existing literature on the subject.

# ACKNOWLEDGEMENTS

The authors are grateful to the Director CSIR-CDRI Lucknow, India, for providing the Library facilities.

# REFERENCES

[1]     Champe, H.R.A.P.C.; Fisher, B.D. *Lippincott'sIllustrated Reviews: Microbiology*; Lippincott Williams & Wilkins: Philadelphia, **2007**.

[2]     He, H. Vaccines and antiviral agents. *Viral. Gene.Biotech. Appl.,* **2013**, *2013*, 239-250.

[3]     De Clercq, E.; Li, G. Approved antiviral drugs over the past 50 years. *Clin. Microbiol. Rev.,* **2016**, *29*(3), 695-747.
        [http://dx.doi.org/10.1128/CMR.00102-15] [PMID: 27281742]

[4]     Saxena, S.K.; Saxena, S.; Saxena, R. Emerging trends, challenges and prospects in anti viral therapeutics and drug development for infectious diseases. *Electr. J. Biol.,* **2010**, *6*, 26-31.

[5]     Ryu, W-S. Virus life cycle. *Molec.Virol. Hum. Pathog. Viru.,* **2017**, *2017*, 31-45.

[6]     Connolly, S.A.; Jackson, J.O.; Jardetzky, T.S.; Longnecker, R. Fusing structure and function: A structural view of the herpesvirus entry machinery. *Nat. Rev. Microbiol.,* **2011**, *9*(5), 369-381.
        [http://dx.doi.org/10.1038/nrmicro2548] [PMID: 21478902]

[7]     Monto, A.S.; Iacuzio, I.A.; LaMontague, J.R. Pandemic influenza: Confronting a re-emergent threat. *Threat. J. Infect. Dis.,* **1997**, *176*, 51.

[8]     Hayden, F.G.; Belshe, R.B.; Clover, R.D.; Hay, A.J.; Oakes, M.G.; Soo, W. Emergence and apparent transmission of rimantadine-resistant influenza a virus in families. *N. Engl. J. Med.,* **1989**, *321*(25), 1696-1702.
        [http://dx.doi.org/10.1056/NEJM198912213212502]

[9]     Hay, A.J.; Wolstenholme, A.J.; Skehel, J.J.; Smith, M.H. The molecular basis of the specific anti-influenza action of amantadine. *EMBO J.,* **1985**, *4*(11), 3021-3024.
        [http://dx.doi.org/10.1002/j.1460-2075.1985.tb04038.x] [PMID: 4065098]

[10]    Hastings, J.C.; Selnick, H.; Wolanski, B.; Tomassini, J.E. Anti-influenza virus activities of 4-substituted 2,4-dioxobutanoic acid inhibitors. *Antimicrob. Agents Chemother.,* **1996**, *40*(5), 1304-1307.
        [http://dx.doi.org/10.1128/AAC.40.5.1304] [PMID: 8723491]

[11]    Mammen, M.; Dahmann, G.; Whitesides, G.M. Effective inhibitors of hemagglutination by influenza virus synthesized from polymers having active ester groups. insight into mechanism of inhibition. *J. Med. Chem.,* **1995**, *38*(21), 4179-4190.
        [http://dx.doi.org/10.1021/jm00021a007] [PMID: 7473545]

[12]    Colman, P.M. *The Influenza Viruses:Influenza Virus Neuraminidase, Enzyme and Antigen*; Krug, R.M., Ed.; Plenum: New York, **1989**, p. 175.
[http://dx.doi.org/10.1007/978-1-4613-0811-9_4]

[13]    Erik De Clercq, E.D. Antiviral drugs: Current state of the art. *J. Clin. Virol.*, **2001**, *22*, 73.
[http://dx.doi.org/10.1016/S1386-6532(01)00167-6] [PMID: 11418355]

[14]    Ryan, D.M.; Ticehurst, J.; Dempsey, M.H. GG167 (4-guanidino-2,4-dideoxy-2,3-dehydro-N-acetylneuraminic acid) is a potent inhibitor of influenza virus in ferrets. *Antimicrob. Agents. Chemother.*, **1995**, *39*(11), 2583-2584.
[http://dx.doi.org/10.1128/AAC.39.11.2583] [PMID: 8585752]

[15]    Kiso, M.; Mitamura, K.; Sakai-Tagawa, Y.; Shiraishi, K.; Kawakami, C.; Kimura, K.; Hayden, F.G.; Sugaya, N.; Kawaoka, Y. Resistant influenza A viruses in children treated with oseltamivir: Descriptive study. *Lancet*, **2004**, *364*(9436), 759-765.
[http://dx.doi.org/10.1016/S0140-6736(04)16934-1] [PMID: 15337401]

[16]    Puthavathana, P.; Auewarkul, P.; Charoenying, P.C.; Sangsiriwut, K.; Pooruk, P.; Boonnak, K.; Khanyak, R.; Thawachsupa, P.; Kijpliati, R. Molecular characterization of the complete genome of human influenza H5N1 virus isolates from Thailand. *J. Gen. Virol.*, **2005**, *86*, 423.
[http://dx.doi.org/10.1099/vir.0.80368-0] [PMID: 15659762]

[17]    Le, Q.M.; Kiso, M.; Someya, K.; Sakai, Y.T.; Nguyen, T.H.; Nguyen, K.H.L.; Pham, N.D.; Ngyen, H.H.; Yamada, S.; Muramoto, Y.; Horimoto, T.; Takada, A.; Goto, H.; Suzuki, T.; Suzuki, Y.; Kawaoka, Y. Isolation of drug-resistant H5N1 virus. *Nature*, **2005**, *437*(7062), 1108.
[http://dx.doi.org/10.1038/4371108a] [PMID: 16228009]

[18]    Hatakeyama, S.; Sugaya, N.; Ito, M.; Yamazaki, M.; Ichikawa, M.; Kimura, K.; Kiso, M.; Shimizu, H.; Kawakami, C.; Koike, K.; Mitamura, K.; Kawaoka, Y. Emergence of influenza B viruses with reduced sensitivity to neuraminidase inhibitors. *JAMA*, **2007**, *297*(13), 1435-1442.
[http://dx.doi.org/10.1001/jama.297.13.1435] [PMID: 17405969]

[19]    Hoofnagle, J.H. Hepatitis C: The clinical spectrum of disease. *Hepatology*, **1997**, *26*(S3) 1, 15S-20S.
[http://dx.doi.org/10.1002/hep.510260703] [PMID: 9305658]

[20]    Szabó, E.; Lotz, G.; Páska, C.; Kiss, A.; Schaff, Z. Viral hepatitis: New data on hepatitis C infection. *Pathol. Oncol. Res.*, **2003**, *9*(4), 215-221.
[http://dx.doi.org/10.1007/BF02893380] [PMID: 14688826]

[21]    Lake-Bakaar, G. Current and future therapy for chronic hepatitis C virus liver disease. *Curr. Drug Targets Infect. Disord.*, **2003**, *3*(3), 247-253.
[http://dx.doi.org/10.2174/1568005033481132] [PMID: 14529357]

[22]    Fried, M.W.; Shiffman, M.L.; Reddy, K.R.; Smith, C.; Marinos, G.; Gonçales, F.L., Jr; Häussinger, D.; Diago, M.; Carosi, G.; Dhumeaux, D.; Craxi, A.; Lin, A.; Hoffman, J.; Yu, J. Peginterferon Alfa-2a plus ribavirin for chronic hepatitis C Virus infection. *N. Engl. J. Med.*, **2002**, *347*(13), 975-982.
[http://dx.doi.org/10.1056/NEJMoa020047]

[23]    Hadziyannis, S.J.; Sette, H., Jr; Morgan, T.R.; Balan, V.; Diago, M.; Marcellin, P.; Ramadori, G.; Bodenheimer, H., Jr; Bernstein, D.; Rizzetto, M.; Zeuzem, S.; Pockros, P.J.; Lin, A.; Ackrill, A.M. Peginterferon-alpha2a and ribavirin combination therapy in chronic hepatitis C: A randomized study of treatment duration and ribavirin dose. *Ann. Intern. Med.*, **2004**, *140*(5), 346-355.
[http://dx.doi.org/10.7326/0003-4819-140-5-200403020-00010] [PMID: 14996676]

[24]    Manns, M.P.; McHutchison, J.G.; Gordon, S.C.; Rustgi, V.K.; Shiffman, M.; Reindollar, R.; Goodman, Z.D.; Koury, K.; Ling, M.H.; Albrecht, J.K. Peginterferon alfa-2b plus ribavirin compared with interferon alfa-2b plus ribavirin for initial treatment of chronic hepatitis C: A randomised trial. *Lancet*, **2001**, *358*(9286), 958-965.
[http://dx.doi.org/10.1016/S0140-6736(01)06102-5] [PMID: 11583749]

[25]    Maddrey, W.C. Hepatitis B--an important public health issue. *Clin. Lab.*, **2001**, *47*(1-2), 51-55.

[PMID: 11214223]

[26]  Lok, A.S.F. Hepatitis B infection: Pathogenesis and management. *J. Hepatol.,* **2000**, *32*(1), 89-97.
[http://dx.doi.org/10.1016/S0168-8278(00)80418-3] [PMID: 10728797]

[27]  Perrillo, R.P.; Schiff, E.R.; Davis, G.L.; Bodenheimer, H.C., Jr; Lindsay, K.; Payne, J.; Dienstag, J.L.;
O'Brien, C.; Tamburro, C.; Jacobson, I.M.; Sampliner, R.; Feit, D.; Lefkowitch, J.; Kuhns, M.;
Meschievitz, C.; Sanghvi, B.; Albrecht, J.; Gibas, A. A randomized, controlled trial of interferon alfa-
2b alone and after prednisone withdrawal for the treatment of chronic hepatitis B. *N. Engl. J. Med.,*
**1990**, *323*(5), 295-301.
[http://dx.doi.org/10.1056/NEJM199008023230503]

[28]  Behrens, S.E.; Tomei, L.; De Francesco, R. Identification and properties of the RNA-dependent RNA
polymerase of hepatitis C virus. *EMBO J.,* **1996**, *15*(1), 12-22.
[http://dx.doi.org/10.1002/j.1460-2075.1996.tb00329.x] [PMID: 8598194]

[29]  Takamizawa, A.; Mori, C.; Fuke, I.; Manabe, S.; Murakami, S.; Fujita, J.; Onishi, E.; Andoh, T.;
Yoshida, I.; Okayama, H. Structure and organization of the hepatitis C virus genome isolated from
human carriers. *J. Virol.,* **1991**, *65*(3), 1105-1113.
[http://dx.doi.org/10.1128/jvi.65.3.1105-1113.1991] [PMID: 1847440]

[30]  Rotbart, H.A. Treatment of picornavirus infections. *Antiviral Res.,* **2002**, *53*(2), 83-98.
[http://dx.doi.org/10.1016/S0166-3542(01)00206-6] [PMID: 11750935]

[31]  Barnard, D. Current status of anti-picornavirus therapies. *Curr. Pharm. Des.,* **2006**, *12*(11), 1379-1390.
[http://dx.doi.org/10.2174/138161206776361129] [PMID: 16611122]

[32]  Senior, K. FDA panel rejects common cold treatment. *Lancet Infect. Dis.,* **2002**, *2*(5), 264.
[http://dx.doi.org/10.1016/S1473-3099(02)00277-3] [PMID: 12062983]

[33]  Lamb, R.A.; Kolakofsky, D. Paramyxoviridae and their replication.*Fields Virology,* 3rd; Fields, B.N.;
Knipe, D.M.; Howley, P.M., Eds.; Lippincott-Raven Publishers: Philadelphia, **1996**, p. 1177.

[34]  Morris, J.A.; Blount, R.E., Jr; Savage, R.E. Recovery of cytopathogenic agent from chimpanzees with
goryza. *Exp. Biol. Med.,* **1956**, *92*(3), 544-549.
[http://dx.doi.org/10.3181/00379727-92-22538]

[35]  Gelfand, E.; McCurdy, D.; Rao, C.P.; Middleton, P. Ribavirin treatment of viral pneumonitis in severe
combined immunodeficiency disease. *Lancet,* **1983**, *322*(8352), 732-733.
[http://dx.doi.org/10.1016/S0140-6736(83)92265-1]

[36]  Elizaga, J.; Olavarria, E.; Apperley, J.F.; Goldman, J.M.; Ward, K.N. Parainfluenza virus 3 infection
after stem cell transplant: Relevance to outcome of rapid diagnosis and ribavirin treatment. *Clin.
Infect. Dis.,* **2001**, *32*(3), 413-418.
[http://dx.doi.org/10.1086/318498] [PMID: 11170949]

[37]  Canonico, P.G.; Kende, M.; Huggins, J.W.; Smith, R. A.; Knight, V.; Smith, A. D. *Academic Press:
Orlando, FL, 1984, 65.; J. Med. Chem, 2001, 44, 4561*;

[38]  Turner, B.G.; Summers, M.F. Structural biology of HIV. *J. Mol. Biol.,* **1999**, *285*(1), 1-32.
[http://dx.doi.org/10.1006/jmbi.1998.2354] [PMID: 9878383]

[39]  De Clercq, E. Targets and strategies for the antiviral chemotherapy of AIDS. *Trends Pharmacol. Sci.,*
**1990**, *11*(5), 198-205.
[http://dx.doi.org/10.1016/0165-6147(90)90115-O] [PMID: 2188403]

[40]  De Clercq, E. New approaches toward anti-HIV chemotherapy. *J. Med. Chem.,* **2005**, *48*(5), 1297-
1313.
[http://dx.doi.org/10.1021/jm040158k] [PMID: 15743172]

[41]  Rashad, A.E.; Ali, M.A. Synthesis and antiviral screening of some thieno[2,3- *d* ]Pyrimidine
Nucleosides. *Nucleo. Nucleo. Nucl. Acids.,* **2006**, *25*(1), 17-28.
[http://dx.doi.org/10.1080/15257770500377730]

[42]   Tanka, H.; Baba, M.; Hayakawa, H.; Sakamaki, T.; Miyasaka, T.; Shigeta, S.; Walker, R.T.; Balzarini, J.; Declercq, E. A new class of HIV-1-specific 6-substituted acyclouridine derivatives: Synthesis and anti-HIV-1 activity of 5- or 6-substituted analogues of 1-[(2-hydroxyethoxy)methyl--6-(phenylthio)thymine (HEPT). *J. Med. Chem.,* **1991**, *34*, 349.
       [http://dx.doi.org/10.1021/jm00105a055] [PMID: 1992136]

[43]   Kaufman, H.E. Clinical cure of herpes simplex keratitis by 5-iodo-2-deoxyuridine. *Exp. Biol. Med.,* **1962**, *109*(2), 251-252.
       [http://dx.doi.org/10.3181/00379727-109-27169] [PMID: 14454445]

[44]   Prusoff, W.H. Synthesis and biological activities of iododeoxyuridine, an analog of thymidine. *Biochim. Biophys. Acta,* **1959**, *32*(1), 295-296.
       [http://dx.doi.org/10.1016/0006-3002(59)90597-9] [PMID: 13628760]

[45]   De Clercq, E.; Descamps, J.; De Somer, P.; Barr, P.J.; Jones, A.S.; Walker, R.T. (E)-5--2-Bromovinyl)-2'-deoxyuridine: A potent and selective anti-herpes agent. *Proc. Natl. Acad. Sci.,* **1979**, *76*(6), 2947-2951.
       [http://dx.doi.org/10.1073/pnas.76.6.2947] [PMID: 223163]

[46]   De Clercq, E.; Hol_y, A.; Rosenberg, I.; Sakuma, T.; Balzarini, J.; Maudgal, P. C. A novel selective broad-spectrum anti-DNA virus agent. *Nature,* **1986**, *323*, 464.
       [PMID: 3762696]

[47]   Balzarini, J.; Hol_y, A.; Jindrich, J.; Naesens, L.; Snoeck, R.; Schols, D.; De Clercq, E. Differential antiherpesvirus and antiretrovirus effects of the (S) and (R) enantiomers of acyclic nucleoside phosphonates: Potent and selective *in vitro* and *in vivo* antiretrovirus activities of (R)-9--2-phosphonomethoxypropyl)-2,6-diaminopurine. *Antimicrob. Agents Chemother.,* **1993**, *37*, 332.
       [http://dx.doi.org/10.1128/AAC.37.2.332] [PMID: 8452366]

[48]   Hol_y, A.; Kre_cmerov_a, M.; Pohl, R.; Masojı´, R.; dkov_a, M.; Andrei, G.; Naesens, L.; Neyts, J.; Balzarini, J.; De Clercq, E.; Snoeck, R. *J. Med. Chem.,* **2007**, *50*, 5765.

[49]   Privat de Garilhe, M.; de Rudder, J.C.R. Biotechnological potential of marine sponges. *Acad. Sci. Paris,* **1964**, *259*, 2725.

[50]   Davies, W.L.; Grunert, R.R.; Haff, R.F.; McGahen, J.W.; Neumayer, E.M.; Paulshock, M.; Watts, J.C.; Wood, T.R.; Hermann, E.C.; Hoffmann, C.E. Antiviral activity of 1-adamantanamine (amantadine). *Science,* **1964**, *144*(3620), 862-863.
       [http://dx.doi.org/10.1126/science.144.3620.862] [PMID: 14151624]

[51]   Sidwell, R.W.; Huffman, J.H.; Khare, G.P.; Allen, L.B.; Witkowski, J.T.; Robins, R.K. Broad-spectrum antiviral activity of Virazole: 1-beta-D-ribofuranosyl-1,2,4-triazole-3-carboxamide. *Science,* **1972**, *177*(4050), 705-706.
       [http://dx.doi.org/10.1126/science.177.4050.705] [PMID: 4340949]

[52]   Schaeffer, H.J.; Beauchamp, L.; de Miranda, P.; Elion, G.B.; Bauer, D.J.; Collins, P. 9-(--Hydroxyethoxymethyl)guanine activity against viruses of the herpes group. *Nature,* **1978**, *272*(5654), 583-585.
       [http://dx.doi.org/10.1038/272583a0] [PMID: 205792]

[53]   De Clercq, E.; Descamps, J.; De Somer, P.; Holý, A. ( S )-9-(2,3-Dihydroxypropyl)adenine: An aliphatic nucleoside analog with broad-spectrum antiviral activity. *Science,* **1978**, *200*(4341), 563-565.
       [http://dx.doi.org/10.1126/science.200.4341.563] [PMID: 17839440]

[54]   Fyfe, J.A.; Keller, P.M.; Furman, P.A.; Miller, R.L.; Elion, G.B. Thymidine kinase from herpes simplex virus phosphorylates the new antiviral compound, 9-(2-hydroxyethoxymethyl)guanine. *J. Biol. Chem.,* **1978**, *253*(24), 8721-8727.
       [http://dx.doi.org/10.1016/S0021-9258(17)34236-9] [PMID: 214430]

[55]   McGuigan, C.; Barucki, H.; Blewett, S.; Carangio, A.; Erichsen, J.T.; Andrei, G.; Snoeck, R.; De Clercq, E.; Balzarini, J. Highly potent and selective inhibition of varicella-zoster virus by bicyclic

furopyrimidine nucleosides bearing an aryl side chain. *J. Med. Chem.,* **2000**, *43*(26), 4993-4997.
[http://dx.doi.org/10.1021/jm000210m] [PMID: 11150169]

[56]   De Clercq, E.; Field, H.J. Antiviral prodrugs - the development of successful prodrug strategies for antiviral chemotherapy. *Br. J. Pharmacol.,* **2006**, *147*(1), 1-11.
[http://dx.doi.org/10.1038/sj.bjp.0706446] [PMID: 16284630]

[57]   De Clercq, E.; Andrei, G.; Snoeck, R.; De Bolle, L.; Naesens, L.; Degr_eve, B.; Balzarini, J.; Zhang, Y.; Schols, D.; Leyssen, P.; Ying, C. Acyclic/carbocyclic guanosine analogues as anti-herpesvirus agents. *J. Nucleic Acids,* **2001**, *20*, 271.
[http://dx.doi.org/10.1081/NCN-100002298]

[58]   Erice, A.; Jordan, M.C.; Chace, B.A.; Fletcher, C.; Chinnock, B.J.; Balfour, H.H., Jr Ganciclovir treatment of cytomegalovirus disease in transplant recipients and other immunocompromised hosts. *JAMA,* **1987**, *257*(22), 3082-3087.
[http://dx.doi.org/10.1001/jama.1987.03390220080025] [PMID: 3035246]

[59]   Anderson, R.D.; Griffy, K.G.; Jung, D.; Door, A.; Hulse, J.D.; Smith, R.B. Ganciclovir absolute bioavailability and steady-state pharmacokinetics after oral administration of two 3000-mg/d dosing regimens in human immunodeficiency virus— and cytomegalovirus-seropositive patients. *Clin. Ther.,* **1995**, *17*(3), 425-432.
[http://dx.doi.org/10.1016/0149-2918(95)80107-3] [PMID: 7585846]

[60]   Boyd, M.R.; Bacon, T.H.; Sutton, D.; Cole, M. Antiherpesvirus activity of 9-(4-hydroxy-3-hydoxy-methylbut-1-yl)guanine (BRL 39123) in cell culture. *Antimicrob. Agents Chemother.,* **1987**, *31*(8), 1238-1242.
[http://dx.doi.org/10.1128/AAC.31.8.1238]

[61]   Tyring, S.; Barbarash, R.A.; Nahlik, J.E.; Cunningham, A.; Marley, J.; Heng, M.; Jones, T.; Rea, T.; Boon, R.; Saltzman, R. Famciclovir for the treatment of acute herpes zoster: Effects on acute disease and postherpetic neuralgia. A randomized, double-blind, placebo-controlled trial. *Ann. Intern. Med.,* **1995**, *123*(2), 89-96.
[http://dx.doi.org/10.7326/0003-4819-123-2-199507150-00002] [PMID: 7778840]

[62]   Safrin, S.; Crumpacker, C.; Chatis, P.; Davis, R.; Hafner, R.; Rush, J.; Kessler, H.A.; Landry, B.; Mills, J. A controlled trial comparing foscarnet with vidarabine for acyclovir-resistant mucocutaneous herpes simplex in the acquired immunodeficiency syndrome. *N. Engl. J. Med.,* **1991**, *325*(8), 551-555.
[http://dx.doi.org/10.1056/NEJM199108223250805] [PMID: 1649971]

[63]   Huggins, J.W.; Hsiang, C.M.; Cosgriff, T.M.; Guang, M.Y.; Smith, J.I.; Wu, Z.O.; LeDuc, J.W.; Zheng, Z.M.; Meegan, J.M.; Wang, Q.N.; Oland, D.D.; Gui, X.E.; Gibbs, P.H.; Yuan, G.H.; Zhang, T.M. Prospective, double-blind, concurrent, placebo-controlled clinical trial of intravenous ribavirin therapy of hemorrhagic fever with renal syndrome. *J. Infect. Dis.,* **1991**, *164*(6), 1119-1127.
[http://dx.doi.org/10.1093/infdis/164.6.1119] [PMID: 1683355]

[64]   Taylor, K.; Fritz, K.; Parmar, M. Lamivudine.*StatPearls*; StatPearls Publishing: Treasure Island, FL, **2020**.

[65]   Dolin, R.; Reichman, R.C.; Madore, H.P.; Maynard, R.; Linton, P.N.; Webber-Jones, J. A controlled trial of amantadine and rimantadine in the prophylaxis of influenza A infection. *N. Engl. J. Med.,* **1982**, *307*(10), 580-584.
[http://dx.doi.org/10.1056/NEJM198209023071002] [PMID: 7050702]

[66]   Balfour, H.H., Jr Resistance of herpes simplex to acyclovir. *Ann. Intern. Med.,* **1983**, *98*(3), 404-406.
[http://dx.doi.org/10.7326/0003-4819-98-3-404] [PMID: 6299155]

[67]   Baba, M.; Tanaka, H.; De Clercq, E.; Pauwels, R.; Balzarini, J.; Schols, D.; Nakashima, H.; Perno, C.F.; Walker, R.T.; Miyasaka, T. Highly specific inhibition of human immunodeficiency virus type 1 by a novel 6-substituted acyclouridine derivative. *Biochem. Biophys. Res. Commun.,* **1989**, *165*(3), 1375-1381.
[http://dx.doi.org/10.1016/0006-291X(89)92756-3] [PMID: 2575380]

[68] Miyasaka, T.; Tanaka, H.; Baba, M.; Hayakawa, H.; Walker, R.T.; Balzarini, J.; De Clercq, E. A novel lead for specific anti-HIV-1 agents: 1-[(2-hydroxyethoxy)methyl]-6-(phenylthio)thymine. *J. Med. Chem.,* **1989**, *32*(12), 2507-2509.
[http://dx.doi.org/10.1021/jm00132a002] [PMID: 2479745]

[69] De Clercq, E. The AMD3100 story: The path to the discovery of a stem cell mobilizer *(Mozobil)*. *Biochem. Pharmacol.,* **2009**, *77*(11), 1655-1664.
[http://dx.doi.org/10.1016/j.bcp.2008.12.014] [PMID: 19161986]

[70] De Clercq, E. The bicyclam AMD3100 story. *Nat. Rev. Drug Discov.,* **2003**, *2*(7), 581-587.
[http://dx.doi.org/10.1038/nrd1134] [PMID: 12815382]

[71] De Clercq, E. Therapeutic potential of HPMPC as an antiviral drug. *Rev. Med. Virol.,* **1993**, *3*(2), 85-96.
[http://dx.doi.org/10.1002/rmv.1980030205]

[72] De Clercq, E. Therapeutic potential of Cidofovir *(HPMPC, Vistide)* for the treatment of DNA virus (i.e. herpes-, papova-, pox- and adenovirus) infections. *Acad. Geneesk. Belg,* **1996**, *58*, 19-47.

[73] De Clercq, E. Highlights in the discovery of antiviral drugs: A personal retrospective. *J. Med. Chem.,* **2010**, *53*(4), 1438-1450.
[http://dx.doi.org/10.1021/jm900932g] [PMID: 19860424]

[74] Geerinck, K.; Lukito, G.; Snoeck, R.; De Vos, R.; De Clercq, E.; Vanrenterghem, Y.; Degreef, H.; Maes, B. A case of human Orf in an immunocompromised patient treated successfully with cidofovir cream. *J. Med. Virol.,* **2001**, *64*(4), 543-549.
[http://dx.doi.org/10.1002/jmv.1084] [PMID: 11468742]

[75] Frediansyah, A.; Tiwari, R.; Sharun, K.; Dhama, K.; Harapan, H. Antivirals for COVID-19: A critical review. *Clin. Epidemiol. Glob. Health,* **2021**, *9*, 90-98.
[http://dx.doi.org/10.1016/j.cegh.2020.07.006] [PMID: 33521390]

[76] Jomah, S.; Asdaq, S.M.B.; Al-Yamani, M.J. Clinical efficacy of antivirals against novel coronavirus (COVID-19): A review. *J. Infect. Public Health,* **2020**, *13*(9), 1187-1195.
[http://dx.doi.org/10.1016/j.jiph.2020.07.013] [PMID: 32773212]

[77] Jasenosky, L.D.; Cadena, C.; Mire, C.E. *Science,* **2019**, *19*, 1279-1290.

[78] Rossignol, J.F. Nitazoxanide, a new drug candidate for the treatment of Middle East respiratory syndrome coronavirus. *J. Infect. Public Health,* **2016**, *9*(3), 227-230.
[http://dx.doi.org/10.1016/j.jiph.2016.04.001] [PMID: 27095301]

[79] Yoshimura, Y.; Kano, F.; Miyazaki, S.; Ashida, N.; Sakata, S.; Haraguchi, K.; Itoh, Y.; Tanaka, H.; Miyasaka, T. Synthesis and biological evaluation of 1′- *c* -cyano-pyrimidine nucleosides. *Nucleo. Nucleot.,* **1996**, *15*(1-3), 305-324.
[http://dx.doi.org/10.1080/07328319608002386]

[80] Yoshimura, Y.; Kitano, K.; Yamada, K.; Sakata, S.; Miura, S.; Ashida, N.; Machida, H. Synthesis and biological activities of 2′-deoxy-2′-fluoro-4′-thioarabinofuranosylpyrimidine and -purine nucleosides. *Bioorg. Med. Chem.,* **2000**, *8*(7), 1545-1558.
[http://dx.doi.org/10.1016/S0968-0896(00)00065-1] [PMID: 10976503]

[81] Hantz, O.; Allaudeen, H.S.; Ooka, T.; De Clercq, E.; Trepo, C. Inhibition of human and woodchuck hepatitis virus DNA polymerase by the triphosphates of acyclovir, 1-(2′-deoxy-2′-fluo-o-β-d-arabinofuranosyl)-5-iodocytosine and E-5-(2-bromovinyl)-2′-deoxyuridine. *Antiviral Res.,* **1984**, *4*(4), 187-199.
[http://dx.doi.org/10.1016/0166-3542(84)90017-2] [PMID: 6541455]

[82] Kumar, R.; Nath, M.; Tyrrell, D.L.J. Design and synthesis of novel 5-substituted acyclic pyrimidine nucleosides as potent and selective inhibitors of hepatitis B virus. *J. Med. Chem.,* **2002**, *45*(10), 2032-2040.
[http://dx.doi.org/10.1021/jm010410d] [PMID: 11985471]

[83]  Lee, B.; Luo, W.X.; Suzuki, S.; Robins, M.J.; Tyrrell, D.L. *In vitro* and *in vivo* comparison of the abilities of purine and pyrimidine 2′,3′-dideoxynucleosides to inhibit duck hepadnavirus. *Antimicrob. Agents Chemother.,* **1989**, *33*(3), 336-339.
[http://dx.doi.org/10.1128/AAC.33.3.336] [PMID: 2729928]

[84]  Tuttleman, J.S.; Pugh, J.C.; Summers, J.W. *In vitro* experimental infection of primary duck hepatocyte cultures with duck hepatitis B virus. *J. Virol.,* **1986**, *58*(1), 17-25.
[http://dx.doi.org/10.1128/jvi.58.1.17-25.1986] [PMID: 3512855]

[85]  Srivastav, N.C.; Shakya, N.; Mak, M.; Agrawal, B.; Tyrrell, D.L.; Kumar, R. Antiviral activity of various 1-(2′-deoxy-β-D-lyxofuranosyl), 1-(2′-fluoro-β-D-xylofuranosyl), 1-(3′-fluoro-β-D-arabinofuranosyl), and 2′-fluoro-2′,3′-didehydro-2′,3′-dideoxyribose pyrimidine nucleoside analogues against duck hepatitis B virus (DHBV) and human hepatitis B virus (HBV) replication. *J. Med. Chem.,* **2010**, *53*(19), 7156-7166.
[http://dx.doi.org/10.1021/jm100803c] [PMID: 20857959]

[86]  Stuyver, L.J.; Lostia, S.; Adams, M.; Mathew, J.S.; Pai, B.S.; Grier, J.; Tharnish, P.M.; Choi, Y.; Chong, Y.; Choo, H.; Chu, C.K.; Otto, M.J.; Schinazi, R.F. Antiviral activities and cellular toxicities of modified 2′,3′-dideoxy-2′,3′-didehydrocytidine analogues. *Antimicrob. Agents Chemother.,* **2002**, *46*(12), 3854-3860.
[http://dx.doi.org/10.1128/AAC.46.12.3854-3860.2002] [PMID: 12435688]

[87]  Escuret, V.; Aucagne, V.; Joubert, N.; Durantel, D.; Rapp, K.L.; Schinazi, R.F.; Zoulim, F.; Agrofoglio, L.A. Synthesis of 5-haloethynyl- and 5-(1,2-dihalo)vinyluracil nucleosides: Antiviral activity and cellular toxicity. *Bioorg. Med. Chem.,* **2005**, *13*(21), 6015-6024.
[http://dx.doi.org/10.1016/j.bmc.2005.06.021] [PMID: 16023859]

[88]  El-Brollosy, N.R.; Jørgensen, P.T.; Dahan, B.; Boel, A.M.; Pedersen, E.B.; Nielsen, C. Synthesis of novel N-1 (allyloxymethyl) analogues of 6-benzyl-1-(ethoxymethyl)-5-isopropyluracil (MKC-442, emivirine) with improved activity against HIV-1 and its mutants. *J. Med. Chem.,* **2002**, *45*(26), 5721-5726.
[http://dx.doi.org/10.1021/jm020949r] [PMID: 12477355]

[89]  El-Brollosy, N.R.; Pedersen, E.B.; Nielsen, C. Synthesis of Novel MKC-442 Analogues with Potent Activities against HIV-1. *Arch. Pharm.,* **2003**, *336*(45), 236-241.
[http://dx.doi.org/10.1002/ardp.200300742]

[90]  Wamberg, M.; Pedersen, E.B.; El-Brollosy, N.R.; Nielsen, C. Synthesis of 6-arylvinyl analogues of the HIV drugs SJ-3366 and Emivirine. *Bioorg. Med. Chem.,* **2004**, *12*(5), 1141-1149.
[http://dx.doi.org/10.1016/j.bmc.2003.11.032] [PMID: 14980626]

[91]  Zhan, P.; Liu, X.; Cao, Y.; Wang, Y.; Pannecouque, C.; De Clercq, E. 1,2,3-Thiadiazole thioacetanilides as a novel class of potent HIV-1 non-nucleoside reverse transcriptase inhibitors. *Bioorg. Med. Chem. Lett.,* **2008**, *18*(20), 5368-5371.
[http://dx.doi.org/10.1016/j.bmcl.2008.09.055] [PMID: 18824350]

[92]  Yu, M.; Liu, X.; Li, Z.; Liu, S.; Pannecouque, C.; Clercq, E.D. Synthesis and biological evaluation of novel 2-(substituted phenylaminocarbonylmethylthio)-6-(2,6-dichlorobenzyl)-pyrimidin-4(3H)-ones as potent HIV-1 NNRTIs. *Bioorg. Med. Chem.,* **2009**, *17*(22), 7749-7754.
[http://dx.doi.org/10.1016/j.bmc.2009.09.035] [PMID: 19819705]

[93]  Reverse Transcriptase Assay. *Colorimetric kit, Roche Diagnostics GmbH, Roche Applied Science;*

[94]  Pauwels, R.; Balzarini, J.; Baba, M.; Snoeck, R.; Schols, D.; Herdewijn, P.; Desmyter, J.; De Clercq, E. Rapid and automated tetrazolium-based colorimetric assay for the detection of anti-HIV compounds. *J. Virol. Methods,* **1988**, *20*(4), 309-321.
[http://dx.doi.org/10.1016/0166-0934(88)90134-6] [PMID: 2460479]

[95]  Balzarini, J.; Karlsson, A.; Perez-perez, M-J.; Vrang, L.; Walbers, J.; Zhang, H.; O̎berg, B.; Vandamme, A.-M.; Camarasa, M.-J.; DeClercq, E. HIV-1-specific reverse transcriptase inhibitors show differential activity against HIV-1 mutant strains containing different amino acid substitutions in

the reverse transcriptase. *Virology,* **1993**, *192*, 246.
[http://dx.doi.org/10.1006/viro.1993.1027] [PMID: 7685964]

[96]   Rawal, R.K.; Tripathi, R.; Katti, S.B.; Pannecouque, C.; De Clercq, E. Synthesis and evaluation of 2-
      (2,6-dihalophenyl)-3-pyrimidinyl-1,3-thiazolidin-4-one analogues as anti-HIV-1 agents. *Bioorg. Med.
      Chem.,* **2007**, *15*(9), 3134-3142.
      [http://dx.doi.org/10.1016/j.bmc.2007.02.044] [PMID: 17349793]

[97]   Meng, G.; Chen, F.E.; De Clercq, E.; Balzarini, J.; Pannecouque, C. Nonnucleoside HIV-1 reverse
      transcriptase inhibitors: Part I. Synthesis and structure-activity relationship of 1-alkoxymethyl-5-al-
      yl-6-naphthylmethyl uracils as HEPT analogues. *Chem. Pharm. Bull.,* **2003**, *51*(7), 779-789.
      [http://dx.doi.org/10.1248/cpb.51.779] [PMID: 12843582]

[98]   Pauwels, R.; Baba, M.; Snoeck, R.; Schols, D.; Herdewijn, P.; Desmyster, J.; De, E.; Balzarini, J.
      Rapid and automated tetrazolium-based colorimetric assay for the detection of anti-HIV compounds.
      *Clercq,* **1988**, *20*, 309-321.

[99]   He, Y.; Chen, F.; Yu, X.; Wang, Y.; De Clercq, E.; Balzarini, J.; Pannecouque, C. Nonnucleoside
      HIV-1 reverse transcriptase inhibitors; part 3. Synthesis and antiviral activity of 5-alkyl-2-[(aryl and
      alkyloxyl-carbonylmethyl)thio]-6-(1-naphthylmethyl) pyrimidin-4(3H)-ones. *Bioorg. Chem.,* **2004**,
      *32*(6), 536-548.
      [http://dx.doi.org/10.1016/j.bioorg.2004.05.007] [PMID: 15530994]

[100]  Holy, A.; Votruba, I.; Masoj_idkova, M.; Andrei, G.; Snoeck, R.; Naesens, L.; De Clercq, E.;
      Balzarini, J. 6-[2-(Phosphonomethoxy)alkoxy]pyrimidines with antiviral activity. *J. Med. Chem.,*
      **2002**, *45*, 1918.
      [PMID: 11960502]

[101]  Balzarini, J.; Pannecouque, C.; De Clercq, E.; Aquaro, S.; Perno, C.F.; Egberink, H.; Holý, A.
      Antiretrovirus activity of a novel class of acyclic pyrimidine nucleoside phosphonates. *Antimicrob.
      Agents Chemother.,* **2002**, *46*(7), 2185-2193.
      [http://dx.doi.org/10.1128/AAC.46.7.2185-2193.2002] [PMID: 12069973]

[102]  Hocková, D.; Holý, A.; Masojídková, M.; Andrei, G.; Snoeck, R.; De Clercq, E.; Balzarini, J.
      Synthesis and antiviral activity of 2,4-diamino-5-cyano-6-[2-(phosphonomethoxy)ethoxy]pyrimidine
      and related compounds. *Bioorg. Med. Chem.,* **2004**, *12*(12), 3197-3202.
      [http://dx.doi.org/10.1016/j.bmc.2004.04.002] [PMID: 15158787]

[103]  Garaci, E.; Palamara, A.T.; Di Francesco, P.; Favalli, C.; Ciriolo, M.R.; Rotilio, G. Glutathione
      inhibits replication and expression of viral proteins in cultured cells infected with sendai virus.
      *Biochem. Biophys. Res. Commun.,* **1992**, *188*(3), 1090-1096.
      [http://dx.doi.org/10.1016/0006-291X(92)91343-O] [PMID: 1332709]

[104]  Saladino, R.; Crestini, C.; Palamara, A.T.; Danti, M.C.; Manetti, F.; Corelli, F.; Garaci, E.; Botta, M.
      Synthesis, biological evaluation, and pharmacophore generation of uracil, 4(3H)-pyrimidinone, and
      uridine derivatives as potent and selective inhibitors of parainfluenza 1 (Sendai) virus. *J. Med. Chem.,*
      **2001**, *44*(26), 4554-4562.
      [http://dx.doi.org/10.1021/jm010938i] [PMID: 11741474]

[105]  Kumar, R.; Wiebe, L.I.; Knaus, E.E. Synthesis and antiviral activity of novel 5-(1-azido-2-haloethyl)
      and 5-(1-azido-, amino-, or methoxyethyl) analogs of 2'-deoxyuridine. *J. Med. Chem.,* **1993**, *36*(17),
      2470-2474.
      [http://dx.doi.org/10.1021/jm00069a004] [PMID: 8394933]

[106]  Kumar, R.; Rai, D.; Sharma, S.K.; Saffran, H.A.; Blush, R.; Tyrrell, D.L.J. Synthesis and antiviral
      activity of novel 5-(1-cyanamido-2-haloethyl) and 5-(1-hydroxy(or methoxy)-2-azidoethyl) analogues
      of uracil nucleosides. *J. Med. Chem.,* **2001**, *44*(21), 3531-3538.
      [http://dx.doi.org/10.1021/jm010226s] [PMID: 11585457]

[107]  Kumar, R.; Sharma, N.; Nath, M.; Saffran, H.A.; Tyrrell, D.L.J. Synthesis and antiviral activity of
      novel acyclic nucleoside analogues of 5-(1-azido-2-haloethyl)uracils. *J. Med. Chem.,* **2001**, *44*(24),

4225-4229.
[http://dx.doi.org/10.1021/jm010227k] [PMID: 11708924]

[108]   De Clercq, E.; Descamps, J.; Verhelst, G.; Walker, R.T.; Jones, A.S.; Torrence, P.F.; Shugar, D. Comparative efficacy of antiherpes drugs against different strains of herpes simplex virus. *J. Infect. Dis.,* **1980**, *141*(5), 563-574.
[http://dx.doi.org/10.1093/infdis/141.5.563] [PMID: 6246180]

[109]   De Clercq, E.; Sakuma, T.; Baba, M.; Pauwels, R.; Balzarini, J.; Rosenberg, I.; Holy, A. Antiviral activity of phosphonylmethoxyalkyl derivatives of purine and pyrimidines. *Antiviral Res.,* **1987**, *8*, 261-272.
[http://dx.doi.org/10.1016/S0166-3542(87)80004-9] [PMID: 3451698]

[110]   Balzarini, J.; Naesens, L.; Slachmuylders, J.; Niphuis, H.; Rosenberg, I.; Hol, A.; Schellekens, H.; Clercq, E.D. 9-(2-phosphonylmethoxyethyl)adenine (PMEA) effectively inhibits retrovirus replication *in vitro* and simian immunodeficiency virus infection in rhesus monkeys. *AIDS,* **1991**, *5*(1), 21-28.
[http://dx.doi.org/10.1097/00002030-199101000-00003] [PMID: 2059358]

[111]   Stuyver, L.J.; Lostia, S.; Adams, M.; Mathew, J.S.; Pai, B.S.; Grier, J.; Tharnish, P.M.; Choi, Y.; Chong, Y.; Choo, H.; Chu, C.K.; Otto, M.J.; Schinazi, R.F. Antiviral activities and cellular toxicities of modified 2′,3′-dideoxy-2′,3′-didehydrocytidine analogues. *Antimicrob. Agents Chemother.,* **2002**, *46*(12), 3854-3860.
[http://dx.doi.org/10.1128/AAC.46.12.3854-3860.2002] [PMID: 12435688]

[112]   Holý, A.; Votruba, I.; Masojídková, M.; Andrei, G.; Snoeck, R.; Naesens, L.; De Clercq, E.; Balzarini, J. 6-[2-(Phosphonomethoxy)alkoxy]pyrimidines with antiviral activity. *J. Med. Chem.,* **2002**, *45*(9), 1918-1929.
[http://dx.doi.org/10.1021/jm011095y] [PMID: 11960502]

[113]   Qiu, Y.L.; Ksebati, M.B.; Ptak, R.G.; Fan, B.Y.; Breitenbach, J.M.; Lin, J.S.; Cheng, Y.C.; Kern, E.R.; Drach, J.C.; Zemlicka, J. (Z)- and (E)-2-((hydroxymethyl)cyclopropylidene)methyladenine and -guanine. New nucleoside analogues with a broad-spectrum antiviral activity. *J. Med. Chem.,* **1998**, *41*(1), 10-23.
[http://dx.doi.org/10.1021/jm9705723] [PMID: 9438017]

[114]   Chen, J.J.; Wei, Y.; Drach, J.C.; Townsend, L.B. Synthesis and antiviral evaluation of trisubstituted indole N-nucleosides as analogues of 2,5,6-trichloro-1-(beta-D-ribofuranosyl)benzimidazole (TCRB). *J. Med. Chem.,* **2000**, *43*(12), 2449-2456.
[http://dx.doi.org/10.1021/jm990320x] [PMID: 10882372]

[115]   Zhou, S.; Kern, E.R.; Gullen, E.; Cheng, Y.C.; Drach, J.C.; Matsumi, S.; Mitsuya, H.; Zemlicka, J. (Z)- and (E)-[2-Fluoro-2-(hydroxymethyl)cyclopropylidene]methylpurines and -pyrimidines, a new class of methylenecyclopropane analogues of nucleosides: synthesis and antiviral activity. *J. Med. Chem.,* **2004**, *47*(27), 6964-6972.
[http://dx.doi.org/10.1021/jm040093l] [PMID: 15615545]

[116]   Weinberg, A.; Bate, B.J.; Masters, H.B.; Schneider, S.A.; Clark, J.C.; Wren, C.G.; Allaman, J.A.; Levin, M.J. *In vitro* activities of penciclovir and acyclovir against herpes simplex virus types 1 and 2. *Antimicrob. Agents Chemother.,* **1992**, *36*(9), 2037-2038.
[http://dx.doi.org/10.1128/AAC.36.9.2037] [PMID: 1329640]

[117]   Biron, K.K.; Elion, G.B. *In vitro* susceptibility of varicella-zoster virus to acyclovir. *Antimicrob. Agents Chemother.,* **1980**, *18*(3), 443-447.
[http://dx.doi.org/10.1128/AAC.18.3.443] [PMID: 6252836]

[118]   Calvani, F.; Macchia, M.; Rossello, A.; Gismondo, M.R.; Drago, L.; Fassina, M.C.; Cisternino, M.; Domiano, P. Synthesis and antiviral activity of dihydroxycyclohexyl pyrimidine and purine carbocyclic nucleosides. *Bioorg. Med. Chem. Lett.,* **1995**, *5*(21), 2567-2572.
[http://dx.doi.org/10.1016/0960-894X(95)00439-Z]

[119]   Prekupec, S.; Makuc, D.; Janez Plavec, J.; Lidija Sÿuman, L.; Marijeta Kralj, M.; Kresimir Pavelic,

K.; Balzarini, J.; Clercq, E.D.; Mladen Mintas, M. Novel C-6 fluorinated acyclic side chain pyrimidine derivatives: Synthesis, (1)H and (13)C NMR conformational studies, and antiviral and cytostatic evaluations. *J. Med. Chem.,* **2007**, *50*, 3037.
[http://dx.doi.org/10.1021/jm0614329]

[120] Pérez-Pérez, M.J.; De Clercq, E.; Herdewijn, P. Synthesis and antiviral activity of 2-deoxy-1-5-anhydro-D-mannitol nucleosides containing a pyrimidine base moiety. *Bioorg. Med. Chem. Lett.,* **1996**, *6*(13), 1457-1460.
[http://dx.doi.org/10.1016/S0960-894X(96)00244-2]

[121] Farrow, S.N.; Jones, A.S.; Kumar, A.; Walker, R.T.; Balzarini, J.; De Clercq, E. Synthesis and biological properties of novel phosphotriesters: A new approach to the introduction of biologically active nucleotides into cells. *J. Med. Chem.,* **1990**, *33*(5), 1400-1406.
[http://dx.doi.org/10.1021/jm00167a019] [PMID: 2329561]

[122] Miyasaka, T.; Tanaka, H.; Baba, M.; Hayakawa, H.; Walker, R.T.; Balzarini, J.; De Clercq, E. A novel lead for specific anti-HIV-1 agents: 1-[(2-hydroxyethoxy)methyl]-6-(phenylthio)thymine. *J. Med. Chem.,* **1989**, *32*(12), 2507-2509.
[http://dx.doi.org/10.1021/jm00132a002] [PMID: 2479745]

[123] Amblard, F.; Aucagne, V.; Guenot, P.; Schinazi, R.F.; Agrofoglio, L.A.; Agrofoglio, L.A. Synthesis and antiviral activity of novel acyclic nucleosides in the 5-alkynyl- and 6-alkylfuro[2,3-d]pyrimidine series. *Bioorg. Med. Chem.,* **2005**, *13*(4), 1239-1248.
[http://dx.doi.org/10.1016/j.bmc.2004.11.057] [PMID: 15670933]

[124] Dymock, B.W. Emerging therapies for hepatitis C virus infection. *Expert Opin. Emerg. Drugs,* **2001**, *6*(1), 13-42.
[PMID: 15989494]

[125] Fried, M.W.; Shiffman, M.L.; Reddy, K.R.; Smith, C.; Marinos, G.; Gonçales, F.L., Jr; Häussinger, D.; Diago, M.; Carosi, G.; Dhumeaux, D.; Craxi, A.; Lin, A.; Hoffman, J.; Yu, J. Peginterferon alfa-2a plus ribavirin for chronic hepatitis C virus infection. *N. Engl. J. Med.,* **2002**, *347*(13), 975-982.
[http://dx.doi.org/10.1056/NEJMoa020047] [PMID: 12324553]

[126] Fried, M.W. Side effects of therapy of hepatitis C and their management. *Hepatology,* **2002**, *36*(5) 1, S237-S244.
[PMID: 12407599]

[127] Lohmann, V.; Körner, F.; Koch, J.O.; Herian, U.; Theilmann, L.; Bartenschlager, R. Replication of subgenomic hepatitis C virus RNAs in a hepatoma cell line. *Science,* **1999**, *285*(5424), 110-113.
[http://dx.doi.org/10.1126/science.285.5424.110] [PMID: 10390360]

[128] Bartenschlager, R. Hepatitis C virus replicons: Potential role for drug development. *Nat. Rev. Drug Discov.,* **2002**, *1*(11), 911-916.
[http://dx.doi.org/10.1038/nrd942] [PMID: 12415250]

[129] Koch, U.; Attenni, B.; Malancona, S.; Colarusso, S.; Conte, I.; Di Filippo, M.; Harper, S.; Pacini, B.; Giomini, C.; Thomas, S.; Incitti, I.; Tomei, L.; De Francesco, R.; Altamura, S.; Matassa, V.G.; Narjes, F. 2-(2-Thienyl)-5,6-dihydroxy-4-carboxypyrimidines as inhibitors of the hepatitis C virus NS5B polymerase: discovery, SAR, modeling, and mutagenesis. *J. Med. Chem.,* **2006**, *49*(5), 1693-1705.
[http://dx.doi.org/10.1021/jm051064t] [PMID: 16509585]

[130] Korba, B.E.; Boyd, M.R. Penciclovir is a selective inhibitor of hepatitis B virus replication in cultured human hepatoblastoma cells. *Antimicrob. Agents Chemother.,* **1996**, *40*(5), 1282-1284.
[http://dx.doi.org/10.1128/AAC.40.5.1282] [PMID: 8723485]

[131] Sells, M.A.; Chen, M.L.; Acs, G. Production of hepatitis B virus particles in Hep G2 cells transfected with cloned hepatitis B virus DNA. *Proc. Natl. Acad. Sci.,* **1987**, *84*(4), 1005-1009.
[http://dx.doi.org/10.1073/pnas.84.4.1005] [PMID: 3029758]

[132] Srivastav, N.C.; Shakya, N.; Mak, M.; Liang, C.; Tyrrell, D.L.J.; Agrawal, B.; Kumar, R. Synthesis and *in vitro* antiviral activities of 3'-fluoro (or chloro) and 2',3'-difluoro 2',3'-dideoxynucleoside

analogs against hepatitis B and C viruses. *Bioorg. Med. Chem.,* **2010**, *18*(21), 7542-7547.
[http://dx.doi.org/10.1016/j.bmc.2010.08.048] [PMID: 20869253]

[133] Kumar, R.; Semaine, W.; Johar, M.; Tyrrell, D.L.J.; Agrawal, B. Effect of various pyrimidines possessing the 1-[(2-hydroxy-1-(hydroxymethyl)ethoxy)methyl] moiety, able to mimic natural 2'-deoxyribose, on wild-type and mutant hepatitis B virus replication. *J. Med. Chem.,* **2006**, *49*(12), 3693-3700.
[http://dx.doi.org/10.1021/jm060102l] [PMID: 16759112]

[134] Lee, B.; Luo, W.X.; Suzuki, S.; Robins, M.J.; Tyrrell, D.L. *In vitro and in vivo* comparison of the abilities of purine and pyrimidine 2',3'-dideoxynucleosides to inhibit duck hepadnavirus. *Antimicrob. Agents Chemother.,* **1989**, *33*(3), 336-339.
[http://dx.doi.org/10.1128/AAC.33.3.336] [PMID: 2729928]

[135] Tuttleman, J.S.; Pugh, J.C.; Summers, J.W. *In vitro* experimental infection of primary duck hepatocyte cultures with duck hepatitis B virus. *J. Virol.,* **1986**, *58*(1), 17-25.
[http://dx.doi.org/10.1128/jvi.58.1.17-25.1986] [PMID: 3512855]

[136] Shaw, T.; Amor, P.; Civitico, G.; Boyd, M.; Locarnini, S. *In vitro* antiviral activity of penciclovir, a novel purine nucleoside, against duck hepatitis B virus. *Antimicrob. Agents Chemother.,* **1994**, *38*(4), 719-723.
[http://dx.doi.org/10.1128/AAC.38.4.719] [PMID: 8031035]

[137] Kim, H.O.; Schinazi, R.F.; Nampalli, S.; Shanmuganathan, K.; Cannon, D.L.; Alves, A.J.; Jeong, L.S.; Beach, J.W.; Chu, C.K. 1,3-Dioxolanylpurine nucleosides (2R,4R) and (2R,4S) with selective anti-HIV-1 activity in human lymphocytes. *J. Med. Chem.,* **1993**, *36*(1), 30-37.
[http://dx.doi.org/10.1021/jm00053a004] [PMID: 8421287]

[138] Schinazi, R.F.; Chu, C.K.; Peck, A.; McMillan, A.; Mathis, R.; Cannon, D.; Jeong, L.S.; Beach, J.W.; Choi, W.B.; Yeola, S.; Liotta, D.C. Activities of the four optical isomers of 2',3'-dideoxy--'-thiacytidine (BCH-189) against human immunodeficiency virus type 1 in human lymphocytes. *Antimicrob. Agents Chemother.,* **1992**, *36*(3), 672-676.
[http://dx.doi.org/10.1128/AAC.36.3.672] [PMID: 1320365]

[139] Furman, P.A.; Davis, M.; Liotta, D.C.; Paff, M.; Frick, L.W.; Nelson, D.J.; Dornsife, R.E.; Wurster, J.A.; Wilson, L.J.; Fyfe, J.A.; Miller, W.H.; Condreay, L.; Avereet, D.R.; Schinazi, R.F.; Painter, G.R. The anti-hepatitis B virus activities, cytotoxicities, and anabolic profiles of the (-) and (+) enantiomers of cis-5-fluoro-1-[2-(hydroxymethyl)-1,3-oxathiolan-5-yl]cytosine. *Antimicrob. Agents Chemother.,* **1992**, *36*(12), 2686-2692.
[http://dx.doi.org/10.1128/AAC.36.12.2686] [PMID: 1336341]

[140] Schinazi, R.F.; McMillan, A.; Cannon, D.; Mathis, R.; Lloyd, R.M.; Peck, A.; Sommadossi, J.P.; St Clair, M.; Wilson, J.; Furman, P.A.; Painter, G.; Choi, W.B.; Liotta, D.C. Selective inhibition of human immunodeficiency viruses by racemates and enantiomers of cis-5-fluoro--[2-(hydroxymethyl)-1,3-oxathiolan-5-yl]cytosine. *Antimicrob. Agents Chemother.,* **1992**, *36*(11), 2423-2431.
[http://dx.doi.org/10.1128/AAC.36.11.2423] [PMID: 1283296]

[141] Du, J.; Surzhykov, S.; Lin, J.S.; Newton, M.G.; Cheng, Y.C.; Schinazi, R.F.; Chu, C.K. Synthesis, anti-human immunodeficiency virus and anti-hepatitis B virus activities of novel oxaselenolane nucleosides. *J. Med. Chem.,* **1997**, *40*(19), 2991-2993.
[http://dx.doi.org/10.1021/jm9703698] [PMID: 9301659]

[142] Lin, T.S.; Luo, M.Z.; Liu, M.C.; Pai, S.B.; Dutschman, G.E.; Cheng, Y.C. Synthesis and biological evaluation of 2',3'-dideoxy-L-pyrimidine nucleosides as potential antiviral agents against human immunodeficiency virus (HIV) and hepatitis B virus (HBV). *J. Med. Chem.,* **1994**, *37*(6), 798-803.
[http://dx.doi.org/10.1021/jm00032a013] [PMID: 8145230]

[143] Lin, T-S. Luo, M-Z.; Man-Chin Liu, M.C. *Tetrahedron,* **1995**, *51*, 1055.
[http://dx.doi.org/10.1016/0040-4020(94)00997-9]

[144] Semaine, W.; Johar, M.; Tyrrell, D.L.J.; Kumar, R.; Agrawal, B. Inhibition of hepatitis B virus (HBV) replication by pyrimidines bearing an acyclic moiety: effect on wild-type and mutant HBV. *J. Med. Chem.,* **2006**, *49*(6), 2049-2054.
[http://dx.doi.org/10.1021/jm058271d] [PMID: 16539393]

[145] Artico, M.; Massa, S.; Mai, A.; Marongiu, M.E.; Piras, G.; Tramontano, E.; la Colla, P. 3,4-Dihydro-2-Alkoxy-6-Benzyl-4-Oxopyrimidines (DABOs): A New Class of Specific Inhibitors of Human Immunodeficiency Virus Type 1. *Antivir. Chem. Chemother.,* **1993**, *4*(6), 361-368.
[http://dx.doi.org/10.1177/095632029300400608]

[146] Ragno, R.; Mai, A.; Sbardella, G.; Artico, M.; Massa, S.; Musiu, C.; Mura, M.; Marturana, F.; Cadeddu, A.; La Colla, P. Computer-aided design, synthesis, and anti-HIV-1 activity *in vitro* of 2-alkylamino-6-[1-(2,6-difluorophenyl)alkyl]-3,4-dihydro-5-alkylpyrimidin-4(3H)-ones as novel potent non-nucleoside reverse transcriptase inhibitors, also active against the Y181C variant. *J. Med. Chem.,* **2004**, *47*(4), 928-934.
[http://dx.doi.org/10.1021/jm0309856] [PMID: 14761194]

[147] Mai, A.; Artico, M.; Ragno, R.; Sbardella, G.; Massa, S.; Musiu, C.; Mura, M.; Marturana, F.; Cadeddu, A.; Maga, G.; Colla, P.L. 5-Alkyl-2-alkylamino-6-(2,6-difluorophenylalk-l)-3,4-dihydropyrimidin-4(3H)-ones, a new series of potent, broad-spectrum non-nucleoside reverse transcriptase inhibitors belonging to the DABO family. *Bioorg. Med. Chem.,* **2005**, *13*(6), 2065-2077.
[http://dx.doi.org/10.1016/j.bmc.2005.01.005] [PMID: 15727860]

[148] Danel, K.; Larsen, L.M.; Pedersen, E.B.; Sanna, G.; La Colla, P.; Loddo, R. Synthesis and antiviral activity of new dimeric inhibitors against HIV-1. *Bioorg. Med. Chem.,* **2008**, *16*(1), 511-517.
[http://dx.doi.org/10.1016/j.bmc.2007.09.015] [PMID: 17904371]

[149] He, Y.; Chen, F.; Yu, X.; Wang, Y.; De Clercq, E.; Balzarini, J.; Pannecouque, C. Nonnucleoside HIV-1 reverse transcriptase inhibitors; part 3. Synthesis and antiviral activity of 5-alkyl-2-[(aryl and alkyloxyl-carbonylmethyl)thio]-6-(1-naphthylmethyl) pyrimidin-4(3H)-ones. *Bioorg. Chem.,* **2004**, *32*(6), 536-548.
[http://dx.doi.org/10.1016/j.bioorg.2004.05.007] [PMID: 15530994]

[150] Wang, Y.P.; Chen, F.E.; De Clercq, E.; Balzarini, J.; Pannecouque, C. Synthesis and biological evaluation of novel 6-substituted 5-alkyl-2-(arylcarbonylmethylthio)pyrimidin-4(3H)-ones as potent non-nucleoside HIV-1 reverse transcriptase inhibitors. *Bioorg. Med. Chem.,* **2008**, *16*(7), 3887-3894.
[http://dx.doi.org/10.1016/j.bmc.2008.01.039] [PMID: 18267363]

[151] Reverse Transcriptase Assay. *Reverse Transcriptase Assay, Colorimetric kit, Roche Diagnostics GmbH, Roche Applied Science;*

[152] Chen, H.; Bai, J.; Jiao, L.; Guo, Z.; Yin, Q.; Li, X. Design, microwave-assisted synthesis and HIV-RT inhibitory activity of 2-(2,6-dihalophenyl)-3-(4,6-dimethyl-5-(un)substituted-pyimidin-2-yl)thiazolidin-4-ones. *Bioorg. Med. Chem.,* **2009**, *17*(11), 3980-3986.
[http://dx.doi.org/10.1016/j.bmc.2009.04.024] [PMID: 19411176]

[153] Danel, K.; Larsen, E.; Pedersen, E.B. Easy synthesis of 5,6-disubstituted acyclouridine derivatives. *Synthesis,* **1995**, *1995*(8), 934-936.
[http://dx.doi.org/10.1055/s-1995-4022]

[154] Lu, X.; Chen, Y.; Guo, Y.; Liu, Z.; Shi, Y.; Xu, Y.; Wang, X.; Zhang, Z. The design and synthesis of N-1-alkylated-5-aminoaryalkylsubstituted-6-methyluracils as potential non-nucleoside HIV-1 RT inhibitors. *Bioorg. Med. Chem.,* **2007**, *15*, 7399.
[http://dx.doi.org/10.1016/j.bmc.2007.07.058] [PMID: 17870545]

[155] Mai, A.; Artico, M.; Sbardella, G.; Massa, S.; Novellino, E.; Greco, G.; Loi, A.G.; Tramontano, E.; Marongiu, M.E.; La Colla, P. 5-Alkyl-2-(alkylthio)-6-(2,6-dihalophenylmethyl)-3, 4-dihydropyrimidin-4(3H)-ones: novel potent and selective dihydro-alkoxy-benzyl-oxopyrimidine derivatives. *J. Med. Chem.,* **1999**, *42*(4), 619-627.
[http://dx.doi.org/10.1021/jm980260f] [PMID: 10052969]

[156] Armand-Ugón, M.; Clotet-Codina, I.; Tintori, C.; Manetti, F.; Clotet, B.; Botta, M.; Esté, J.A. The anti-HIV activity of ADS-J1 targets the HIV-1 gp120. *Virology,* **2005**, *343*(1), 141-149.
[http://dx.doi.org/10.1016/j.virol.2005.08.007] [PMID: 16168454]

[157] Maga, G.; Amacker, M.; Ruel, N.; Hübscher, U.; Spadari, S. Resistance to nevirapine of HIV-1 reverse transcriptase mutants: loss of stabilizing interactions and thermodynamic or steric barriers are induced by different single amino acid substitutions. *J. Mol. Biol.,* **1997**, *274*(5), 738-747.
[http://dx.doi.org/10.1006/jmbi.1997.1427] [PMID: 9405155]

[158] Mai, A.; Artico, M.; Rotili, D.; Tarantino, D.; Clotet-Codina, I.; Armand-Ugo, M.; Rino Ragno, R.; Simeoni, S.; Sbardella, G.; Nawrozkij, M.B.; Samuele, A.; Maga, G.; Jose´, A. Synthesis and biological properties of novel 2-aminopyrimidin-4(3H)-ones highly potent against HIV-1 mutant strains. *J. Med. Chem.,* **2007**, *50*, 5412-5424.
[http://dx.doi.org/10.1021/jm070811e] [PMID: 17910429]

[159] Hazuda, D.J.; Felock, P.; Witmer, M.; Wolfe, A.; Stillmock, K.; Grobler, J.A.; Espeseth, A.; Gabryelski, L.; Schleif, W.; Blau, C.; Miller, M.D. Inhibitors of strand transfer that prevent integration and inhibit HIV-1 replication in cells. *Science,* **2000**, *287*(5453), 646-650.
[http://dx.doi.org/10.1126/science.287.5453.646] [PMID: 10649997]

[160] Zhuang, L.; Wai, J.S.; Embrey, M.W.; Fisher, T.E.; Egbertson, M.S.; Payne, L.S.; Guare, J.P., Jr; Vacca, J.P.; Hazuda, D.J.; Felock, P.J.; Wolfe, A.L.; Stillmock, K.A.; Witmer, M.V.; Moyer, G.; Schleif, W.A.; Gabryelski, L.J.; Leonard, Y.M.; Lynch, J.J., Jr; Michelson, S.R.; Young, S.D. Design and synthesis of 8-hydroxy-[1,6]naphthyridines as novel inhibitors of HIV-1 integrase *in vitro* and in infected cells. *J. Med. Chem.,* **2003**, *46*(4), 453-456.
[http://dx.doi.org/10.1021/jm025553u] [PMID: 12570367]

[161] Vacca, J.P.; Dorsey, B.D.; Schleif, W.A.; Levin, R.B.; McDaniel, S.L.; Darke, P.L.; Zugay, J.; Quintero, J.C.; Blahy, O.M.; Roth, E.; Sardana, V.V.; Schlabach, A.J.; Graham, P.I.; Condra, J.H.; Gotlib, L.; Holloway, M.K.; Lin, J.; Chen, I.; Vastag, K.; Ostovic, D.; Anderson, P.S.; Emini, E.A.; Huff, J.R. L-735,524: An orally bioavailable human immunodeficiency virus type 1 protease inhibitor. *Proc. Natl. Acad. Sci.,* **1994**, *91*(9), 4096-4100.
[http://dx.doi.org/10.1073/pnas.91.9.4096] [PMID: 8171040]

[162] Pace, P.; Francesco, M.E.D.; Gardelli, C.; Harper, S.; Muraglia, E.; Nizi, E.; Orvieto, F.; Petrocchi, A.; Marco Poma, M.; Rowley, M.; Scarpelli, R.; Laufer, R.; Paz, O.G.; Monteagudo, E.; Bonelli, F.; Hazuda, D.; Stillmock, K.A. Dihydroxypyrimidine-4-carboxamides as novel potent and selective HIV integrase inhibitors. *J. Med. Chem.,* **2007**, *50*, 2225.
[http://dx.doi.org/10.1021/jm070027u] [PMID: 17428043]

[163] Ohrui, H.; Kohgo, S.; Kitano, K.; Sakata, S.; Kodama, E.; Yoshimura, K.; Matsuoka, M.; Shigeta, S.; Mitsuya, H. Syntheses of 4'-C-ethynyl-beta-D-arabino- and 4'-C-ethynyl-2'-deoxy-beta-D-ribo-pentofuranosylpyrimidines and -purines and evaluation of their anti-HIV activity. *J. Med. Chem.,* **2000**, *43*(23), 4516-4525.
[http://dx.doi.org/10.1021/jm000209n] [PMID: 11087576]

[164] Choo, H.; Chong, Y.; Choi, Y.; Mathew, J.; Schinazi, R.F.; Chu, C.K. Synthesis, anti-HIV activity, and molecular mechanism of drug resistance of L-2',3'-didehydro-2',3'-dideoxy-2'-floro-4'-thionucleosides. *J. Med. Chem.,* **2003**, *46*(3), 389-398.
[http://dx.doi.org/10.1021/jm020376i] [PMID: 12540238]

[165] Mitsuya, H.; Weinhold, K.J.; Furman, P.A.; St Clair, M.H.; Lehrman, S.N.; Gallo, R.C.; Bolognesi, D.; Barry, D.W.; Broder, S. 3'-Azido-3'-deoxythymidine (BW A509U): An antiviral agent that inhibits the infectivity and cytopathic effect of human T-lymphotropic virus type III/lymphadenopathy-associated virus *in vitro*. *Proc. Natl. Acad. Sci.,* **1985**, *82*(20), 7096-7100.
[http://dx.doi.org/10.1073/pnas.82.20.7096] [PMID: 2413459]

[166] Tsai, C.C.; Follis, K.; Beck, T.W.; Sabo, A.; Bischofberger, N.; Dailey, P.J. Effects of (R)-9--2-phosphonylmethoxypropyl)adenine monotherapy on chronic SIV infection in macaques. *AIDS Res. Hum. Retroviruses,* **1997**, *13*(8), 707-712.

[http://dx.doi.org/10.1089/aid.1997.13.707] [PMID: 9168239]

[167] Baba, M.; Konno, K.; Shigeta, S.; De Clercq, E. *In vitro* activity of (S)-9-(3-hydroxy-2-phosphonylmethoxypropyl)-adenine against newly isolated clinical varicella-zoster viras strains. *Eur. J. Clin. Microbiol. Infect. Dis.,* **1987**, *6*, 158-160.

[168] Hocková, D.; Holý, A.; Masojídková, M.; Andrei, G.; Snoeck, R.; De Clercq, E.; Balzarini, J. 5-Substituted-2,4-diamino-6-[2-(phosphonomethoxy)ethoxy]pyrimidines-acyclic nucleoside phosphonate analogues with antiviral activity. *J. Med. Chem.,* **2003**, *46*(23), 5064-5073.
[http://dx.doi.org/10.1021/jm030932o] [PMID: 14584956]

[169] Marquez, V.E.; Lim, M.I.; Treanor, S.P.; Plowman, J.; Priest, M.A.; Markovac, A.; Khan, M.S.; Kaskar, B.; Driscoll, J.S. Cyclopentenylcytosine. A carbocyclic nucleoside with antitumor and antiviral properties. *J. Med. Chem.,* **1988**, *31*(9), 1687-1694.
[http://dx.doi.org/10.1021/jm00117a004] [PMID: 3411597]

[170] Song, G.Y.; Paul, V.; Choo, H.; Morrey, J.; Sidwell, R.W.; Schinazi, R.F.; Chu, C.K. Enantiomeric synthesis of D- and L-cyclopentenyl nucleosides and their antiviral activity against HIV and West Nile virus. *J. Med. Chem.,* **2001**, *44*(23), 3985-3993.
[http://dx.doi.org/10.1021/jm010256v] [PMID: 11689085]

[171] Pauwels, R.; Balzarini, J.; Baba, M.; Snoeck, R.; Schols, D.; Herdewijn, P.; Desmyter, J.; De Clercq, E. Rapid and automated tetrazolium-based colorimetric assay for the detection of anti-HIV compounds. *J. Virol. Methods,* **1988**, *20*(4), 309-321.
[http://dx.doi.org/10.1016/0166-0934(88)90134-6] [PMID: 2460479]

[172] Rawal, R.K.; Tripathi, R.; Katti, S.B.; Pannecouque, C.; De Clercq, E. Synthesis and evaluation of 2-(2,6-dihalophenyl)-3-pyrimidinyl-1,3-thiazolidin-4-one analogues as anti-HIV-1 agents. *Bioorg. Med. Chem.,* **2007**, *15*(9), 3134-3142.
[http://dx.doi.org/10.1016/j.bmc.2007.02.044] [PMID: 17349793]

[173] Main, J.; McCarron, B.; Thomas, H.C. Treatment of chronic viral hepatitis. *Antivir. Chem. Chemother.,* **1998**, *9*(6), 449-460.
[http://dx.doi.org/10.1177/095632029800900601] [PMID: 9865383]

[174] Kumar, R.; Tyrrell, D.L.J. Novel 5-vinyl pyrimidine nucleosides with potent anti-hepatitis B virus activity. *Bioorg. Med. Chem. Lett.,* **2001**, *11*(22), 2917-2920.
[http://dx.doi.org/10.1016/S0960-894X(01)00589-3] [PMID: 11677126]

[175] Shaw, T.; Amor, P.; Civitico, G.; Boyd, M.; Locarnini, S. In vitro antiviral activity of penciclovir, a novel purine nucleoside, against duck hepatitis B virus. *Antimicrob. Agents Chemother.,* **1994**, *38*(4), 719-723.
[http://dx.doi.org/10.1128/AAC.38.4.719] [PMID: 8031035]

[176] Holy, A. *Advances in Antiviral Drug Design*; Clercq, E.D., Ed.; JAI: Greenwich, CT, **1994**, p. 179.

[177] Holy, A. *Recent Advances in Nucleosides:Chemistry and Chemotherapy*; Chu, C.K., Ed.; Elsevier, **2002**, p. 167.
[http://dx.doi.org/10.1016/B978-044450951-2/50007-2]

[178] Naesens, L.; Snoeck, R.; Andrei, G.; Balzarini, J.; Neyts, J.; De Clercq, E. HPMPC (cidofovir), PMEA (adefovir) and Related acyclic nucleoside phosphonate analogues: A review of their pharmacology and clinical potential in the treatment of viral infections. *Antivir. Chem. Chemother.,* **1997**, *8*(1), 1-23.
[http://dx.doi.org/10.1177/095632029700800101]

[179] Ying, C.; De Clercq, E.; Neyts, J. Lamivudine, adefovir and tenofovir exhibit long-lasting anti-hepatitis B virus activity in cell culture. *J. Viral Hepat.,* **2000**, *7*(1), 79-83.
[http://dx.doi.org/10.1046/j.1365-2893.2000.00192.x] [PMID: 10718947]

[180] Perrillo, R.; Schiff, E.; Yoshida, E.; Statler, A.; Hirsch, K.; Wright, T.; Gutfreund, K.; Lamy, P.; Murray, A. Adefovir dipivoxil for the treatment of lamivudine-resistant hepatitis B mutants. *Hepatology,* **2000**, *32*(1), 129-134.

[http://dx.doi.org/10.1053/jhep.2000.8626] [PMID: 10869300]

[181] Gilson, R.J.C.; Chopra, K.B.; Newell, A.M.; Murray-Lyon, I.M.; Nelson, M.R.; Rice, S.J.; Tedder, R.S.; Toole, J.; Jaffe, H.S.; Weller, I.V.D. A placebo-controlled phase I/II study of adefovir dipivoxil in patients with chronic hepatitis B virus infection. *J. Viral Hepat.,* **1999**, *6*(5), 387-395.
[http://dx.doi.org/10.1046/j.1365-2893.1999.00182.x] [PMID: 10607255]

[182] Srinivas, R.V.; Fridland, A. Antiviral activities of 9-R-2-phosphonomethoxypropyl adenine (PMPA) and bis(isopropyloxymethylcarbonyl)PMPA against various drug-resistant human immunodeficiency virus strains. *Antimicrob. Agents Chemother.,* **1998**, *42*(6), 1484-1487.
[http://dx.doi.org/10.1128/AAC.42.6.1484] [PMID: 9624498]

[183] Van Rompay, K.K.A.; Miller, M.D.; Marthas, M.L.; Margot, N.A.; Dailey, P.J.; Canfield, D.R.; Tarara, R.P.; Cherrington, J.M.; Aguirre, N.L.; Bischofberger, N.; Pedersen, N.C. Prophylactic and therapeutic benefits of short-term 9-[2-(R)-(phosphonomethoxy)propyl]adenine (PMPA) administration to newborn macaques following oral inoculation with simian immunodeficiency virus with reduced susceptibility to PMPA. *J. Virol.,* **2000**, *74*(4), 1767-1774.
[http://dx.doi.org/10.1128/JVI.74.4.1767-1774.2000] [PMID: 10644348]

[184] Hockov, D.; Holy, A.; Masojıdkova, M.; Graciela Andrei, G.; Robert Snoeck, R.; Clercq, E.D.; Balzarin, J. Synthesis and antiviral activity of 2,4-diamino-5-cyano-6-[2-(phosphonomethoxy)ethoxy]pyrimidine and related compounds. *Bioorg. Med. Chem.,* **2004**, *12*, 3197.
[http://dx.doi.org/10.1016/j.bmc.2004.04.002] [PMID: 15158787]

[185] Lennerstrand, J.; Chu, C.K.; Schinazi, R.F. Biochemical studies on the mechanism of human immunodeficiency virus type 1 reverse transcriptase resistance to 1-(beta-D-dioxolane)thymine triphosphate. *Antimicrob. Agents Chemother.,* **2007**, *51*(6), 2078-2084.
[http://dx.doi.org/10.1128/AAC.00119-07] [PMID: 17403997]

[186] Chu, C.K.; Yadav, V.; Chong, Y.H.; Schinazi, R.F. Anti-HIV activity of (-)-(2R,4R)-1- (2-hydroxymethyl-1,3-dioxolan-4-yl)-thymine against drug-resistant HIV-1 mutants and studies of its molecular mechanism. *J. Med. Chem.,* **2005**, *48*(12), 3949-3952.
[http://dx.doi.org/10.1021/jm050060l] [PMID: 15943470]

[187] Schinazi, R.F.; Sommadossi, J.P.; Saalmann, V.; Cannon, D.L.; Xie, M.Y.; Hart, G.C.; Smith, G.A.; Hahn, E.F. Activities of 3'-azido-3'-deoxythymidine nucleotide dimers in primary lymphocytes infected with human immunodeficiency virus type 1. *Antimicrob. Agents Chemother.,* **1990**, *34*(6), 1061-1067.
[http://dx.doi.org/10.1128/AAC.34.6.1061] [PMID: 2393266]

[188] Schinazi, R.F.; Cannon, D.L.; Arnold, B.H.; Martino-Saltzman, D. Combinations of isoprinosine and 3'-azido-3'-deoxythymidine in lymphocytes infected with human immunodeficiency virus type 1. *Antimicrob. Agents Chemother.,* **1988**, *32*(12), 1784-1787.
[http://dx.doi.org/10.1128/AAC.32.12.1784] [PMID: 2469387]

[189] Liang, Y.; Sharon, A.; Grier, J.P.; Rapp, K.L.; Schinazi, R.F.; Chu, C.K. 5'-O-Aliphatic and amino acid ester prodrugs of (−)-β-d-(2R,4R)-dioxolane-thymine (DOT): Synthesis, anti-HIV activity, cytotoxicity and stability studies. *Bioorg. Med. Chem.,* **2009**, *17*(3), 1404-1409.
[http://dx.doi.org/10.1016/j.bmc.2008.10.078] [PMID: 19153047]

[190] Turk, G.; Moroni, G.; Pampuro, S.; Briñón, M.C.; Salomón, H. Antiretroviral activity and cytotoxicity of novel zidovudine (AZT) derivatives and the relation to their chemical structure. *Int. J. Antimicrob. Agents,* **2002**, *20*(4), 282-288.
[http://dx.doi.org/10.1016/S0924-8579(02)00191-7] [PMID: 12385685]

[191] Ravetti, S.; Gualdesi, M.S.; Trinchero-Hernández, J.S.; Turk, G.; Briñón, M.C. Synthesis and anti-HIV activity of novel 2',3'-dideoxy-3'-thiacytidine prodrugs. *Bioorg. Med. Chem.,* **2009**, *17*(17), 6407-6413.
[http://dx.doi.org/10.1016/j.bmc.2009.07.032] [PMID: 19660957]

[192]    Keith, K.A.; Wan, W.B.; Ciesla, S.L.; Beadle, J.R.; Hostetler, K.Y.; Kern, E.R. Inhibitory activity of alkoxyalkyl and alkyl esters of cidofovir and cyclic cidofovir against orthopoxvirus replication *in vitro. Antimicrob. Agents Chemother.,* **2004**, *48*(5), 1869-1871.
[http://dx.doi.org/10.1128/AAC.48.5.1869-1871.2004] [PMID: 15105146]

[193]    Fan, X.; Zhang, X.; Longhu Zhou, L.; Kathy, A.; Keith, K. A.; Earl, R.; Kern, E. R.; Paul, F.; Torrencea, P.F. A pyrimidine-pyrazolone nucleoside chimera with potent *in vitro* anti-orthopoxvirus activity. *Bioorg. Med. Chem. Lett.,* **2006**, *16*, 3224-3228.
[http://dx.doi.org/10.1016/j.bmcl.2006.03.043] [PMID: 16603351]

[194]    Verheggen, I.; Van Aerschot, A.; Toppet, S.; Snoeck, R.; Janssen, G.; Balzarini, J.; De Clercq, E.; Herdewijn, P. Synthesis and antiherpes virus activity of 1,5-anhydrohexitol nucleosides. *J. Med. Chem.,* **1993**, *36*(14), 2033-2040.
[http://dx.doi.org/10.1021/jm00066a013] [PMID: 8393114]

[195]    Verheggen, I.; Van Aerschot, A.; Van Meervelt, L.; Rozenski, J.; Wiebe, L.; Snoeck, R.; Andrei, G.; Balzarini, J.; Claes, P.; De Clercq, E. Synthesis, biological evaluation, and structure analysis of a series of new 1,5-anhydrohexitol nucleosides. *J. Med. Chem.,* **1995**, *38*(5), 826-835.
[http://dx.doi.org/10.1021/jm00005a010] [PMID: 7877148]

[196]    Ostrowski, T.; Wroblowski, B.; Busson, R.; Rozenski, J.; De Clercq, E.; Bennett, M.S.; Champness, J.N.; Summers, W.C.; Sanderson, M.R.; Herdewijn, P. 5-Substituted pyrimidines with a 1,5-anhydr-2, 3-dideoxy-D-arabino-hexitol moiety at N-1: Synthesis, antiviral activity, conformational analysis, and interaction with viral thymidine kinase. *J. Med. Chem.,* **1998**, *41*(22), 4343-4353.
[http://dx.doi.org/10.1021/jm980287z] [PMID: 9784109]

[197]    Johan Wouters, J.; Herdewijn, P. 5-Substituted pyrimidine 1,5-anhydrohexitols: Conformational analysis and interaction with viral thymidine kinase. *Bioorg. Med. Chem. Lett.,* **1999**, *9*, 1563.
[http://dx.doi.org/10.1016/S0960-894X(99)00225-5] [PMID: 10386936]

[198]    Vedula, M.S.; Jennepalli, S.; Aryasomayajula, R.; Rondla, S.R.; Musku, M.R.; Kura, R.R.; Bandi, P.R. Novel nucleosides as potent influenza viral inhibitors. *Bioorg. Med. Chem.,* **2010**, *18*(17), 6329-6339.
[http://dx.doi.org/10.1016/j.bmc.2010.07.017] [PMID: 20674371]

[199]    Saladino, R.; Bernini, R.; Crestini, C.; Mincione, E.; Bergamini, A.; Marini, S.; Teresa Palamara, A.; Palamarac, T.A. Studies on the chemistry of pyrimidine derivatives with dimethyldioxirane: synthesis, cytotoxic effect and antiviral activity of new 5,6-oxiranyl-5,6-dihydro and 5-hydroxy-5,6-dihydo-6-substituted uracil derivatives and pyrimidine nucleosides. *Tetrahedron,* **1995**, *51*(27), 7561-7578.
[http://dx.doi.org/10.1016/0040-4020(95)00380-Q]

[200]    Farag, R.S.; Shalaby, A.S.; El-Baroty, G.A.; Ibrahim, N.A.; Ali, M.A.; Hassan, E.M. Chemical and biological evaluation of the essential oils of differentMelaleuca species. *Phytother. Res.,* **2004**, *18*(1), 30-35.
[http://dx.doi.org/10.1002/ptr.1348] [PMID: 14750197]

[201]    Rashad, A.E.; Hegab, M.I.; Abdel-Megeid, R.E.; Micky, J.A.; Abdel-Megeid, F.M.E. Synthesis and antiviral evaluation of some new pyrazole and fused pyrazolopyrimidine derivatives. *Bioorg. Med. Chem.,* **2008**, *16*(15), 7102-7106.
[http://dx.doi.org/10.1016/j.bmc.2008.06.054] [PMID: 18635363]

[202]    McGuigan, C.; Yarnold, C.J.; Jones, G.; Vela' zquez, S.; Barucki, H.; Brancale, A.; Andrei, G.; Snoeck, R.; De Clercq, E.; Balzarini, J. Potent and selective inhibition of varicella-zoster virus (VZV) by nucleoside analogues with an unusual bicyclic base. *J. Med. Chem.,* **1999**, *42*, 4479.
[http://dx.doi.org/10.1021/jm990346o] [PMID: 10579812]

[203]    Andrei, G.; Snoeck, R.; Reymen, D.; Liesnard, C.; Goubau, P.; Desmyter, J.; De Clercq, E. Comparative activity of selected antiviral compounds against clinical isolates of varicella-zoster virus. *Eur. J. Clin. Microbiol. Infect. Dis.,* **1995**, *14*(4), 318-329.
[http://dx.doi.org/10.1007/BF02116525] [PMID: 7649195]

[204]    Sienaert, R.; Naesens, L.; Brancale, A.; De Clercq, E.; McGuigan, C. BSpecific recognition of the

bicyclic pyrimidine nucleoside analogs, a new class of highly potent and selective inhibitors of varicella-zoster virus (VZV), by the VZV-encoded thymidine kinase. *J. Mol. Pharmacol.,* **2002**, *61,* 249.
[http://dx.doi.org/10.1124/mol.61.2.249]

[205] Snoeck, R.; Andrei, G.; Bodaghi, B.; Lagneaux, L.; Daelemans, D.; de Clercq, E.; Neyts, J.; Schols, D.; Naesens, L.; Michelson, S.; Bron, D.; Otto, M.J.; Bousseau, A.; Nemecek, C.; Roy, C. 2-chloro-3-pyridin-3-yl-5,6,7,8-tetrahydroindolizine-1-carboxamide (CMV423), a new lead compound for the treatment of human cytomegalovirus infections. *Antiviral Res.,* **2002**, *55*(3), 413-424.
[http://dx.doi.org/10.1016/S0166-3542(02)00074-8] [PMID: 12206879]

[206] McGuigan, C.; Brancale, A.; Andrei, G.; Snoeck, R.; De Clercq, E.; Balzarini, J. Novel bicyclic furanopyrimidines with dual anti-VZV and -HCMV activity. *Bioorg. Med. Chem. Lett.,* **2003**, *13*(24), 4511-4513.
[http://dx.doi.org/10.1016/j.bmcl.2003.08.028] [PMID: 14643358]

[207] McGuigan, C.; Barucki, H.; Brancale, A.; Blewett, S.; Carangio, A.; Jones, G.; Pathirana, R.; Srinivasan, S.; Vela'zquez, S.; Yarnold, C.J.; Alvarez, R.; Andrei, G.; Snoeck, R.; De Clercq, E.; Balzarini, J. *Drugs Future,* **2000**, *25,* 1151.
[http://dx.doi.org/10.1358/dof.2000.025.11.858698]

[208] McGuigan, C.; Brancale, A.; Barucki, H.; Srinivasan, S.; Jones, G.; Pathirana, R.; Carangio, A.; Blewett, S.; Luoni, G.; Bidet, O.; Jukes, A.; Jarvis, C.; Andrei, G.; Snoeck, R.; De Clercq, E.; Balzarini, J. Furano pyrimidines as novel potent and selective anti-VZV agents. *Antivir. Chem. Chemother.,* **2001**, *12,* 77.
[http://dx.doi.org/10.1177/095632020101200201] [PMID: 11527045]

[209] McGuigan, C.; Pathirana, R.N.; Snoeck, R.; Andrei, G.; De Clercq, E.; Balzarini, J. Discovery of a new family of inhibitors of human cytomegalovirus (HCMV) based upon lipophilic alkyl furano pyrimidine dideoxy nucleosides: Action *via* a novel non-nucleosidic mechanism. *J. Med. Chem.,* **2004**, *47*(7), 1847-1851.
[http://dx.doi.org/10.1021/jm030857h] [PMID: 15027877]

[210] Balzarini, J.; McGuigan, C. Bicyclic pyrimidine nucleoside analogues *(BCNAs)* as highly selective and potent inhibitors of varicella-zoster virus replication. *J. Antimicrob. Chemother.,* **2002**, *50*(1), 5-9.
[http://dx.doi.org/10.1093/jac/dkf037] [PMID: 12096000]

[211] Clercq, E.D. Highly potent and selective inhibition of varicella-zoster virus replication by bicyclic furo[2,3-d]pyrimidine nucleoside analogues. *Med. Res. Rev.,* **2003**, *23*(3), 253-274.
[http://dx.doi.org/10.1002/med.10035] [PMID: 12647310]

[212] Robins, M.J.; Miranda, K.; Rajwanshi, V.K.; Peterson, M.A.; Andrei, G.; Snoeck, R.; De Clercq, E.; Balzarini, J. Synthesis and biological evaluation of 6-(alkyn-1-yl)furo[2,3-d]pyrimidin-2(3H)-one base and nucleoside derivatives. *J. Med. Chem.,* **2006**, *49*(1), 391-398.
[http://dx.doi.org/10.1021/jm050867d] [PMID: 16392824]

[213] Migliore, M.D.; Zonta, N.; McGuigan, C.; Henson, G.; Andrei, G.; Snoeck, R.; Balzarini, J. Synthesis and antiviral activity of the carbocyclic analogue of the highly potent and selective anti-VZV bicyclo furano pyrimidines. *J. Med. Chem.,* **2007**, *50*(26), 6485-6492.
[http://dx.doi.org/10.1021/jm070357e] [PMID: 18052321]

[214] Schinazi, R.F.; Sommadossi, J.P.; Saalmann, V.; Cannon, D.L.; Xie, M.Y.; Hart, G.C.; Smith, G.A.; Hahn, E.F. Activities of 3'-azido-3'-deoxythymidine nucleotide dimers in primary lymphocytes infected with human immunodeficiency virus type 1. *Antimicrob. Agents Chemother.,* **1990**, *34*(6), 1061-1067.
[http://dx.doi.org/10.1128/AAC.34.6.1061] [PMID: 2393266]

[215] Stuyver, L.J.; Lostia, S.; Adams, M.; Mathew, J.S.; Pai, B.S.; Grier, J.; Tharnish, P.M.; Choi, Y.; Chong, Y.; Choo, H.; Chu, C.K.; Otto, M.J.; Schinazi, R.F. Antiviral activities and cellular toxicities of modified 2',3'-dideoxy-2',3'-didehydrocytidine analogues. *Antimicrob. Agents Chemother.,* **2002**, *46*(12), 3854-3860.

[http://dx.doi.org/10.1128/AAC.46.12.3854-3860.2002] [PMID: 12435688]

[216] Kifli, N.; De Clercq, E.; Balzarini, J.; Simons, C. Novel imidazo[1,2-c]pyrimidine base-modified nucleosides: Synthesis and antiviral evaluation. *Bioorg. Med. Chem.,* **2004**, *12*(15), 4245-4252.
[http://dx.doi.org/10.1016/j.bmc.2004.05.017] [PMID: 15246100]

[217] Andrea Brancale, A.; Christopher McGuigan, C.; Berthe Algain, B.; Pascal Savy, P.; Rachid Benhida, R.; Jean-Louis Fourrey, J-L.; Graciela Andrei, G.; Robert Snoeck, R.; Erik De Clercq, E.D.; Jan Balzarini, J. Bicyclic anti-VZV nucleosides: Thieno analogues retain full antiviral activity. *Bioorg. Med. Chem. Lett.,* **2001**, *11*, 2507.
[http://dx.doi.org/10.1016/S0960-894X(01)00471-1] [PMID: 11549457]

[218] Robins, M.J.; Nowak, I.; Rajwanshi, V.K.; Miranda, K.; Cannon, J.F.; Peterson, M.A.; Andrei, G.; Snoeck, R.; De Clercq, E.; Balzarini, J.; Balzarini, J. Synthesis and antiviral evaluation of 6-(alky--heteroaryl)furo[2,3-d]pyrimidin-2(3H)-one nucleosides and analogues with ethynyl, ethenyl, and ethyl spacers at C6 of the furopyrimidine core. *J. Med. Chem.,* **2007**, *50*(16), 3897-3905.
[http://dx.doi.org/10.1021/jm070210n] [PMID: 17622128]

[219] McGuigan, C.; Barucki, H.; Blewett, S.; Carangio, A.; Erichsen, J.T.; Andrei, G.; Snoeck, R.; De Clercq, E.; Balzarini, J. Highly potent and selective inhibition of varicella-zoster virus by bicyclic furopyrimidine nucleosides bearing an aryl side chain. *J. Med. Chem.,* **2000**, *43*(26), 4993-4997.
[http://dx.doi.org/10.1021/jm000210m] [PMID: 11150169]

[220] McGuigan, C.; Bidet, O.; Derudas, M.; Andrei, G.; Snoeck, R.; Balzarini, J. Alkenyl substituted bicyclic nucleoside analogues retain nanomolar potency against Varicella Zoster Virus. *Bioorg. Med. Chem.,* **2009**, *17*(8), 3025-3027.
[http://dx.doi.org/10.1016/j.bmc.2009.03.022] [PMID: 19328697]

[221] Davies, W.L.; Grunert, R.R.; Haff, R.F.; McGahen, J.W.; Neumayer, E.M.; Paulshock, M.; Watts, J.C.; Wood, T.R.; Hermann, E.C.; Hoffmann, C.E. Antiviral activity of 1-adamantanamine (amantadine). *Science,* **1964**, *144*(3620), 862-863.
[http://dx.doi.org/10.1126/science.144.3620.862] [PMID: 14151624]

[222] Mazel, P.; La-Du, B.N.; Mandel, G.H. *Fundamentals of Drug Metabolism and Drug Disposition*; Leong Way, E. The Williams and Wilkins Co.: Baltimore, **1971**, p. 527.

[223] Sznaidman, M.L.; Meade, E.A.; Beauchamp, L.M.; Russell, S.; Tisdale, M. The antiinfluenza activity of pyrrolo[2,3-d]pyrimidines. *Bioorg. Med. Chem. Lett.,* **1996**, *6*(5), 565-568.
[http://dx.doi.org/10.1016/0960-894X(96)00070-4]

[224] Otto, M.J.; Fox, M.P.; Fancher, M.J.; Kuhrt, M.F.; Diana, G.D.; McKinlay, M.A. *In vitro* activity of WIN 51711, a new broad-spectrum antipicornavirus drug. *Antimicrob. Agents Chemother.,* **1985**, *27*(6), 883-886.
[http://dx.doi.org/10.1128/AAC.27.6.883] [PMID: 2992365]

[225] Chern, J-H.; Kak-Shan Shia, K-S.; Hsu, T-A.; Chia-Liang Tai, C-L.; Chung-Chi Lee, C-C.; Yen-Chun Lee, Y-C.; Chang, C-S.; Sung-Nien Tseng, S-N.; Shin-Ru Shih, S-R. Design, synthesis, and structure-activity relationships of pyrazolo[3,4-d]pyrimidines: A novel class of potent enterovirus inhibitors. *Bioorg. Med. Chem. Lett.,* **2004**, *14*, 2519.
[http://dx.doi.org/10.1016/j.bmcl.2004.02.092] [PMID: 15109643]

[226] Makarov, V.A.; Riabova, O.B.; Granik, V.G.; Dahse, H.M.; Stelzner, A.; Wutzler, P.; Schmidtke, M. Anti-coxsackievirus B3 activity of 2-amino-3-nitropyrazolo[1,5-a]pyrimidines and their analogs. *Bioorg. Med. Chem. Lett.,* **2005**, *15*(1), 37-39.
[http://dx.doi.org/10.1016/j.bmcl.2004.10.043] [PMID: 15582406]

[227] Pauwels, R.; Balzarini, J.; Baba, M.; Snoeck, R.; Schols, D.; Herdewijn, P.; Desmyter, J.; De Clercq, E. Rapid and automated tetrazolium-based colorimetric assay for the detection of anti-HIV compounds. *J. Virol. Methods,* **1988**, *20*(4), 309-321.
[http://dx.doi.org/10.1016/0166-0934(88)90134-6] [PMID: 2460479]

[228] Zeng, Z.S.; He, Q.Q.; Liang, Y.H.; Feng, X.Q.; Chen, F.E.; Clercq, E.D.; Balzarini, J.; Pannecouque,

C. Hybrid diarylbenzopyrimidine non-nucleoside reverse transcriptase inhibitors as promising new leads for improved anti-HIV-1 chemotherapy. *Bioorg. Med. Chem.,* **2010**, *18*(14), 5039-5047.
[http://dx.doi.org/10.1016/j.bmc.2010.05.081] [PMID: 20598556]

[229] Monto, A.S.; Iacuzio, I.A.; LaMontague, J.R. Pandemic influenza: Confronting a Re-emergent threat. *Threat. J. Infect. Dis.,* **1997**, *176*, 51.

[230] Zhu, W.; Gumina, G.; Schinazi, R.F.; Chu, C.K. Synthesis and anti-HIV activity of 1-β-3'-C-c-ano-2',3'-unsaturated nucleosides and 1-3'-C-cyano-3'-deoxyribonucleosides. *Tetrahedron,* **2003**, *59*(34), 6423-6431.
[http://dx.doi.org/10.1016/S0040-4020(03)01074-3]

[231] Sun, C.; Zhang, X.; Huang, H.; Zhou, P. Synthesis and evaluation of a new series of substituted acyl(thio)urea and thiadiazolo [2,3-a] pyrimidine derivatives as potent inhibitors of influenza virus neuraminidase. *Bioorg. Med. Chem.,* **2006**, *14*(24), 8574-8581.
[http://dx.doi.org/10.1016/j.bmc.2006.08.034] [PMID: 16979342]

[232] Mohamed, S.F.; Flefel, E.M.; Amr, A.E.G.E.; Abd El-Shafy, D.N. Anti-HSV-1 activity and mechanism of action of some new synthesized substituted pyrimidine, thiopyrimidine and thiazolopyrimidine derivatives. *Eur. J. Med. Chem.,* **2010**, *45*(4), 1494-1501.
[http://dx.doi.org/10.1016/j.ejmech.2009.12.057] [PMID: 20110135]

# CHAPTER 4

# Drugs and Phytochemicals Targeting Cancer

**Garima Tripathi**[1], **Anil Kumar Singh**[2,*] and **Abhijeet Kumar**[2,*]

*[1] Department of Chemistry, T.N. B. College, TMBU, Bhagalpur, Bihar, India*

*[2] Department of Chemistry, School of Physical Sciences, Mahatma Gandhi Central University, Motihari, Bihar-845401, India*

**Abstract:** Cancer which is basically uncontrolled cell division and, thereby, the formation of tumors, has been a prominent cause of death across the world. More than 10 million people have lost their lives due to different types of cancer such as breast, lung, prostate, gastrointestinal, *etc.* Several pathways, including metabolic, signalling, *etc.*, get altered to support uncontrolled cell division and their growth in case of cancer. Despite an increasing understanding of this disease over the period of time, still, specific causes could not be held responsible for the occurrence. Therefore, various different strategies mainly focused on preventing and killing cancerous cells have been explored. This chapter will primarily focus on the different drugs, including different types of chemotherapeutic agents such as DNA-alkylating agents like nitrogen mustard, cyclophosphamide, drug-peptide, drug-steroid conjugates, antimetabolites, antibiotics, *etc.* In addition to that, phytochemicals, which have also been investigated for their anti-cancerous activities and are under clinical trial, have also been discussed.

**Keywords:** Alkylators, Antimetabolite, Berberine, Cancer, Chemotherapeutic agent, Curcumin, Isothiocyanate, Phytochemicals, Quercetin, Resveratrol.

## 1. INTRODUCTION

Owing to mutation, some of the cells start proliferating uncontrollably, lose the ability to differentiate and may lead to the formation of tumors which could be *cancerous* or *benign*. Although the evidence suggests that the existence of cancer was there even before the existence of humans on the earth but in humans, it is as old as 3000 B.C., as some evidence has been found related to breast cancer [1]. Earlier supernatural powers and events were considered to be the real cause of cancer. But in 400 B.C., Hippocrates revealed that it occurs due to biological reasons and mainly due to the excess production of *black bile* in the body [2, 3].

* **Corresponding authors Abhijeet Kumar and Anil Kumar Singh:** Department of Chemistry, School of Physical Sciences, Mahatma Gandhi Central University, Motihari, Bihar-845401, India; E-mails: abhijeetkumar@mgcub.ac.in, anilkumarsingh@mgcub.ac.in

**Ashok Kumar Jha & Ravi S. Singh (Eds.)**

According to the American Cancer Society (ACS), cancer could be defined as *a group of diseases characterized by uncontrolled growth and spread of abnormal cells.* Abnormal function, uncontrolled rate of proliferation and tendency to invade nearby tissues are some of the important characteristics of the cancerous cells. In general, such an abnormally higher rate of proliferation leads to the formation of *tumors* that could be *benign* in nature and may remain confined to the area where it originates and does not spread to other tissues, whereas *cancerous or malignant tumors* may also invade other nearby tissues and could also spread to the other parts of the body through a process known as *metastasis* [4]. Although the term *cancer* is used to refer to a group of diseases having similar characteristics, such as uncontrolled cell division, growth and invasion of other tissues, it gets its name depending on the area of origin and the name of the organ. Importantly each type of cancer has its own characteristic features, and therefore, they vary in their behavior and responses to the treatment. Even after metastasis, it continues to maintain its properties [5].

**Table 1. The most common types of cancer and estimated new cancer cases and death as projected for the year 2022 in the United States [6].**

| Type | Estimated New Cases | Estimated Death (Approx.) |
|---|---|---|
| All sites | 1918030 | 609360 |
| Breast | 290560 | 43780 |
| Prostate | 268490 | 34500 |
| Lung and Bronchus | 236740 | 130180 |
| Colorectal | 151030 | 52580 |
| Lymphoma | 89010 | 21170 |
| Skin Melanoma | 108480 | 11990 |
| Urinary Bladder | 81180 | 17100 |
| Leukemia | 60650 | 24000 |

Carcinoma *(Skin or epithelial tissues),* Sarcoma *(supportive and connective tissue),* Myeloma *(Plasma Cell of bone marrow),* Leukemia *(Blood Cancer),* Lymphoma *(gland and lymph nodes)* are a few major categories of cancer. 80-90% of the total cases fall in the category of *carcinoma.* More than 19 million new cases and over 10 million deaths have been reported worldwide in 2020. As per the data produced in *CA: A Cancer Journal for Clinicians,* a journal published by the *American Cancer Society,* 609 360 million deaths and more than 19 million new cases have been estimated to be registered only in the United States in 2022 (Table **1**) [7]. Among the different types of cancer, lung and bronchus cancer is one of the leading types of cancer, which itself accounts for more than one lakh death each year and as per the data, it is almost equally common in both males and females. In males, lung, along with prostrate and colorectal cancer, accounts for almost 42% of all types of cancer, whereas in females, breast cancer (~26%) remained the most diagnosed type of cancer in 2020. Lung, colorectal and cervical cancer remained another prominently diagnosed cancer type in females [6].

## 2. CAUSE AND RISK FACTORS LEADING TO CANCER

Unlike various other diseases, especially pathogen caused ailments where the causative agent is known, in the case of cancer, there is no such single reason or therapeutic target which could be held responsible for the occurrence of cancer. In fact, it is the result of a diverse range of factors, including environmental, hormonal, occupational, pharmaceutical, dietary, *etc.*, which could contribute to this disease [8]. Although smoking and the use of tobacco-based products are a well-established reason that contributes to a wide range of cancers almost at all sites of the body, various other lesser known facts are there which may contribute to cancer [9, 10]. Any agents which are capable of causing cancer are termed *carcinogens* and these could be chemical, physical or biological in nature. Exposure time, amount of exposure and genetic background of a person are some of the key factors which determine the occurrence of cancer. Some of the examples have been discussed below.

### 2.1. Chemical Carcinogens

Several chemicals which could be of natural origin or could be synthesized have been found to exhibit carcinogenic effects. For example, Aflatoxin $B_1$ (Fig. **1**), which is an example of aflatoxin produced by fungi *such as Aspergillus flavus*, has been found to be carcinogenic in nature and may cause liver cancer [11, 12]. Similarly, other polyaromatic hydrocarbons (PAH), such as benzo[$\alpha$] pyrene, benzo [$\alpha$] anthracene, *etc.*, are well-known examples of carcinogens. Similarly, other organic compounds, such as 4-(4-aminophenyl) aniline and *N*-nitrosodimethylamine (NDMA), also exhibit carcinogenicity. In addition to that, several organic solvents, such as benzene, toluene, carbon tetrachloride, *etc.*, also display a carcinogenic effect [13]. Apart from the well-documented organic compounds, various inorganic compounds, such as $Ni(CO)_4$, and heavy metals, such as arsenic (As) and cadmium (Cd), are a few important examples of inorganic carcinogens [14]. In particular, Arsenic contamination in drinking water has been considered a major cause of cancer in the Indo – Gangetic region of Bihar in India.

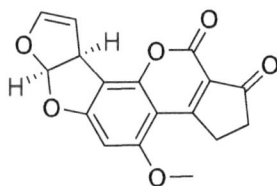

Aflatoxin $B_1$

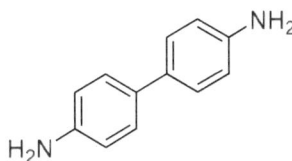

4-(4-aminophenyl)aniline

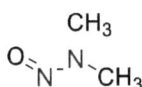

N-Nitrosodimethylamine
(NDMA)

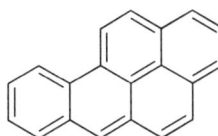

Benzo[a]pyrene

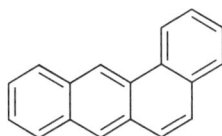

benzo[a]anthracene

**Fig. (1).** Representative examples of organic compounds as carcinogens.

## 2.2. Physical Carcinogens

In addition to chemicals, various other factors are known which induce cancer. For example, electromagnetic radiations of high energy, such as UV-rays, γ-rays, X-rays, *etc.*, are known to damage DNA which may lead to cancer [15]. Apart from the radiations, different types of materials, which are fibrous or non-fibrous, as well as gel in nature, have also been considered carcinogens. For example, various metals and their alloys, different types of polymers, *etc.*, have also shown carcinogenicity.

## 2.3. Biological Carcinogens

It has also been found that some of the viral infections could also lead to different types of cancer. For example, infection due to *Epstein-Barr Virus* (EBV) may cause mutations in human B cells which may lead to different types of cancer such as Burkett's lymphoma, and Hodgkin's disease. Similarly, different *Human papilloma viruses* (HPV), mainly high risk viruses, such as HPV 16 and HPV 18, are known to cause different types of cancer, such as cervical, oropharyngeal, anal, vaginal cancers, *etc.* [16]. Similarly, *human herpes virus 8* (HHV-8) is considered as a causative agent of Kaposi Sarcoma which is a type of skin related cancer. Likewise, *Hepatitis Band C* (HBV and HCV) viruses are known to cause hepatocellular carcinoma (HCC) [17]. In addition to aforementioned carcinogens, various reports are available in the literature which indicates that long term use of the drugs such as ranitidine, losartan, valsartans, *etc.*, may cause cancer probably due to the presence of *N*-Nitrosodimethylamine (NDMA), which is a known carcinogen [18, 19]. Various other factors such as obesity, lack of physical exercises, use of food material cooked at high temperature are also some of the causes which are known to contribute to cancer.

## 3. DIFFERENT APPROACHES TOWARDS THE TREATMENT OF CANCER

Unlike various other diseases, in particular, pathogenic diseases where targets are known, in the case of cancer, there is not a single target as this disease involves several important deviations from the normal cellular behaviors such as genetic aberration, ability to proliferate uncontrollably, dysregulation in various metabolic pathways, avoiding apoptosis, *etc.*

Therefore, in order to curb the progression of tumorigenesis and control the disease, various different therapeutic approaches have been developed (Fig. **2**). This chapter will mainly focus on the treatment using small molecules, *i.e.*, *chemotherapy* as well as also on the phytochemicals which have also exhibited potential anti-cancerous properties.

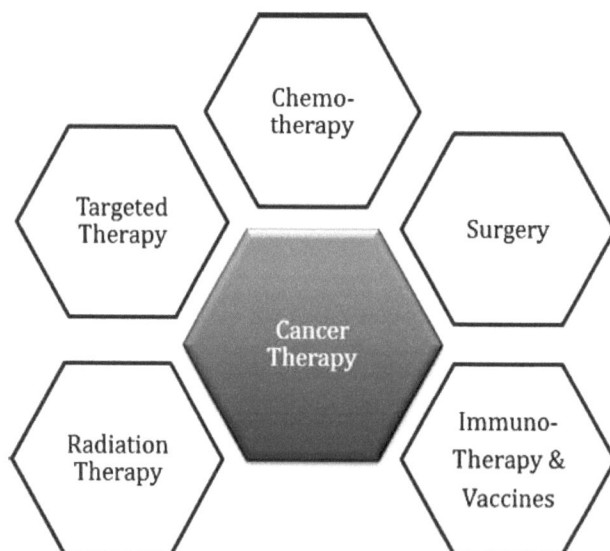

**Fig. (2).** Different Approaches for Cancer Treatment.

## 3.1. Radiation Therapy

In ancient times, the treatment of cancer was mostly based on having a proper balanced diet, and use of the plant extract, such as extract of poppy (*Papaversomniferum*), *etc.* The discovery of X-rays in 1896 by Wilhelm Conrad Röntgen and later their application for the treatment of breast cancer by Emil H. Grubbé in the same year opened up the path of radiotherapy for the treatment of this disease. Later on, in 1899, Marie and Pierre Curie also demonstrated the application of X-Ray for the treatment of tumors. However, modern radiation therapy is considered to begin only in 1920 when Claudius Regaud applied radiation in different fractions instead of continuous ones to minimize the side effect on the healthy cell. Radiation therapy involves the use of high energy electromagnetic waves such as X-rays and ϒ-rays, *etc.*, which lead to the death of cancerous cells due to the damage to their DNA. The mode and types of it, such as external, internal and systematic radiation, could vary with the type site [20, 21].

## 3.2. Chemotherapy and Different Types of ChemotherapeuticAgents

It is basically the treatment of tumor cells using chemicals which are generally organic compounds of natural or synthetic origin. A vast number of organic compounds extracted from the plants, such as paclitaxel (Taxol), Irinotecan, *etc.*, are a few drugs which have been isolated from the plant and used as anti-cancerous drugs [22]. In addition to that, a large number of compounds have been synthesized and their anti-cancerous effect, as well as their role as anti-cancerous drugs, has been explored. As per the data available, till 01 February 2022, 284 drugs have received a license from different agencies such as FDA, EMA, *etc.* Out of that, 257 have got approved by FDA [23]. Fig. (**3**) shows examples of some of the best-selling organic compounds which are being used for chemotherapy.

Different types of organic compounds have been explored for the treatment of different types of cancer. Mainly these could be classified into three major categories, including alkylating agents, antimetabolites, and antibiotics. In addition to that, targeted therapy is another modern approach towards the treatment of cancer. In the following sections, each of them will be discussed separately.

### 3.2.1. Nitrogen Mustards Alkylators

Alkylating agents are compounds which directly interact with DNA and damage it by alkylating the nitrogenous base of DNA that leads to the formation of inter strand cross-link (ICL) between both strands of DNA (Fig. **4**) [24 - 26].

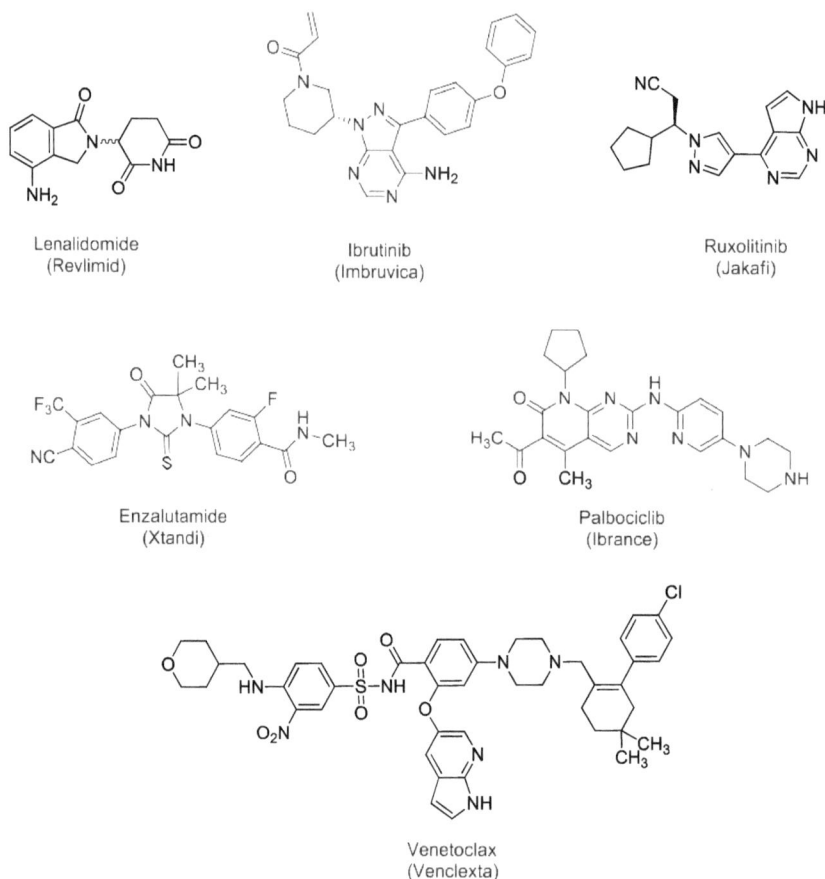

**Fig. (3).** Examples of Top Selling Drugs for Cancer Treatment.

Thereafter other important processes, such as DNA replication, transcription, *etc.* get hampered, and finally, it leads to cell death [27]. The clue of the potential application of a chemical in the treatment of cancer got revealed accidentally during World War II when a large number of people who got exposed to mustard gas could not survive due to the toxic effect on bone marrow cells leading to the drastic reduction in the number of white blood cells. Later on in 1942, the efficacies of Mechlorethamine (Fig. **5**), the first Nitrogen mustard were demonstrated for the treatment of different types of lymphomas by Alfred Gilman and Louis Goodman from Yale University [26]. In 1949, Mechlorethamine hydrochloride got approval from US FDA, and was the first nitrogen mustard which exhibited its anti-cancerous potential by alkylating one of the nitrogen (N7) of guanine base present in DNA and thereby inhibiting the process of DNA replication which is essential for further growth. It exhibited its efficacy against different types of lymphoid malignancies. Mechlorethamine gel (Valchlor) has also been approved by US FDA for the treatment of mycosis fungoides which is a type of cutaneous T-cell lymphoma [28]. Although the instability of this drug in a water medium poses a problem for its oral use as it reacts with water and loses its active form. Therefore, it is administered intravenously. Some of the prominent side effect associated with this drug includes vomiting, nausea, fatigue, *etc.* [29].

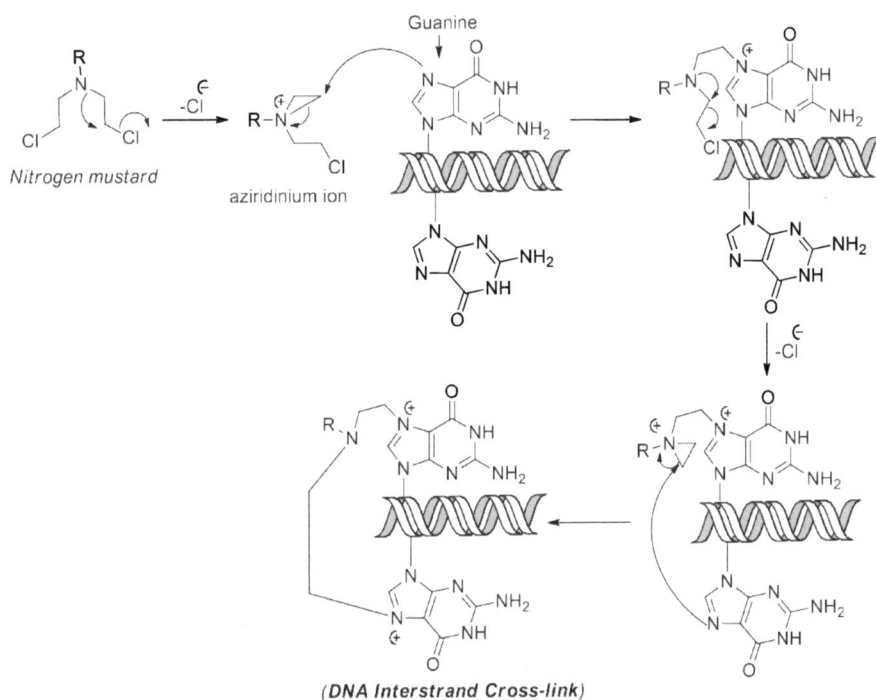

**Fig. (4).** Mechanism of alkylation of DNA and formation of inter-strand cross-link.

In order to enhance the bioavailability and decrease the reactivity of Mechlorethamine, various other nitrogen mustard alkylators were developed by replacing the methyl group attached to $N$ with different aromatic and hetero aromatic groups, which is considered to decrease the electron density of Nitrogen and consequently minimizes the chances of formation of aziridinium ring that is how nitrogen replaces chlorine. This led to the development *of second generation nitrogen mustard* as an alkylator [24]. *Chlorambucil, melphalan, bendamustine* (Fig. **5**) are some of the commercially available examples of this category. Due to relatively less reactive nature of these alternatives compared to mechlorethamine, these could also be administered orally. Chlorambucil which is *4-(4-(bis- (2-chloroethyl)amino)phenyl)butanoicacid* and a lesser toxic alternative of mechlorethamine received approval from USFDA in 1957 for the treatment of

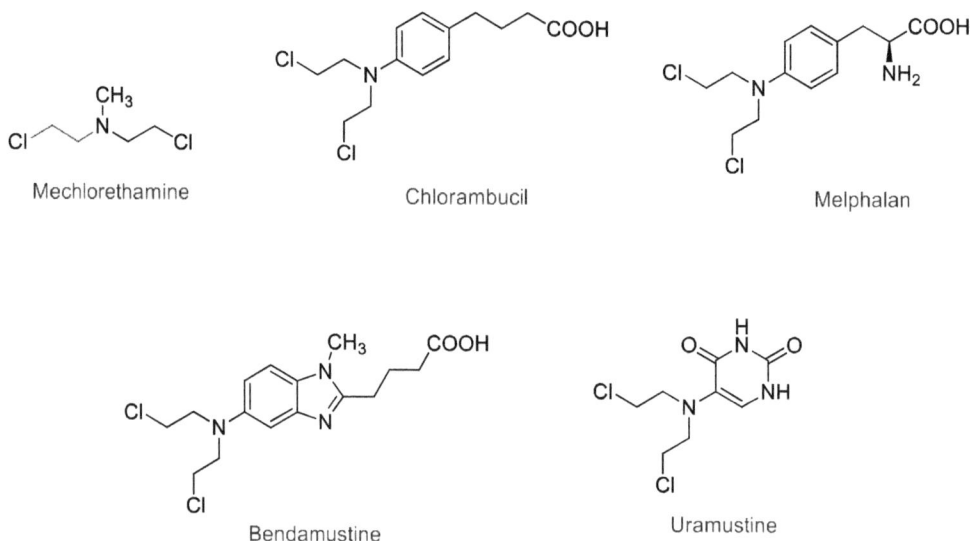

**Fig. (5).** Representative examples of Nitrogen mustard as alkylating agents.

different types of cancer, such as malignant lymphoma, lymphosarcoma, Hodgkin's disease *etc.* [30]. Similarly, another nitrogen mustard known as Melphalan (2-amino-3-[4-(bis[2-chloroethyl]amino)phenyl]propanoic acid) got approval from FDA in 1964 [31]. Similar to other alkylators, it also acts by forming inter-strand cross linking between the different strands of DNA and there by hampers the further growth of cells. It has displayed efficacy against a vast range of cancer such as breast cancer, multiple myelomaetc. Another example of nitrogen mustard is Bendamustine (4-[5-[bis(2-chloroethyl) amino]-1-methylbenzimidazol-2-yl] butanoicacid) which was synthesized in 1963 but received approval from US FDA in 2008 [32]. It is used for the treatment of multiple myeloma and indolent B-cellnon-Hodgkin lymphoma, chronic lymphocytic leukemia, *etc.* The presence of benzimidazole moiety in bendamustine makes it safer compared to other nitrogen mustard. In addition to that, metabolites formed after the hydrolysis has also shown lower cytotoxicity. Apart from the useful effect, some adverse effects, such as genotoxic and neurotoxic effects, have also been reported from some of the patients. Likewise, nitrogen mustard with a uracil moiety called uramustine or uracil mustard has also been developed for the treatment of different types of leukemia, such as chronic myelogenous leukemia and also for different types of lymphoma [33]. In addition to that, it has also been used for the treatment of breast and ovarian cancer. The activity of this drug is considered to be through the formation of ethylenimmonium ion.

### 3.2.2. Phosphoramide Mustard

In order to minimize the adverse effect of nitrogen mustard, a non-toxic pro-drug was developed in the form of phosphoramide mustards containing oxazaphosphorine rings which convert into their active and cytotoxic form under the enzymatic actions inside the cell. Similar to nitrogen mustard, this class of drug also exhibited their cytotoxic effect through the alkylation of N7 present on guanine in the two different strands of DNA that leads to the formation of inter as well as intra-strand cross link that finally leads to the cell death [34].

*Cyclophosphamide* Fig. (**6**) is an example of such phosphoramide mustard, which was synthesized for the first time in 1958 and got FDA approval in 1959 for the treatment of various types of cancer such as malignant lymphomas, multiplemyeloma, breast cancer, *etc.* [34]. This drug was initially developed with the assumption that the drug will easily release nitrogen mustard by the phosphamidase catalysed cleavage of the P-N bond of the oxazaphosphorine ring [26]. It has been observed that in some cancer cells, the concentration of phosphamidase is higher therefore, cyclophosphamide could be a suitable drug in such cases. But later, it was realised that cyclophosphamide itself is a pro-drug which lies in an inactive form and directly does not display its anti-cancerous effect on cancer cells; it requires some sort of activation which mainly could be enzymatic to be converted into its active form to exert its anti-cancerous effect. The metabolic pathway (Fig. **7**) for the conversion of cyclophosphamide to its active form begins with the *cytochrome P-450* catalysed hydroxylation of the cyclophosphphosphamide which leads to the formation of 4-hydroxy cyclophosphamide. This cyclichydroxy-metabolite along with its tautomer *aldophosphamide* remains in equilibrium which is the open chain tautomer of 4-hydroxyphosphamide that easily diffuses inside the cell but does not display cytotoxicity. Aldophosphamide converts into the actual active form of phosphoramide mustard with the elimination of acrolein, through the β-elimination process. In the case of some hematopoietic stem cells (HSC), *aldophosphamide* could also be oxidized into *carboxyphosphamide*, an inactive metabolite, under the enzymatic action of aldehyde dehydrogenase as these cells contain a higher concentration of this enzyme [34].

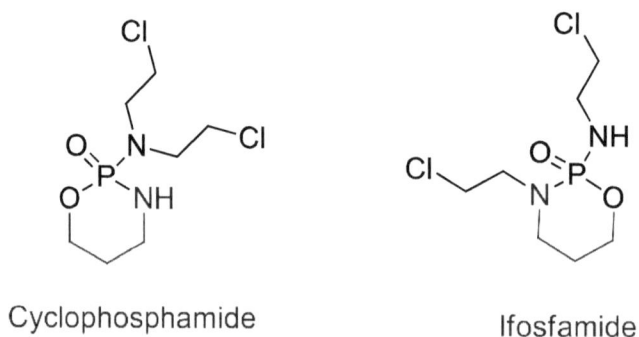

Cyclophosphamide                                    Ifosfamide

**Fig. (6).**  Representative examples of phosphoramide mustard.

Similar to cyclophosphamide, *ifosfamide* Ifex, Fig. (**6**) is another example of oxazaphosphorine rings containing mustard. Like cyclophosphamide gets metabolized to 4-hydroxy ifosfamide under the enzymatic action of different iso forms of cytochrome 450 enzymes, enzymes such as CYP3A4 and CYP2B6 also get hydroxylated to produce 4-hydroxyifosfamide. It further gets converted into 4-ketoifosfamide, which does not exhibit cytotoxic properties. Similar to cyclophosphamide, non-enzymatic $\beta$-elimination leads to the elimination of acrolein and the formation of an active component with a cytotoxic effect.

### 3.2.3. Drug-Conjugates as Alkylator

In addition to aforementioned nitrogen mustard, various drug conjugates have also been explored for their application in the treatment of cancer. For example, melphalanflufenamide (melflufen/pepaxto) Fig. (**8**) is an example of such a drug which is a dipeptide of meplhalan which itself is an example of second-generation nitrogen mustard and (*S*)-ethyl2-amino-3-(4-fluorophenyl) propanoate is an example of peptide-drug conjugate [35]. This peptide-drug conjugate helps in enhancing the lipophilicity of the actual drug and consequently enhances the concentration of the actual alkylator inside the cell, where it cleaves into the drug under the action of peptidases. In general, the concentration of peptidase enzyme is higher in tumor cells. Due to enhanced lipophilicity and, thereby, increased concentration of alkylator inside the cell, this conjugate exhibits almost 50 times higher potency in myeloma cells and leads to rapid damaging of DNA [36].

Melflufen, in combination with dexamethasone, received accelerated approval from the FDA for the treatment of a patient with *relapsed multiple myeloma* in February 2021 but later, in October 2021, the oncopeptide company decided to withdraw the drug from the U.S. market [37]. Likewise, estramustine phosphate (Fig. **8**) is a conjugate of estradiol which is basically a sex hormone and mechlorethamine which is connected through carbamate linkage. The attachment of estradiol to the alkylator leads to the higher uptake of the drug inside the hormone sensitive cell such as prostate cancer cells, and therefore, it is used for the palliative treatment of prostate cancer, which is in the metastatic stage [38].

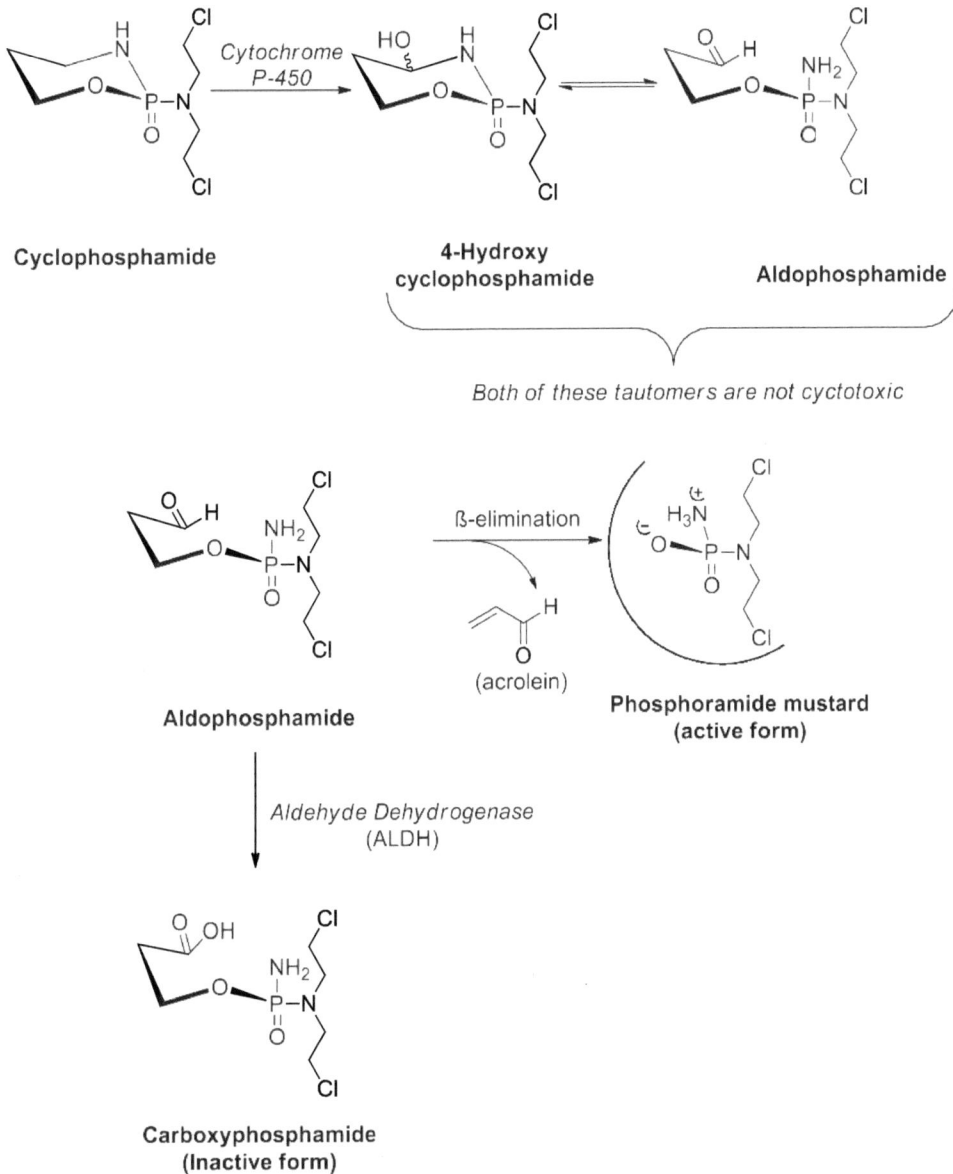

**Fig. (7).** Metabolic pathways for the transformation of cyclophosphamide to the active and cytotoxic form.

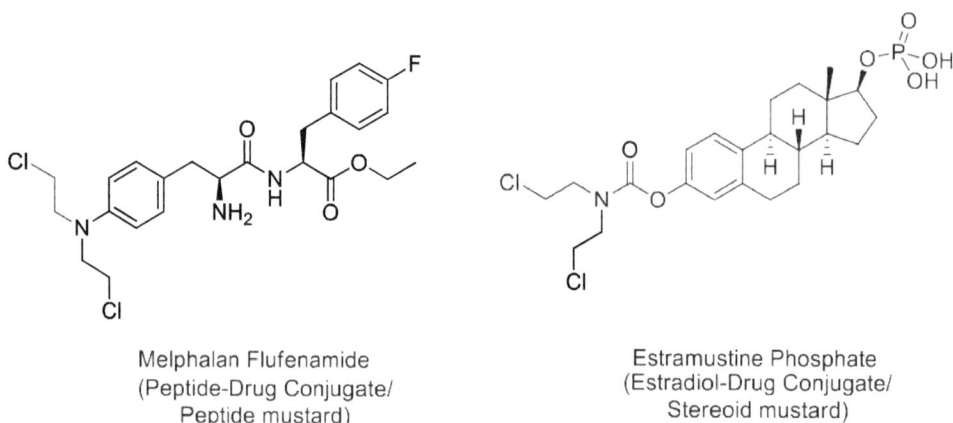

Melphalan Flufenamide
(Peptide-Drug Conjugate/
Peptide mustard)

Estramustine Phosphate
(Estradiol-Drug Conjugate/
Stereoid mustard)

**Fig. (8).** Drug-Conjugates as anti-cancerous agents.

## 3.2.4. Antimetabolites

In addition to above-discussed alkylators, various other chemotherapeutic agents have also been explored for the treatment of different types of cancer. Antimetabolites could be defined as drugs having structural similarity with essential metabolites, which are required for the proper growth of the cell, but unlike these metabolites, they interfere with the desired metabolic processes and thereby obstruct the growth of cancer cells [39]. Due to the structural resemblance, these antimetabolites also participate in the enzymatic pathway similar to their natural analogues and block the pathway, which leads to hampering the production of desired metabolites such as purine, pyrimidines, *etc.* For example, folic acid is an important dietary supplement required for the synthesis of nucleic acid and amino acids, and thereby functions as a nutrient for the fast-growing cells. Therefore, in order to restrict cellular division and growth, several anti-folates have been developed, and their anti-cancerous effect has also been studied. For example, *aminopterin* and *methotrexate (amethopterin)* Fig. (**9**) are examples of drugs which are also known as anti-folates as these resemble structurally with folic acids but exhibit antagonistic effects, therefore, these are also known as *folic acid-antagonist* [40]. The medicinal importance of aminopterin was realized in 1948 when Farber et al. reported the remission of leukaemia by using *aminopterin* [41]. Later on, several antimetabolites have been developed and their applications in the treatment of different diseases have also been demonstrated.

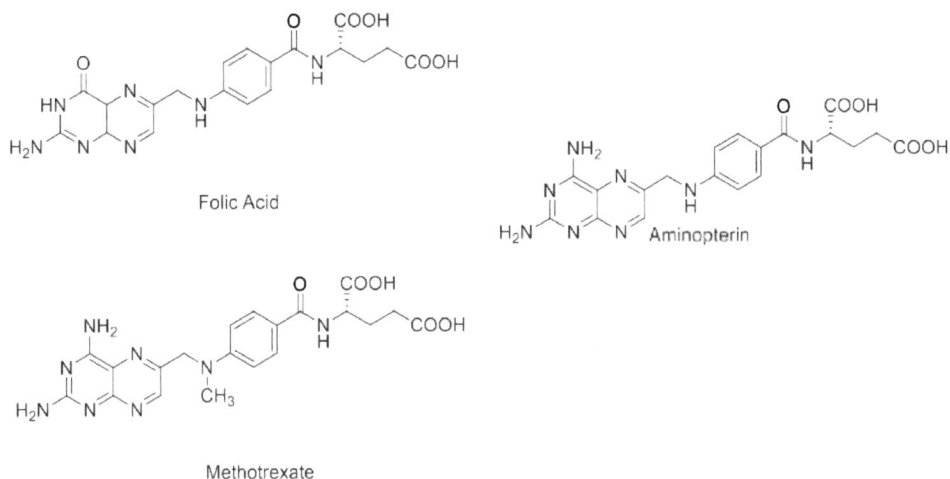

**Fig. (9).** Folic acid antagonist as a chemotherapeutic agent.

*Methotraxate* (MTX) Fig. (**10**) is another example of anti-folate, which is basically used to treat different forms of arthritis [42]. Methotrexatemono glutamate converts into its polyglutmate form, which forms under folylpolyglutamate synthase (FPGS) catalyzed transformation.

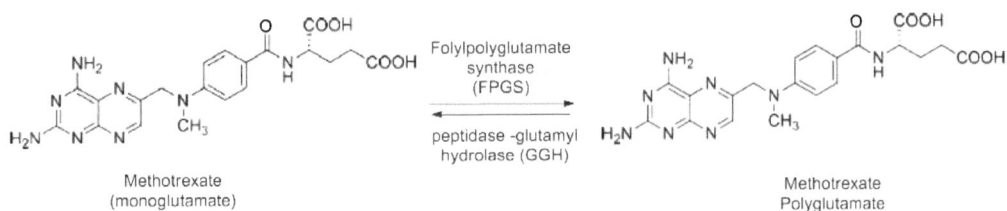

**Fig. (10).** Enzymatic conversion of methotrexate mono glutamate to polyglutamate.

Methotraxatepolyglutamate is considered to be the active form of drug that inhibits the enzymatic activities of various enzymes such as *5-aminoimidazole-4-carboxamideribonucleotide(AICAR) transformylase (ATIC), dihydrofolate reductase (DHFR), thymidylate synthase (TYMS) methylenetetrahydrofolate reductase(MTHFR), etc.*, involved in the biosynthesis of nucleo bases such as purine and pyrimidine which are essential substrate in the synthesis of nucleic acids. In particular, the binding of methotrexate with *dihydrofolate reductase (DHFR)* enzyme causes an inhibitory effect on the production of purine and other important metabolites required for cell division and growth that finally promotes apoptosis. Methotrexate has been found to be efficient in limiting the growth of different types of tumors. Similarly, various purine derivatives such as 6-mercaptopurine (6-MP), 6-thioguanine (6-TG) and pyrimidine derivatives such as 5-fluorouracil (5-FU), capecitabine, and gemcitabine have also displayed remarkable anti-cancerous effects [43]. Due to the structural similarity with natural nucleo bases, these drugs compete with them and inhibit various enzymatic reactions required for the synthesis of DNA and RNA. In particular, 6-MP (Fig. **11**) has been found to be efficient for the treatment of different types of leukemia such as *acute lymphocytic leukemia (ALL) and acute myeloid leukemia (AML)*. Likewise, 5-FU Fig. (**11**) displayed favorable effects in the case of colorectal cancer. Under the enzymatic action of thymidine phosphorylase, Capecitabine converts into its active and cytotoxic form, fluorouracil, which further converts into other active metabolites such as *5-fluoro-2-deoxyuridine monophosphate (FdUMP)* and *5-fluorouridine triphosphate (FUTP)*. These two metabolites, FdUMP and FUTP, inhibit the synthesis of DNA and RNA, respectively.

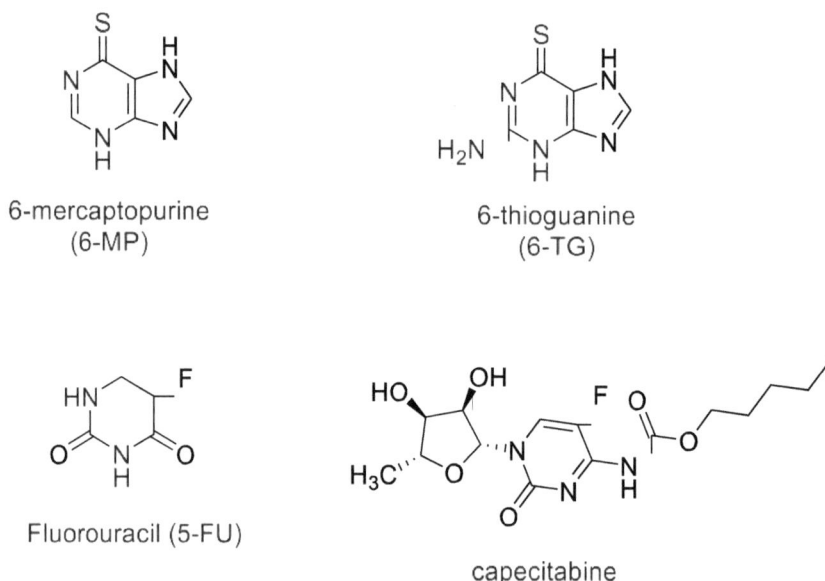

6-mercaptopurine
(6-MP)

6-thioguanine
(6-TG)

Fluorouracil (5-FU)

capecitabine

**Fig. (11).** Examples of purine and pyrimidine based anti-metabolites.

### 3.2.5. Antibiotics as Chemotherapeutic Agents

In addition to that, various antibiotics have also been investigated for their cytotoxic effect and for the treatment of cancer. Like earlier mentioned drugs, they also target DNA synthesis. *Puromycin* was the first antibiotic that was used as an anti-tumor agent [44, 45]. But due to higher toxicity and non-selectivity, it was not used later. Later, antibiotics belonging to anthracyclines such as daunorubicin and doxorubicin Fig. (**12**) have displayed promising efficacy against different types of cancer, and currently, these are being prescribed as chemotherapy drugs which are also similar to other drug targets of DNA, and other enzymes, such as topoisomerase II, are required for the relaxing of DNA which consequently prevents the further process of replication and transcription [44, 46].

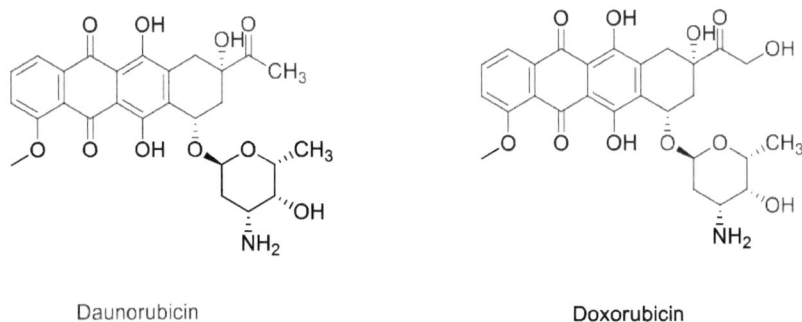

Daunorubicin                                Doxorubicin

**Fig. (12).** Examples of anthracyclines antibiotics as chemotherapeutic agents.

Similarly, bleomycin is another example of antibiotic which has been used as a chemotherapy drug for the treatment of different types of cancer, including lymphoma, cervical and various other cancers.

## 3.3. Metal Salts as a Chemotherapeutic Agent

In addition to organic compounds, various inorganic complexes, mainly the complexes of Pt such as cisplatin, carboplatin, oxaplatin (Fig. **13**), have also been used as chemotherapeutic agents in the treatment of different types of cancer. Similar to most other chemotherapeutic agents, cisplatin also targets DNA and forms intra-strand DNA adduct and thereby activates various signal transduction pathways, and finally, it results in apoptosis [47].

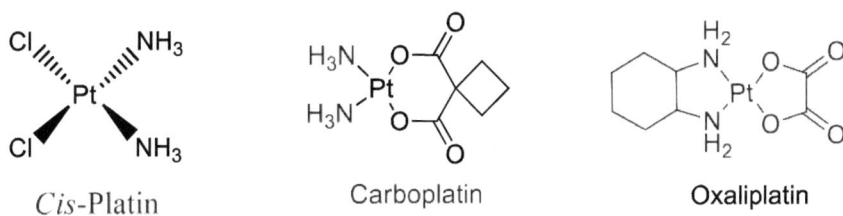

*Cis*-Platin                    Carboplatin                    Oxaliplatin

**Fig. (13).** Representative examples of Metal-complexes as chemotherapeutic agents.

## 4. PHYTOCHEMICALS AND THEIR ROLE IN THE REGULATION OF CANCER METABOLISM

The currently available option for cancer treatment is the removal of accumulated biomass of cancer cells by surgery and radiation therapy followed by systemic chemotherapeutic treatment. The typical chemotherapeutic treatment includes DNA interactive agents like, *cis*-platin and doxorubicin, antimetabolites such as methotrexate, anti-tubulin agents (taxanes) and other molecular targeting agents [48]. All these chemotherapeutic agents have several drawbacks, including, recurrence of cancer, drug resistance and immense side effects on non-targeted tissues, which harshly affect the patient's quality of life. To overcome these disadvantages, there is always a need for the discovery of promising anti-cancer drug candidates which are more compatible with the human body with less side effects.

Phytochemicals and their derivatives are promising agents for the treatment of cancer with increased efficacy and decreased adverse effects on the health of the patient. The active ingredients of phytochemicals are naturally occurring and can be isolated with the aid of modern separation processes and are well characterized by advanced spectroscopic techniques. Furthermore, these phytochemicals are tested *in-vitro* and *in-vivo* for assessment of their anticancer potentials. A number of phytochemicals have significant anti-cancer properties. It is estimated that approximately, 50% of the total anticancer drugs used from 1940 to 2014 are either plant derived products or originated from natural products [49]. Phytochemicals may possess complementary or overlapped mechanisms which reduce the effect of carcinogens, including free radical scavenging [50], suppression of proliferative cancerous cells [51], and reducing invasiveness or angiogenesis in tumor cells [52].

A large number of phytochemicals have been evaluated for their anticancer properties in preclinical and clinical trials. The major aspects which are being evaluated for phytochemicals as efficient anticancer drug candidates include, the improvement of *in vitro* and *in vivo* response of cancer cell lines towards standard chemo- and radiotherapy, minimizing the adverse side effects, and undesirable interaction of phytochemicals with standard chemotherapy. Several preclinical studies advocate the effectiveness of various phytochemicals such as curcumin, resveratrol, lycopene, quercetin, sulforaphane, green tea, catechins, including EGCG, berberines, *etc.* (Fig. **14**). Some of them are briefly described below:

### 4.1. Curcumin

Curcumin belongs to the class polyphenols (diferuloylmethane, *bis-α, β*-unsaturated β-diketone) isolated from the rhizome of Curcuma Longa (Fig. **14**).

Curcuma Longa belongs to the family *Zingiberaceae* and commonly known as *turmeric*. It is a herb cultivated in Southern Asiatic regions like India and China as a major ingredient of spices. The yellow pigmented part of turmeric contains curcuminoids: curcumin I (the main component), demethoxy curcumin (curcumin II), bisdemethoxycurcumin (curcumin III) and cyclocurcumin (Fig. **15**).

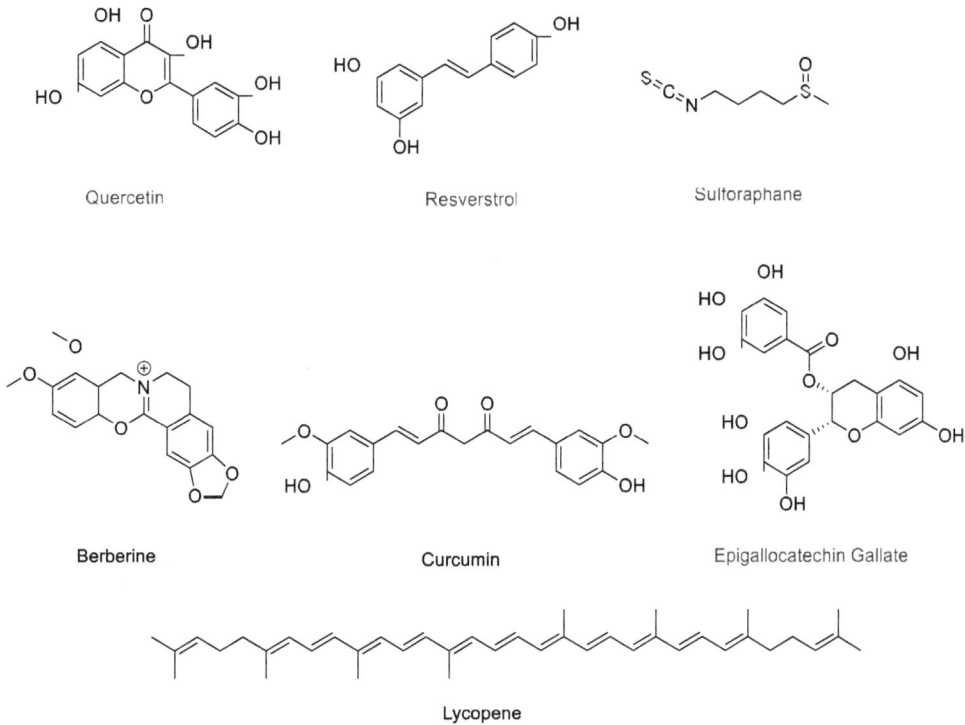

**Fig. (14).** Structures of some phytochemicals in clinical trials [53].

Curcuminoids have a similar structure and constitute 3-5% of the total mass of turmeric powder. Natural curcuminoids have several therapeutic potentials, such as anticancer, antimicrobial, thrombo-suppressive, hypoglycemic, anti-inflammatory, antiarthritic, hepatoprotective, *etc.* [54, 55]. Several studies have revealed that curcumin and its congeners can prevent proliferation and induce apoptosis in cancer cells of different tissues, such as prostate, epidermis, B and T cells, colon, breast, head and neck squamous cell carcinoma, by arresting the cell progression in the $G_2$/M phase of the cell cycle.

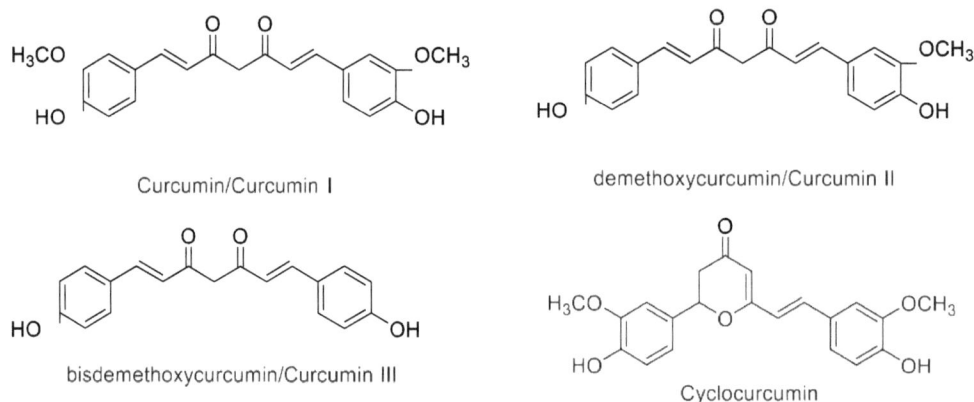

Curcumin/Curcumin I

demethoxycurcumin/Curcumin II

bisdemethoxycurcumin/Curcumin III

Cyclocurcumin

**Fig. (15).** Structure of various curcuminoids.

Curcumin exhibits several modes of action which prevent cancer cell proliferation, including the Warburg effect, apoptosis induction and *via* ROS metabolic pathway. It is well known that cancer cells have different metabolic routes than normal cells. They opt glycolysis pathway rather than oxidative phosphorylation, even in an abundance of oxygen which produces a large quantity of lactate. It is called the Warburg effect. Pyruvate kinase M2 (PKM2) plays a key role in the Warburg effect, and any dysregulation in PKM2 may lead to metabolic disturbance in cancer cells [56, 57]. Siddiqui and co-workers in their studies reported that the treatment of a variety of cancer cell lines with curcumin down-regulates the expression of PKM2 *via* inhibition of the mTOR-HIF1α axis which resulted in the inhibition of glucose uptake and lactate production [58]. They also showed that the overexpression of PKM2 suppresses the effects of curcumin, which is a conclusive evidence for PKM2-mediated inhibition of the Warburg effect by curcumin.

Curcumin induces apoptosis in cancerous cells. The studies on different cancer cell lines reported by Adams and co-workers revealed that curcumin, like EF24 (Fig. **16**), induces the cell cycle arrest in the G2/M phase followed by apoptosis by means of dox-dependent mechanism [59]. They also showed that EF24 induces apoptosis by means of mitochondrial dysfunction, by reaction with glutathione (GSH) and thioredoxin 1, which further leads to the reduction of both intra cellular and oxidized GSH levels in the wild-type and Bcl-xL over expressing HT-29 human colon cancer cells. He and co-workers demonstrated that EF24 induces apoptosis by enhanced accumulation of ROS in both HCT-116 and SW-620 cells which further decreases the mitochondrial membrane potential that results in the release of mitochondrial cytochrome c [60].

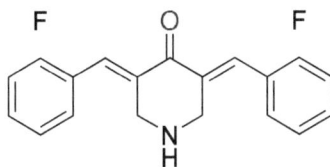

**Fig. (16).** Structure of EF24, a curcumin derivative.

Larasati *et al.* studiedthe anti-cancer effects of curcumin on CML-derived leukemic cells in a xenograft mouse model [61]. They reported that curcumin increases the ROS levels over the threshold by inhibition of ROS metabolic enzymes such as carbonyl reductase, glutathione-S-transferase, glyoxalase, *etc.* and hence modulates the Glutathione (GSH) level. Furthermore, ROS plays a crucial role in curcumin induced DNA damage, apoptosis and cell death. Kocyigit and Guler investigated the effect of curcumin on mouse melanoma cancer cells (B16-F10) and fibroblastic normal cells (L-929). Their results concluded that curcumin reduces mitochondrial membrane potential (MMP) and induces DNA damage, apoptosis and ROS levels in mouse melanoma cancer cells [62].

## 4.2. Resveratrol

Resveratrol ((E)-5-(4-hydroxystyryl)benzene-1,3-diol) (Fig. **14**) is a phytoalex which displays a broad range of pharmacological activities, mainly found in red grapes and red wines. It is known to show beneficial medicinal effects, especially in the case of cancer, diabetes, cardiovascular diseases, *etc.* Many kinds of literature advocate the role of resveratrol on cancer cell metabolism. Resveratrol is known to alter the lipid metabolism in cancer cells and hence affect energy storage. It induces cancer cell apoptosis *via* downregulation of the PI3K/AKT/mTOR pathway. Resveratrol decreases tumor volume and invasiveness *via* reducing serum TAG, VLDL, and LDL levels in cancer patients [63]. Resveratrol is found to dysregulate glucose metabolism in human ovarian cancer cell by reducing the glucose uptake and the production of lactate *via* downregulation of the PI3K/AKT/mTOR pathway. Resveratrol is also known to inhibit the activity of 6-phosphofructo-1-kinase (PFK) in human breast cancer cell MCF-7 which results in decreased glucose consumption and hence less ATP production which leads to cancer cell death and inhibits proliferation [64, 65]. In lung cancer cells, resveratrol dysregulates glucose metabolism by inhibition of HK2, which is mediated by the Akt signaling pathway and ultimately induces apoptosis. Also, resveratrol results in the reduction of glycolytic flux and Glut1 expression *via* ROS mediated HIF-1α induction in lung cancer cell bearing mice [65].

## 4.3. Berberine

Berberine is a protozoan morphinane alkaloid, which is slowly soluble in water and extracted from Berberidaceae, Papaveraceae, and Rutaceaeplant [66]. Berberine has displayed a wide range of biological activity such as anti-inflammation, anti-diabetic, anti-oxidative, anti-tumor, *etc.* [66 - 69]. Berberine showed anti-tumor activity and hence prevented the proliferation of cancer cells *via* different mechanisms [70 - 72].

Various literatures showed that berberines and their derivatives affect the progression of the cell cycle *via* cell cycle arrest at the G1, G0/G1 and G2/M phases [73, 74]. For instance, treatment of T47D and MCF-7 cell lines with berberine results in G2/M and G0/G1 phase arrest, respectively and hence inhibits the cell cycle progression [75]. Berberines are also found to affect the p53 protein, which is a key tumor suppression gene and play a leading role in the process of apoptosis in cancer cells. Some recent studies revealed that berberine up-regulates the expression of p53 *via* inhibition of MDM2 at the post-transcription level [76 - 78]. Berberine also affects tumor proliferation through altering the apoptosis process. Apoptosis is a programmed cell death strictly controlled by a series of genes and proteins, including Bcl-2 and caspase family. Berberine may down-regulate the expression of XIAP, which inhibits the X-linked apoptotic protein, and may induce the apoptosis in leucocyte depleted p53 gene at post transcriptional level [79]. Furthermore, berberine is also found to induce reactive oxygen species (ROS) mediated apoptosis in certain breast cancer cells like MCF-7 and MDA-MBA-231. Several reports advocate the anti-cancer effect of berberine in the human hepatocellular carcinoma (HCC) cell line through the induction of apoptosis. Berberine triggers mitochondrial apoptosis in HCC cells by inducing Bax expression, the formation of permeable transition pores, and cytochrome C release to cytosol, followed by the activation of caspase 3- and 9-signaling pathways [80]. Berberine downregulates the expression of HNF4 alpha and Exo-70, which results in cell cycle arrest in HCC [81]. So there are several evidences that berberine and its analogues possess anti-cancer properties with different targets of action.

More interestingly, berberine and its derivatives have been evaluated *in vivo* and in clinical trials for their anti-tumor properties [53].

## 4.4. Quercetin

Quercetin (Fig. **14**) is a naturally occurring polyphenolic flavonoid with chemical formula 3,3′,4′,5,7-pentahydroxyflavone ($C_{15}H_{10}O_7$), commonly found in different fruits and vegetables like apples, onions, several berries such as cranberries, and lingonberries. The most important properties of quercetin are antioxidants, which display biological activity against various cancers, allergies, viral infections and inflammation [82]. Quercetin exhibits anti-tumor properties with no adverse side effects on the human body. Several *in vitro* and *in vivo* studies have been documented, which showed that quercetin scaffold is well suited against various cancer cell lines such as lung, liver, prostate, colon, breast cancer lines, *etc.* The anti-cancer activity is exerted *via* different mechanisms and modes of action that involve different signaling processes and inhibition of enzymes that are responsible for the activation of carcinogens. It is evident that quercetin binds to various cellular receptors and proteins to inhibit the invasiveness of cancer cells [83, 84].

Quercetin is found to trigger apoptosis and inhibit cell cycle progression in breast cancer cell lines. MCF-7 and MDA-MB-231 cancer cells when treated with quercetin result in G1 phase arrest followed by apoptosis and suppress the expression of Twist, Cyclin D1, p21, and phospho p38 mitogen-activated proteinkinases (p38MAPKs) [85, 86]. Recently, Seo and colleagues reported that quercetin restricts the proliferation and clonogenic survival of breast tumor-474 cells. Also, it is reported that quercetin suppresses the expression of JAK1 and upregulates the levels of cleaved caspase 3 and 8, followed by cleavage of poly(ADP-ribose) polymerase (PARP). Quercetin is reported to inhibit glucose transporter 1 (GLUT1) by binding on exo facial site. GLUT1 is responsible for transportation of glucose across the plasma membrane [87]. Besides binding and inhibiting the action of GLUT1, quercetin also block the process of glycolysis *via* inhibition of other glycolytic enzymes and proteins including Lactate dehdrogenase A (LDHA) and Pyruvate kinase M2 (PMK2) which is directly involved in case of breast cancer cell lines MCF-7andMDA-MB-231 [88]. Consequently, the inhibition of the glycolysis pathway in breast cancer cell lines ultimately causes a reduction in glucose efflux and lactate formation and hence restricts survival, mobility and progression of cancer cell. Quercetin is also known to block Akt-mTOR pathways which leads to autophagy and hence inhibition of metastasis [89].

## 4.5. Isothiocyanates

Secondary metabolites are the important ingredients obtained from vegetables and fruits in our diets which have an immense impact on human health. Sulforaphane (Fig. **14**) is one such secondary metabolite of the compound glucosinolate. Glucosinolates are a large group of sulphur-containing natural products that occur in the members of the Brassicaceae family. Plants use these compounds for their defence against herbivores due to their bitter taste. Isothiocyanates are the group of organic compounds having a -N=C=S group as common structural features. Isothiocyanates are able to inhibit cancer development in animals [90, 91]. The pioneer work which established the efficacy of isothiocyanate as an efficient anti-tumor agent was performed on mice model pre-treated with various carcinogens including ethionine, fluorenyl acetamide, aromatic hydrocarbons, azodyes and several nitrosamines. Studies showed that carcinogens affected organs including the lungs, liver, esophagus, stomach, colon and bladder get faster healing when administrated with isothiocyanates [92, 93].

Studies showed that Benzyl-ITC is able to inhibit benzapyrene induced mouse for stomach cancer [94, 95]. 4-(Methylnitrosamino)-1-(3-pyridyl)-1-butanone (NNK) is the compound which is responsible for lung cancer in smokers. Phenylethyl-ITC (PEITC), BITC and phenyl isothiocyanate (PITC) were found to inhibit lung tumorigenesis in the lung cells from A/J mice treated with NNK [96, 97]. PEIT C also showed the inhibitory activity of *N*-nitrosomethyl benzylamine (NMBA)-induced esophageal carcinogenesis and DNA methylation in rodents. ITCs can regulate the events linked to cell division in leukaemia transformed cells, like cell cycle progression, differentiation and apoptosis. ITCs have been established to exhibit antiproliferative activities against fungi and bacteria. PEITC, Allyl-ITC (AITC) and their cysteine conjugates have been reported to inhibit *in vitro* growth and induce the apoptosis of human leukaemia HL-60 (p53+) and myeloblastic leukaemia-1 cells (p53-) [98]. Studies showed that ITCs can restrict phase I enzymes which are responsible for the activation of several carcinogens, for example, Cytochrome P-450. Cyt P-450 is an important enzyme which is required for normal metabolism in the cell but may also activate certain carcinogens. ITCs have been reported to have the ability to inhibit several members of Cyt. P-450. Sulforaphane (SFN) has the potential to inhibit the catalytic activities of several cyt. enzymes, including Cyt. 1A1, 1A2, 2B1/2, 2E1, and 3A4 [99]. Several factors may play a crucial role which may regulate the potency of isothiocyanate in the inhibition of tumorigenes such as alkyl chain length, substituents and other structural features of the isothiocyanates, the animal species, target tissues, and the specific carcinogen employed [100, 101].

## CONCLUSION

Cancer has been considered as one of the most complex diseases in which there is not a single drug target. Therefore, like several other pathogenic diseases, different therapeutic approaches have been adopted for the treatment. In that, chemotherapy using drugs has been the most adopted approach. Therefore, this chapter mainly focused on the discussion related to different types of chemotherapeutic agents and commercially available drugs. The roles of different types of alkylators, antimetabolites, antibiotics and phytochemicals in the treatment of cancer and their mode of action have been elaborately discussed in this chapter.

# REFERENCES

[1]     Sanchez, G.; Meltzer, E. *The edwin smith papyrus: Updated translation of the trauma treatise and modern medical*; Lockwood Press, **2014**, pp. 1-400.

[2]     Karpozilos, A.; Pavlidis, N. The treatment of cancer in Greek antiquity. *Eur. J. Cancer,* **2004**, *40*(14), 2033-2040.
[http://dx.doi.org/10.1016/j.ejca.2004.04.036] [PMID: 15341975]

[3]     Papavramidou, N.; Papavramidis, T.; Demetriou, T. Ancient Greek and Greco-Roman methods in modern surgical treatment of cancer. *Ann. Surg. Oncol.,* **2010**, *17*(3), 665-667.
[http://dx.doi.org/10.1245/s10434-009-0886-6] [PMID: 20049643]

[4]     Martínez-Reyes, I.; Chandel, N.S. Cancer metabolism: Looking forward. *Nat. Rev. Cancer,* **2021**, *21*(10), 669-680.
[http://dx.doi.org/10.1038/s41568-021-00378-6] [PMID: 34272515]

[5]     DeBerardinis, R.J.; Chandel, N.S. Fundamentals of cancer metabolism. *Sci. Adv.,* **2016**, *2*(5), e1600200-e1600200.
[http://dx.doi.org/10.1126/sciadv.1600200] [PMID: 27386546]

[6]     National cancer institute at the national institutes of health. Available from: Www.Cancer.Gov/Types/Common-Cancers

[7]     Sung, H.; Ferlay, J.; Siegel, R.L.; Laversanne, M.; Soerjomataram, I.; Jemal, A.; Bray, F. Global cancer statistics 2020: Globocan estimates of incidence and mortality worldwide for 36 cancers in 185 countries. *CA Cancer J. Clin.,* **2021**, *71*(3), 209-249.
[http://dx.doi.org/10.3322/caac.21660] [PMID: 33538338]

[8]     Blackadar, C.B. Historical review of the causes of cancer. *World J. Clin. Oncol.,* **2016**, *7*(1), 54-86.
[http://dx.doi.org/10.5306/wjco.v7.i1.54] [PMID: 26862491]

[9]     Danaei, G.; Vander Hoorn, S.; Lopez, A.D.; Murray, C.J.L.; Ezzati, M. Causes of cancer in the world: comparative risk assessment of nine behavioural and environmental risk factors. *Lancet,* **2005**, *366*(9499), 1784-1793.
[http://dx.doi.org/10.1016/S0140-6736(05)67725-2] [PMID: 16298215]

[10]    Ames, B.N.; Gold, L.S.; Willett, W.C. The causes and prevention of cancer. *Proc. Natl. Acad. Sci.,* **1995**, *92*(12), 5258-5265.
[http://dx.doi.org/10.1073/pnas.92.12.5258] [PMID: 7777494]

[11]    U.S. Interagency Staff Group on Carcinogens. Chemical carcinogens: a review of the science and its associated principles. *Environ. Health Perspect.,* **1986**, *67*, 201-282.
[PMID: 3530737]

[12]    Dart, A. The ways in which carcinogens work. *Nat. Rev. Cancer,* **2020**, *20*(12), 695.
[http://dx.doi.org/10.1038/s41568-020-00314-0] [PMID: 33110244]

[13]    Luch, A. The mode of action of organic carcinogens on cellular structures. *EXS,* **2006**, *96*(96), 65-95.
[http://dx.doi.org/10.1007/3-7643-7378-4_4] [PMID: 16383015]

[14]    Martinez, V.D.; Vucic, E.A.; Becker-Santos, D.D.; Gil, L.; Lam, W.L. Arsenic exposure and the induction of human cancers. *J. Toxicol.,* **2011**, *2011*, 1-13.
[http://dx.doi.org/10.1155/2011/431287] [PMID: 22174709]

[15]    El Ghissassi, F.; Baan, R.; Straif, K.; Grosse, Y.; Secretan, B.; Bouvard, V.; Benbrahim-Tallaa, L.; Guha, N.; Freeman, C.; Galichet, L.; Cogliano, V. A review of human carcinogens—Part D: Radiation. *Lancet Oncol.,* **2009**, *10*(8), 751-752.
[http://dx.doi.org/10.1016/S1470-2045(09)70213-X] [PMID: 19655431]

[16]    Das, S.; Kundu, M.; Jena, B.C.; Mandal, M. Chapter 25 - Causes of Cancer: Physical, chemical,biological carcinogens, and viruses.*In: Materials Today*; Kundu, S.C.; Reis, M.; Jena, R.L.B.T.-B. Elsevier, **2020**, pp. 607-641.

[17]     Bouvard, V.; Baan, R.; Straif, K.; Grosse, Y.; Secretan, B.; Ghissassi, F.E.; Benbrahim-Tallaa, L.; Guha, N.; Freeman, C.; Galichet, L.; Cogliano, V. A review of human carcinogens—Part B: Biological agents. *Lancet Oncol.,* **2009**, *10*(4), 321-322.
         [http://dx.doi.org/10.1016/S1470-2045(09)70096-8] [PMID: 19350698]

[18]     Yoon, H.J.; Kim, J.H.; Seo, G.H.; Park, H. Risk of cancer following the use of n-nitrosodimethylamine (ndma) contaminated ranitidine products: A nationwide cohort study in south korea. *J. Clin. Med.,* **2021**, *10*(1), 153.
         [http://dx.doi.org/10.3390/jcm10010153] [PMID: 33466237]

[19]     Adamson, R.H.; Chabner, B.A. The finding of N-Nitrosodimethylamine in common medicines. *Oncologist,* **2020**, *25*(6), 460-462.
         [http://dx.doi.org/10.1634/theoncologist.2020-0142] [PMID: 32267983]

[20]     Demaria, S.; Golden, E.B.; Formenti, S.C. Role of local radiation therapy in cancer immunotherapy. *JAMA Oncol.,* **2015**, *1*(9), 1325-1332.
         [http://dx.doi.org/10.1001/jamaoncol.2015.2756] [PMID: 26270858]

[21]     Baskar, R.; Lee, K.A.; Yeo, R.; Yeoh, K.W. Cancer and radiation therapy: Current advances and future directions. *Int. J. Med. Sci.,* **2012**, *9*(3), 193-199.
         [http://dx.doi.org/10.7150/ijms.3635] [PMID: 22408567]

[22]     Fridlender, M.; Kapulnik, Y.; Koltai, H. Plant derived substances with anti-cancer activity: From folklore to practice. *Front. Plant Sci.,* **2015**, *6*, 799.
         [http://dx.doi.org/10.3389/fpls.2015.00799] [PMID: 26483815]

[23]     Pantziarka, P.; Capistrano I, R.; De Potter, A.; Vandeborne, L.; Bouche, G. An open access database of licensed cancer drugs. *Front. Pharmacol.,* **2021**, *12*, 627574.
         [http://dx.doi.org/10.3389/fphar.2021.627574] [PMID: 33776770]

[24]     Rachid, Z.; Brahimi, F.; Qiu, Q.; Williams, C.; Hartley, J.M.; Hartley, J.A.; Jean-Claude, B.J. Novel nitrogen mustard-armed combi-molecules for the selective targeting of epidermal growth factor receptor overexperessing solid tumors: Discovery of an unusual structure-activity relationship. *J. Med. Chem.,* **2007**, *50*(11), 2605-2608.
         [http://dx.doi.org/10.1021/jm070144p] [PMID: 17472358]

[25]     Deka, B.C.; Bhattacharyya, P.K. Nitrogen mustards: The novel DNA alkylator. *Clin. Cancer Drugs,* **2017**, *4*(1), 10-46.
         [http://dx.doi.org/10.2174/2212697X04666170123120528]

[26]     Lehmann, F.; Wennerberg, J. Evolution of nitrogen-based alkylating anticancer agents. *Processes,* **2021**, *9*(2), 377.
         [http://dx.doi.org/10.3390/pr9020377]

[27]     Ralhan, R.; Kaur, J. Alkylating agents and cancer therapy. *Expert Opin. Ther. Pat.,* **2007**, *17*(9), 1061-1075.
         [http://dx.doi.org/10.1517/13543776.17.9.1061]

[28]     Liner, K.; Brown, C.; McGirt, L. Clinical potential of mechlorethamine gel for the topical treatment of mycosis fungoides-type cutaneous T-cell lymphoma: A review on current efficacy and safety data. *Drug Des. Devel. Ther.,* **2018**, *12*, 241-254.
         [http://dx.doi.org/10.2147/DDDT.S137106] [PMID: 29440874]

[29]     Talpur, R.; Venkatarajan, S.; Duvic, M. Mechlorethamine gel for the topical treatment of stage IA and IB mycosis fungoides-type cutaneous T-cell lymphoma. *Expert Rev. Clin. Pharmacol.,* **2014**, *7*(5), 591-597.
         [http://dx.doi.org/10.1586/17512433.2014.944500] [PMID: 25068889]

[30]     Hillmen, P.; Skotnicki, A.B.; Robak, T.; Jaksic, B.; Dmoszynska, A.; Wu, J.; Sirard, C.; Mayer, J. Alemtuzumab compared with chlorambucil as first-line therapy for chronic lymphocytic leukemia. *J. Clin. Oncol.,* **2007**, *25*(35), 5616-5623.

[http://dx.doi.org/10.1200/JCO.2007.12.9098] [PMID: 17984186]

[31]   Alexanian, R.; Haut, A.; Khan, A.U.; Lane, M.; McKelvey, E.M.; Migliore, P.J.; Stuckey, W.J., Jr;
       Wilson, H.E. Treatment for multiple myeloma. Combination chemotherapy with different melphalan
       dose regimens. *JAMA,* **1969**, *208*(9), 1680-1685.
       [http://dx.doi.org/10.1001/jama.1969.03160090040009] [PMID: 5818682]

[32]   Gandhi, V. Metabolism and mechanisms of action of bendamustine: Rationales for combination
       therapies. *Proc. Semin. oncol.,* **2002**, *29*, 4-11.
       [http://dx.doi.org/10.1053/sonc.2002.34872]

[33]   Bartzatt, R. Potential antineoplastic structural variations of uracil mustard (uramustine) retaining
       cytotoxic activity and drug-likeness suitable for oral administration. *J. Cancer. Tumor. Int.,* **2015**, *2*(2),
       50-58.
       [http://dx.doi.org/10.9734/JCTI/2015/17780]

[34]   Emadi, A.; Jones, R.J.; Brodsky, R.A. Cyclophosphamide and cancer: Golden anniversary. *Nat. Rev.
       Clin. Oncol.,* **2009**, *6*(11), 638-647.
       [http://dx.doi.org/10.1038/nrclinonc.2009.146] [PMID: 19786984]

[35]   Miller, M.L.; Fishkin, N.E.; Li, W.; Whiteman, K.R.; Kovtun, Y.; Reid, E.E.; Archer, K.E.; Maloney,
       E.K.; Audette, C.A.; Mayo, M.F.; Wilhelm, A.; Modafferi, H.A.; Singh, R.; Pinkas, J.; Goldmacher,
       V.; Lambert, J.M.; Chari, R.V.J. A new class of antibody–drug conjugates with potent DNA alkylating
       activity. *Mol. Cancer Ther.,* **2016**, *15*(8), 1870-1878.
       [http://dx.doi.org/10.1158/1535-7163.MCT-16-0184] [PMID: 27216304]

[36]   Miller, M.L.; Shizuka, M.; Wilhelm, A.; Salomon, P.; Reid, E.E.; Lanieri, L.; Sikka, S.; Maloney,
       E.K.; Harvey, L.; Qiu, Q.; Archer, K.E.; Bai, C.; Vitharana, D.; Harris, L.; Singh, R.; Ponte, J.F.;
       Yoder, N.C.; Kovtun, Y.; Lai, K.C.; Ab, O.; Pinkas, J.; Keating, T.A.; Chari, R.V.J. A DNA-
       interacting payload designed to eliminate cross-linking improves the therapeutic index of
       antibody–drug conjugates (ADCs). *Mol. Cancer Ther.,* **2018**, *17*(3), 650-660.
       [http://dx.doi.org/10.1158/1535-7163.MCT-17-0940] [PMID: 29440292]

[37]   Richardson, P.G.; Oriol, A.; Larocca, A.; Bladé, J.; Cavo, M.; Rodriguez-Otero, P.; Leleu, X.;
       Nadeem, O.; Hiemenz, J.W.; Hassoun, H.; Touzeau, C.; Alegre, A.; Paner, A.; Maisel, C.; Mazumder,
       A.; Raptis, A.; Moreb, J.S.; Anderson, K.C.; Laubach, J.P.; Thuresson, S.; Thuresson, M.; Byrne, C.;
       Harmenberg, J.; Bakker, N.A.; Mateos, M.V. Melflufen and dexamethasone in heavily pretreated
       relapsed and refractory multiple myeloma. *J. Clin. Oncol.,* **2021**, *39*(7), 757-767.
       [http://dx.doi.org/10.1200/JCO.20.02259] [PMID: 33296242]

[38]   Kelly, W.K.; Curley, T.; Slovin, S.; Heller, G.; McCaffrey, J.; Bajorin, D.; Ciolino, A.; Regan, K.;
       Schwartz, M.; Kantoff, P.; George, D.; Oh, W.; Smith, M.; Kaufman, D.; Small, E.J.; Schwartz, L.;
       Larson, S.; Tong, W.; Scher, H. Paclitaxel, estramustine phosphate, and carboplatin in patients with
       advanced prostate cancer. *J. Clin. Oncol.,* **2001**, *19*(1), 44-53.
       [http://dx.doi.org/10.1200/JCO.2001.19.1.44] [PMID: 11134194]

[39]   Tiwari, M. Antimetabolites: Established cancer therapy. *J. Cancer Res. Ther.,* **2012**, *8*(4), 510-519.
       [http://dx.doi.org/10.4103/0973-1482.106526] [PMID: 23361267]

[40]   Piper, J.R.; McCaleb, G.S.; Montgomery, J.A.; Kisliuk, R.L.; Gaumont, Y.; Sirotnak, F.M. Syntheses
       and antifolate activity of 5-methyl-5-deaza analogs of aminopterin, methotrexate, folic acid, and N10-
       methylfolic acid. *J. Med. Chem.,* **1986**, *29*(6), 1080-1087.
       [http://dx.doi.org/10.1021/jm00156a029] [PMID: 2423690]

[41]   Meyer, L.M.; Miller, F.R.; Rowen, M.J.; Bock, G.; Rutzky, J. Treatment of acute leukemia with
       amethopterin (4-amino, 10-methyl pteroyl glutamic acid). *Acta Haematol.,* **1950**, *4*(3), 157-167.
       [http://dx.doi.org/10.1159/000203749] [PMID: 14777272]

[42]   Cronstein, B.N.; Aune, T.M. Methotrexate and its mechanisms of action in inflammatory arthritis. *Nat.
       Rev. Rheumatol.,* **2020**, *16*(3), 145-154.
       [http://dx.doi.org/10.1038/s41584-020-0373-9] [PMID: 32066940]

[43]     Karran, P.; Attard, N. Thiopurines in current medical practice: Molecular mechanisms and contributions to therapy-relatedcancer. *Nat. Rev.Cancer,* **2008**, *8*, 24-36.

[44]     Duncan, R.; Kopečková-Rejmanová, P.; Strohalm, J.; Hume, I.; Cable, H.C.; Pohl, J.; Lloyd, J.B.; Kopeček, J. Anticancer agents coupled to N-(2-hydroxypropyl)methacrylamide copolymers. I. Evaluation of daunomycin and puromycin conjugates *in vitro. Br. J. Cancer,* **1987**, *55*(2), 165-174.
[http://dx.doi.org/10.1038/bjc.1987.33] [PMID: 3468994]

[45]     Koh, W.; Jeong, S.J.; Lee, H.J.; Ryu, H.G.; Lee, E.O.; Ahn, K.S.; Bae, H.; Kim, S.H. Melatonin promotes puromycin-induced apoptosis with activation of caspase-3 and 5′-adenosine monophosphate-activated kinase-alpha in human leukemia HL-60 cells. *J. Pineal Res.,* **2011**, *50*(4), 367-373.
[http://dx.doi.org/10.1111/j.1600-079X.2010.00852.x] [PMID: 21244482]

[46]     Jung, J.H.; Sohn, E.J.; Shin, E.A.; Lee, D.; Kim, B.; Jung, D.-B.; Kim, J.-H.; Yun, M.; Lee, H.-J.; Park, Y.K. Melatonin suppresses the expression of 45s preribosomal rna and upstream binding factor and enhances the antitumor activity of puromycin in MDA-MB-231 breast cancer cells.evidence-based complement. *Altern.Med.,* **2013**, *2013*, 879746.

[47]     Siddik, Z.H. Cisplatin: Mode of cytotoxic action and molecular basis of resistance. *Oncogene,* **2003**, *22*(47), 7265-7279.
[http://dx.doi.org/10.1038/sj.onc.1206933] [PMID: 14576837]

[48]     Nussbaumer, S.; Bonnabry, P.; Veuthey, J.L.; Fleury-Souverain, S. Analysis of anticancer drugs: A review. *Talanta,* **2011**, *85*(5), 2265-2289.
[http://dx.doi.org/10.1016/j.talanta.2011.08.034] [PMID: 21962644]

[49]     Newman, D.J.; Cragg, G.M. Natural products as sources of new drugs from 1981 to 2014. *J. Nat. Prod.,* **2016**, *79*(3), 629-661.
[http://dx.doi.org/10.1021/acs.jnatprod.5b01055] [PMID: 26852623]

[50]     Lee, W.L.; Huang, J.Y.; Shyur, L.F. Phytoagents for cancer management: regulation of nucleic acid oxidation, ROS, and related mechanisms. *Oxid. Med. Cell. Longev.,* **2013**, *2013*, 1-22.
[http://dx.doi.org/10.1155/2013/925804] [PMID: 24454991]

[51]     Yan, X-B.; Xie, T.; Wang, S-D.; Wang, Z.; Li, H-Y.; Ye, Z-M. Apigenin Inhibits Proliferation of Human Chondrosarcoma Cells *via* Cell Cycle Arrest and Mitochondrial Apoptosis Induced by ROS Generation-aninVitroandinVivoStudy. *Int. J. Clin. Exp. Med.,* **2018**, *11*, 1615-1631.

[52]     Lu, L.; Zhao, Z.; Liu, L.; Gong, W.; Dong, J. Combination of baicalein and docetaxel additively inhibits the growth of non-small cell lung cancer *in vivo. Trad. Med. Mod. Med.,* **2018**, *1*(3), 213-218.
[http://dx.doi.org/10.1142/S2575900018500131]

[53]     Choudhari, A.S.; Mandave, P.C.; Deshpande, M.; Ranjekar, P.; Prakash, O. Phytochemicals in cancer treatment: From preclinical studies to clinical practice. *Front. Pharmacol.,* **2020**, *10*, 1614.
[http://dx.doi.org/10.3389/fphar.2019.01614] [PMID: 32116665]

[54]     Aggarwal, B.B.; Harikumar, K.B. Potential therapeutic effects of curcumin, the anti-inflammatory agent, against neurodegenerative, cardiovascular, pulmonary, metabolic, autoimmune and neoplastic diseases. *Int. J. Biochem. Cell Biol.,* **2009**, *41*(1), 40-59.
[http://dx.doi.org/10.1016/j.biocel.2008.06.010] [PMID: 18662800]

[55]     Maheshwari, R.K.; Singh, A.K.; Gaddipati, J.; Srimal, R.C. Multiple biological activities of curcumin: A short review. *Life Sci.,* **2006**, *78*(18), 2081-2087.
[http://dx.doi.org/10.1016/j.lfs.2005.12.007] [PMID: 16413584]

[56]     Prakasam, G.; Iqbal, M.A.; Bamezai, R.N.K.; Mazurek, S. Posttranslational modifications of pyruvate kinase M2: Tweaks that benefit cancer. *Front. Oncol.,* **2018**, *8*, 22.
[http://dx.doi.org/10.3389/fonc.2018.00022] [PMID: 29468140]

[57]     Chaneton, B.; Gottlieb, E. Rocking cell metabolism: Revised functions of the key glycolytic regulator PKM2 in cancer. *Trends Biochem. Sci.,* **2012**, *37*(8), 309-316.
[http://dx.doi.org/10.1016/j.tibs.2012.04.003] [PMID: 22626471]

[58]　Siddiqui, F.A.; Prakasam, G.; Chattopadhyay, S.; Rehman, A.U.; Padder, R.A.; Ansari, M.A.; Irshad, R.; Mangalhara, K.; Bamezai, R.N.K.; Husain, M.; Ali, S.M.; Iqbal, M.A. Curcumin decreases Warburg effect in cancer cells by down-regulating pyruvate kinase M2 *via* mTOR-HIF1α inhibition. *Sci. Rep.,* **2018**, *8*(1), 8323.
[http://dx.doi.org/10.1038/s41598-018-25524-3] [PMID: 29844464]

[59]　Adams, B.K.; Cai, J.; Armstrong, J.; Herold, M.; Lu, Y.J.; Sun, A.; Snyder, J.P.; Liotta, D.C.; Jones, D.P.; Shoji, M. EF24, a novel synthetic curcumin analog, induces apoptosis in cancer cells *via* a redox-dependent mechanism. *Anticancer Drugs,* **2005**, *16*(3), 263-275.
[http://dx.doi.org/10.1097/00001813-200503000-00005] [PMID: 15711178]

[60]　He, G.; Feng, C.; Vinothkumar, R.; Chen, W.; Dai, X.; Chen, X.; Ye, Q.; Qiu, C.; Zhou, H.; Wang, Y.; Liang, G.; Xie, Y.; Wu, W. Curcumin analog EF24 induces apoptosis *via* ROS-dependent mitochondrial dysfunction in human colorectal cancer cells. *Cancer Chemother. Pharmacol.,* **2016**, *78*(6), 1151-1161.
[http://dx.doi.org/10.1007/s00280-016-3172-x] [PMID: 27787644]

[61]　Larasati, Y.A.; Yoneda-Kato, N.; Nakamae, I.; Yokoyama, T.; Meiyanto, E.; Kato, J. Curcumin targets multiple enzymes involved in the ROS metabolic pathway to suppress tumor cell growth. *Sci. Rep.,* **2018**, *8*(1), 2039.
[http://dx.doi.org/10.1038/s41598-018-20179-6] [PMID: 29391517]

[62]　Kocyigit, A.; Guler, E.M. Curcumin induce DNA damage and apoptosis through generation of reactive oxygen species and reducing mitochondrial membrane potential in melanoma cancer cells. *Cell. Mol. Biol.,* **2017**, *63*(11), 97-105.
[http://dx.doi.org/10.14715/cmb/2017.63.11.17] [PMID: 29208180]

[63]　Kisková, T.; Kassayová, M. Resveratrol action on lipid metabolism in cancer. *Int. J. Mol. Sci.,* **2019**, *20*(11), 2704.
[http://dx.doi.org/10.3390/ijms20112704] [PMID: 31159437]

[64]　Gomez, L.S.; Zancan, P.; Marcondes, M.C.; Ramos-Santos, L.; Meyer-Fernandes, J.R.; Sola-Penna, M.; Da Silva, D. Resveratrol decreases breast cancer cell viability and glucose metabolism by inhibiting 6-phosphofructo-1-kinase. *Biochimie,* **2013**, *95*(6), 1336-1343.
[http://dx.doi.org/10.1016/j.biochi.2013.02.013] [PMID: 23454376]

[65]　Jung, K.-H.; Lee, J.H.; Thien Quach, C.H.; Paik, J.-Y.; Oh, H.; Park, J.W.; Lee, E.J.; Moon, S.-H.; Lee, K.-H. Resveratrol suppresses cancer cell glucose uptake by targeting reactive oxygen species–mediated hypoxia-inducible factor-1α activation. *J. Nucl. Med.,* **2013**, *54*, 2161-2167.

[66]　Ruan, H.; Zhan, Y.Y.; Hou, J.; Xu, B.; Chen, B.; Tian, Y.; Wu, D.; Zhao, Y.; Zhang, Y.; Chen, X.; Mi, P.; Zhang, L.; Zhang, S.; Wang, X.; Cao, H.; Zhang, W.; Wang, H.; Li, H.; Su, Y.; Zhang, X.K.; Hu, T. Berberine binds RXRα to suppress β-catenin signaling in colon cancer cells. *Oncogene,* **2017**, *36*(50), 6906-6918.
[http://dx.doi.org/10.1038/onc.2017.296] [PMID: 28846104]

[67]　Zou, K.; Li, Z.; Zhang, Y.; Zhang, H.; Li, B.; Zhu, W.; Shi, J.; Jia, Q.; Li, Y. Advances in the study of berberine and its derivatives: A focus on anti-inflammatory and anti-tumor effects in the digestive system. *Acta Pharmacol. Sin.,* **2017**, *38*(2), 157-167.
[http://dx.doi.org/10.1038/aps.2016.125] [PMID: 27917872]

[68]　Yin, J.; Ye, J.; Jia, W. Effects and mechanisms of berberine in diabetes treatment. *Acta Pharm. Sin. B,* **2012**, *2*(4), 327-334.
[http://dx.doi.org/10.1016/j.apsb.2012.06.003]

[69]　Li, Z.; Geng, Y.N.; Jiang, J.D.; Kong, W.J. Antioxidant and anti-inflammatory activities of berberine in the treatment of diabetes mellitus. *Evid. Based Complement. Alternat. Med.,* **2014**, *2014*, 1-12.
[http://dx.doi.org/10.1155/2014/289264] [PMID: 24669227]

[70]　Refaat, A.; Abdelhamed, S.; Saiki, I.; Sakurai, H. Inhibition of p38 mitogen-activated protein kinase potentiates the apoptotic effect of berberine/tumor necrosis factor-related apoptosis-inducing ligand

combination therapy. *Oncol. Lett.,* **2015**, *10*(3), 1907-1911.
[http://dx.doi.org/10.3892/ol.2015.3494] [PMID: 26622773]

[71] Li, D.; Zhang, Y.; Liu, K.; Zhao, Y.; Xu, B.; Xu, L.; Tan, L.; Tian, Y.; Li, C.; Zhang, W.; Cao, H.; Zhan, Y.; Hu, T. Berberine inhibits colitis-associated tumorigenesis *via* suppressing inflammatory responses and the consequent EGFR signaling-involved tumor cell growth. *Lab. Invest.,* **2017**, *97*(11), 1343-1353.
[http://dx.doi.org/10.1038/labinvest.2017.71] [PMID: 28759012]

[72] Shili, L.; Guogai, Z.; Han, C.; Biying, C.; Weimin, L.; Xia, W.; Yifan, F. Synthesis and anti-tumor activities against hepg2 cell *in vitro* of the conjugates of honokiol, quercetin and berberine.youjihuaxue/chinese. ,2018, 1549–1555. **2018**, 1549-1555.

[73] Eo, S.H.; Kim, J.H.; Kim, S.J. Induction of G$_2$/M Arrest by Berberine *via* Activation of PI3K/Akt and p38 in Human Chondrosarcoma Cell Line. *Oncol. Res.,* **2015**, *22*(3), 147-157.
[http://dx.doi.org/10.3727/096504015X14298122915583] [PMID: 26168133]

[74] Gu, M.; Xu, J.; Han, C.; Kang, Y.; Liu, T.; He, Y.; Huang, Y.; Liu, C. Effects of berberine on cellcycle, dna, reactive oxygen species, and apoptosis in l929 murine fibroblast cells. evidence-based complement. *Altern.Med.,* **2015**, *2015*, 796306.
[PMID: 26508985]

[75] Barzegar, E.; Fouladdel, S.; Movahhed, T.K.; Atashpour, S.; Ghahremani, M.H.; Ostad, S.N.; Azizi, E. Effects of berberine on proliferation, cell cycle distribution and apoptosis of human breast cancer T47D and MCF7 cell lines. *Iran. J. Basic Med. Sci.,* **2015**, *18*(4), 334-342.
[PMID: 26019795]

[76] Shukla, S.; Sharma, A.; Pandey, V.K.; Raisuddin, S.; Kakkar, P. Concurrent acetylation of FoxO1/3a and p53 due to sirtuins inhibition elicit Bim/PUMA mediated mitochondrial dysfunction and apoptosis in berberine-treated HepG2 cells. *Toxicol. Appl. Pharmacol.,* **2016**, *291*, 70-83.
[http://dx.doi.org/10.1016/j.taap.2015.12.006] [PMID: 26712469]

[77] Wang, K.; Zhang, C.; Bao, J.; Jia, X.; Liang, Y.; Wang, X.; Chen, M.; Su, H.; Li, P.; Wan, J.B.; He, C. Synergistic chemopreventive effects of curcumin and berberine on human breast cancer cells through induction of apoptosis and autophagic cell death. *Sci. Rep.,* **2016**, *6*(1), 26064.
[http://dx.doi.org/10.1038/srep26064] [PMID: 27263652]

[78] Chrysovergis, A.; Papanikolaou, V.; Tsiambas, E.; Stavraka, C.; Ragos, V.; Peschos, D.; Psyrri, A.; Mastronikolis, N.; Kyrodimos, E. P53/MDM2 co-expression in laryngeal squamous cell carcinoma based on digital image analysis. *Anticancer Res.,* **2019**, *39*(8), 4137-4142.
[http://dx.doi.org/10.21873/anticanres.13572] [PMID: 31366498]

[79] Liu, J.; Zhang, X.; Liu, A.; Liu, S.; Zhang, L.; Wu, B.; Hu, Q. Berberine induces apoptosis in P53-null leukemia cells by down-regulating XIAP atthe post-transcriptional level. *Int.J.Exp.Cell.Physiol. Biochem.Pharmacol.,* **2013**, *32*, 1213-1224.

[80] Wang, N.; Feng, Y.; Zhu, M.; Tsang, C.M.; Man, K.; Tong, Y.; Tsao, S.W. Berberine induces autophagic cell death and mitochondrial apoptosis in liver cancer cells: The cellular mechanism. *J. Cell. Biochem.,* **2010**, *111*(6), 1426-1436.
[http://dx.doi.org/10.1002/jcb.22869] [PMID: 20830746]

[81] Yu, R.; Zhang, Z.; Wang, B.; Jiang, H.; Cheng, L.; Shen, L. Berberine-induced apoptotic and autophagic death of HepG2 cells requires AMPK activation. *Cancer Cell Int.,* **2014**, *14*(1), 49.
[http://dx.doi.org/10.1186/1475-2867-14-49] [PMID: 24991192]

[82] Liu, Y.; Tang, Z.G.; Lin, Y.; Qu, X.G.; Lv, W.; Wang, G.B.; Li, C.L. Effects of quercetin on proliferation and migration of human glioblastoma U251 cells. *Biomed. Pharmacother.,* **2017**, *92*, 33-38.
[http://dx.doi.org/10.1016/j.biopha.2017.05.044] [PMID: 28528183]

[83] Murakami, A.; Ashida, H.; Terao, J. Multitargeted cancer prevention by quercetin. *Cancer Lett.,* **2008**, *269*(2), 315-325.

[http://dx.doi.org/10.1016/j.canlet.2008.03.046] [PMID: 18467024]

[84] Shih, H.; Pickwell, G.V.; Quattrochi, L.C. Differential effects of flavonoid compounds on tumor promoter-induced activation of the human CYP1A2 enhancer. *Arch. Biochem. Biophys.,* **2000**, *373*(1), 287-294.
[http://dx.doi.org/10.1006/abbi.1999.1550] [PMID: 10620351]

[85] Liao, H.; Bao, X.; Zhu, J.; Qu, J.; Sun, Y.; Ma, X.; Wang, E.; Guo, X.; Kang, Q.; Zhen, Y. O-Alkylated derivatives of quercetin induce apoptosis of MCF-7 cells *via* a caspase-independent mitochondrial pathway. *Chem. Biol. Interact.,* **2015**, *242*, 91-98.
[http://dx.doi.org/10.1016/j.cbi.2015.09.022] [PMID: 26415619]

[86] Ranganathan, S.; Halagowder, D.; Sivasithambaram, N.D. Quercetin suppresses twist to induce apoptosis in mcf-7 breast cancer cells. *PLoS One,* **2015**, *10*(10), e0141370.
[http://dx.doi.org/10.1371/journal.pone.0141370] [PMID: 26491966]

[87] Hamilton, K.E.; Rekman, J.F.; Gunnink, L.K.; Busscher, B.M.; Scott, J.L.; Tidball, A.M.; Stehouwer, N.R.; Johncheck, G.N.; Looyenga, B.D.; Louters, L.L. Quercetin inhibits glucose transport by binding to an exofacial site on GLUT1. *Biochimie,* **2018**, *151*, 107-114.
[http://dx.doi.org/10.1016/j.biochi.2018.05.012] [PMID: 29857184]

[88] Srivastava, S.; Somasagara, R.R.; Hegde, M.; Nishana, M.; Tadi, S.K.; Srivastava, M.; Choudhary, B.; Raghavan, S.C. Quercetin, a natural flavonoid interacts with dna, arrests cell cycle and causes tumor regression byactivating mitochondrial pathway of apoptosis. *Sci. Rep.,* **2016**, 6.

[89] Rivera, R.; Castillo-Pichardora, L.; Gerena, Y.; Dharmawardhane, S. Anti-breastcancerpotential of quercetin *via* the akt/ampk/mammalian target of rapamycin (mtor) signaling cascade. *PLoS One,* **2016**, *11*, e0157251.
[http://dx.doi.org/10.1371/journal.pone.0157251] [PMID: 27285995]

[90] Xu, K.; Thornalley, P.J. Signal transduction activated by the cancer chemopreventive isothiocyanates: Cleavage of BID protein, tyrosine phosphorylation and activation of JNK. *Br. J. Cancer,* **2001**, *84*(5), 670-673.
[http://dx.doi.org/10.1054/bjoc.2000.1636] [PMID: 11237388]

[91] Kuroiwa, Y.; Nishikawa, A.; Kitamura, Y.; Kanki, K.; Ishii, Y.; Umemura, T.; Hirose, M. Protective effects of benzyl isothiocyanate and sulforaphane but not resveratrol against initiation of pancreatic carcinogenesis in hamsters. *Cancer Lett.,* **2006**, *241*(2), 275-280.
[http://dx.doi.org/10.1016/j.canlet.2005.10.028] [PMID: 16386831]

[92] Zhang, Y.; Talalay, P. Anticarcinogenic activities of organic isothiocyanates: Chemistry and mechanisms. *Cancer Res.,* **1994**, *54*(7), 1976s-1981s.
[PMID: 8137323]

[93] Hecht, S.S. Chemoprevention by isothiocyanates. *J. Cell. Biochem.,* **1995**, *59*(S22), 195-209.
[http://dx.doi.org/10.1002/jcb.240590825] [PMID: 8538199]

[94] Wattenberg, L.W. Inhibitory effects of benzyl isothiocyanate administered shortly before diethylnitrosamine or benzo[ *a* ]pyrene on pulmonary and forestomach neoplasia in A/J mice. *Carcinogenesis,* **1987**, *8*(12), 1971-1973.
[http://dx.doi.org/10.1093/carcin/8.12.1971] [PMID: 3677323]

[95] Wattenberg, L.W. Inhibition of carcinogenic effects of polycyclic hydrocarbons by benzyl isothiocyanate and related compounds. *J. Natl. Cancer Inst.,* **1977**, *58*(2), 395-398.
[http://dx.doi.org/10.1093/jnci/58.2.395] [PMID: 401894]

[96] Morse, M.A.; Eklind, K.I.; Amin, S.G.; Hecht, S.S.; Chung, F.L. Effects of alkyl chain length on the inhibition of NNK-induced lung neoplasia in A/J mice by arylalkyl isothiocyanates. *Carcinogenesis,* **1989**, *10*(9), 1757-1759.
[http://dx.doi.org/10.1093/carcin/10.9.1757] [PMID: 2766468]

[97] Morse, M.A.; Amin, S.G.; Hecht, S.S.; Chung, F-L. Effects of aromatic isothiocyanates on

tumorigenicity, O6-methylguanine formation, and metabolism of the tobacco-specific nitrosamine 4-(methylnitrosamino)-1-(3-pyridyl)-1-butanone in A/J mouse lung. *Cancer Res.,* **1989**, *49*(11), 2894-2897.
[PMID: 2720649]

[98]    Xu, K.; Thornalley, P.J. Studies on the mechanism of the inhibition of human leukaemia cell growth by dietary isothiocyanates and their cysteine adducts *in vitro. Biochem. Pharmacol.,* **2000**, *60*(2), 221-231.
[http://dx.doi.org/10.1016/S0006-2952(00)00319-1] [PMID: 10825467]

[99]    Fimognari, C.; Lenzi, M.; Hrelia, P. Chemoprevention of cancer by isothiocyanates and anthocyanins: Mechanisms of action and structure-activity relationship. *Curr. Med. Chem.,* **2008**, *15*(5), 440-447.
[http://dx.doi.org/10.2174/092986708783503168] [PMID: 18288999]

[100]   Jiao, D.; Eklind, K.I.; Choi, C.I.; Desai, D.H.; Amin, S.G.; Chung, F.L. Structure-activity relationships of isothiocyanates as mechanism-based inhibitors of 4-(methylnitrosamino)-1-(3-pyridyl)-1-buanone-induced lung tumorigenesis in A/J mice. *Cancer Res.,* **1994**, *54*(16), 4327-4333.
[PMID: 8044780]

[101]   Conaway, C.C.; Jiao, D.; Chung, F.L. Inhibition of rat liver cytochrome P450 isozymes by isothiocyanates and their conjugates: AB structure-activity relationship study. *Carcinogenesis,* **1996**, *17*(11), 2423-2427.
[http://dx.doi.org/10.1093/carcin/17.11.2423] [PMID: 8968058]

# CHAPTER 5

# Harnessing the Neurological Properties of Indian Brain Health Booster Brahmi

**Neerja Tiwari[1], Manju Singh[1], Namita Gupta[1], Kishan Singh[1,2] and Kapil Dev[1,2,\*]**

[1] *Phytochemistry Division, CSIR-Central Institute of Medicinal and Aromatic Plants, Lucknow-226015, India*

[2] *Academy of Scientific and Innovative Research, Ghaziabad-201002, India*

**Abstract:** Brahmi (*Bacopa monnieri* Linn.) is a well-known therapeutic herb used in a broad spectrum of conventional medicines to alleviate various ailments, prominently those involving intellect, anxiety and mental health. In Ayurveda, it is classified as Medhya rasayanas (meaning intellect rejuvenator) and claimed to be a cognitive nutrient and memory enhancer. Although the plant possesses a plethora of compounds, its neurological activity is mainly attributed to its major phytochemical constituents, *i.e.*, bacoside saponins. Majorly isolated compounds are dammarane triterpenoids glycone and aglycones. There are several reports published with neurological activities on *Bacopa monnieri* to validate traditional claims through scientific findings. Some therapeutic formulations containing standardized extracts of *Bacopa monnieri* have also been developed for the betterment of mental health. Besides, being neuroprotective, the plant is reported to possess anti-inflammatory, analgesic, and antipyretic properties and systemic disorders like cardiovascular, hepatic, gastrointestinal, myocardial ischemia, respiratory problems, opioid-related nephrotoxicity and hepatotoxicity. The present chapter described the phytochemical profiling, extraction and isolation, neurological properties, as well as toxicological and clinical studies of the plant.

**Keywords:** *Bacopa monnieri*, Bacoside, Brahmi, Dammarane triterpenes, Neurological disorders, Neurodegenerative disease.

## 1. INTRODUCTION

The Indian nootropic creeper *Bacopa monnieri*(L.) Wettst (Family: Scrophulariaceae), commonly known as Brahmi, is the most important medicinal herb of Ayurveda. The genus bacopa comprises more than 100 species. It is a

---

\* **Corresponding author Kapil Dev:** Phytochemistry Division, CSIR-Central Institute of Medicinal and Aromatic Plants, Lucknow-226015 India; E-mail: kapildeo@cimap.res.in

**Ashok Kumar Jha & Ravi S. Singh (Eds.)**

creeper with succulent, oblong, and 4–6 mm (0.16–0.24 inch) thick leaves. The leaves are oblanceolate and arranged oppositely on the stem.

The flowers of *Bacopa monnieri* (BM) are small, actinomorphic and white, with four to five petals. It is grown in wet and muddy land and distributed throughout the southern and eastern parts of the Indian subcontinent. In the traditional medicinal system, Brahmi is used as a nerve tonic, diuretic, cardiotonic and as therapeutic against insomnia, epilepsy, asthma and rheumatism. Numerous studies on its neuroprotective, anxiolytic and anti-depression properties craftafirm staging to its traditional medicinal usage.

Bacopa has been used as traditional medicine for the management of anxiety, poor cognition, and lack of concentration and other neurodisorders [1]. It has been mentioned in Charaka Samhita (2500 B.C.) and Sushruta Samhita (2300 B.C.) as a medhyarasayana (brain tonic) to sharpen intellect and attenuate mental deficits [2, 3]. Several therapeutic formulations have been prepared to target CNS disorders and manage conditions such as memory impairments, lack of concentration, and anxiety [4]. Besides boosting CNS, it has been reported to treat numerous inflammatory conditions like asthma, bronchitis, dropsy, rheumatism, cardio tonic, nervine, diuretic, *etc.* [5]. Several studies have been published describing the nootropic functions of *Bacopa monnieri* [6, 7].

This renowned ayurvedic medicinal herb contains a vast variety of specialized secondary metabolites, including dammarane triterpenoid glycosides or bacosides, steroids, phenylethanoids, cucurbitacins and alkaloids. However, the pharmacological studies revealed that the neuroprotective effects of BM may be attributed to its most abundant constituents, *i.e.*, dammarane triterpenoids saponins called bacosides. These triterpenoids saponins are further classified as mono-andbi-desmosides on the basis of the linkage of sugar units to attach with aglycones, *i.e.*, at C-3 and C-20 [8].

In the present chapter, we focus on the phytochemical investigation, extraction methods and neurological properties of *B. monnieri*.

## 2. PHYTOCHEMICAL EVALUATION

The brain tonic herb BM contains a wide range of secondary metabolites such as triterpenoids, alkaloids, and aliphatic compounds. Damarane triterpene glycosides (bacosides) (Fig. **1**) are the majorly occurring and responsible compounds for the neurological activity of BM. The isolated and characterized dammarane triterpenoid glycosides possess atetracyclic ring with $\beta$–orientated methyl group at C-8. The most commonly occurring sugar units in dammarane triterpenoid saponins are $\beta$-D-glucopyranosyl, $\alpha$-L-arabinofuranosyl and $\alpha$-L-arabinopyranosyl. Despite the presence of these sugars, three dammarane triterpenoid glycosides are reported to have 6-*O*-sulphonyl-$\beta$-D-glucopyranosyl sugar moiety [9] Chakravarty *et al.*, 2001a, [10] Zhou *et al.*, 2007b). The aglycon moieties of the dammarane triterpenoids are jujubogenin or psuedojujubogenin. The distinctive feature of jujubogenin (**1**) and psuedo jujubogenin(**2**) is the isobutylene linkage to the 23 or 22 positions of the triterpene skeleton, respectively. Different dammarane triterpenoids, alkaloids, steroids, cucurbitacins, and flavonoids have been isolated and characterized from BM and explored for their pharmacological importance.

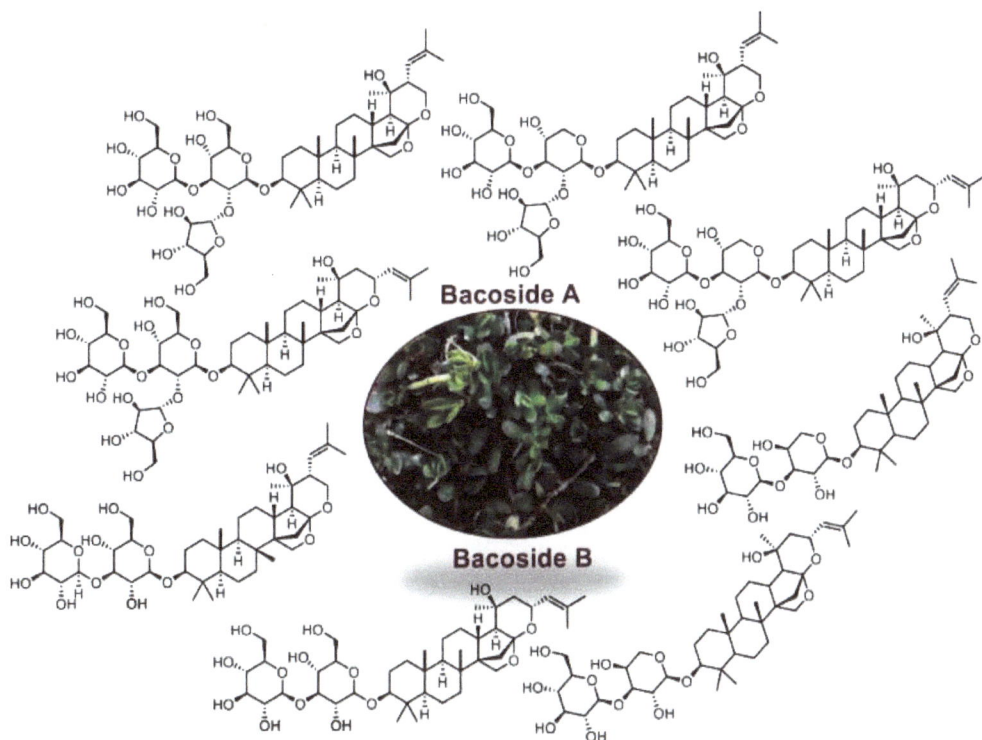

**Fig. (1).** Major dammarane triterpenes of the *B. monnieri*.

In view of the stature of BM in the traditional medicinal system, several research groups have explored this plant for phytochemical characterization and pharmacological evaluations. In 1963, Dutta & Basu isolated a triterpene saponin, monnierin (**3**) [11]. The compound showed a close resemblance of IR spectra with betulinic acid (**4**), no UV absorption and gave a red color with the Libermann-Burchard reagent. The molecular formula of the triterpenoid tetrosidecontains three sugar units, *i.e.*, two arabinoses and one glucose. The physical constants of the compound were in agreement with isolated sapogenin bacogenin A. The structure was confirmed by preparing different derivatives and hydrolysis [12]. In 1965 the major saponin of *B. monnieri* was isolated and named bacoside A. The structure of the compound was elucidated as 3-($\alpha$-L-arabinopyranosyl)-O-$\beta$-D-glucopyranosid-10,20-dihydroxy-16-keto-dammar-24-ene on the basis of the acid hydrolysis product of the compound [13]. It was considered the responsible compound for memory enhancing activity of BM. Previously, it was considered bacoside-A co-exists with bacoside B with different optical rotations [14], which on acidic hydrolysis yielded four different aglycons. These aglycons were characterized as bacogenin A1,A2,A3 and A4 (**5-8**). Bacogenin A1 was identified as 3,18-dihydroxy-20$\rightarrow$25-epoxy-22(or23)-methyl-24-nor-dammar-22-en-16-one while Bacogenin A2 appeared as an isomer of Bacogenin A1. The structure of A3 was supported by different chemical and spectral methods [15]. Bacogenin A4 was the major component of hydrolysis and was identified as beeline lactone pseudo jujubogenin [16 - 18]. Besides these four hydrolysis products, another rearranged compound of psedojujubogenin was also identified and named Bacogenin A5(**9**) [19 - 20].

Subsequent phytochemical studies revealed the identification of Bacoside B. The sugar components and aglycon moiety of bacoside B were found to be the same as that of bacoside A on the basis of analyses of acid hydrolysis products and iodometric, gravimetric as well as colorimetric studies. It was also discovered that Bacoside A and B differ in their optical rotation. This suggested bacoside B is an opticalisomer of bacoside A [15]. However, until 2004, there existed an ambiguity regarding the chemical entities of bacoside A and B [21]. In 2004, Deepak *et al.* separated the constituents of bacoside A. The identities of the individuals of bacosideA were established as bacoside A3 (**10**), bacopaside II (**11**) and bacopasaponin C (**12**) (Fig. **2**) by comparing the NMR data of the isolates with those reported in the literature [21].

Two minor derivatives were identified in the saponin mixture as jujubogenin(3-*O*-[$\alpha$-L-arabinofuranosyl(1$\rightarrow$3)-$\alpha$-L-arabinopyranosyl]   jujubo-genin)   and   pseudojujubogenin(3-$\beta$-[(O-$\alpha$-L-arabinofuranosyl(1$\rightarrow$6)-O-[$\alpha$-L-arabinopyranosyl(1$\rightarrow$5)]-O-$\alpha$-D-glucofuranosyl)oxy]pseudojujubogenin) which later named as Bacoside A1 (**13**) and A2 (**14**), respectively (Fig. **2**). The structures of these compounds were as curtained and confirmed with the help of different spectral experiments [22, 23].The compound BacosideA3(**10**), a constituent of bacoside A was also isolated and identified by Rastogi *et al.* and the structure was established as 3-$\beta$-[O-$\beta$-D-glucopyranosyl (1$\rightarrow$3)-O-[$\alpha$-L- arabinofuranosyl (1$\rightarrow$2)]O-$\beta$-D-glucopyranosyl)oxy] jujubogenin by chemical and spectral analysis. The *cis*-isomer of already reported ebelinlactone was also obtained as an artifact. The structure of ebelinlactone was revised on the basis of spectral analysis [24]. From the aqueous extract of the plant, two dammaranes triterpenes namedbacosideA4 (**15**) and bacosideA5 (**16**) were isolated and characterized as 20-O-α-L-arabinopyranosyl jujubogenin and 3-O-α-L- arabinopyranosyl jujubogenin for bacoside A4 and bacoside A5, respectively [25]. A combination of preparative TLC and column chromatography of the *n*-butanol fraction of methanolic extract of *B.monnieri* leaves yielded three saponins as bacopa saponins A-C (**17-18 &13**). The acid hydrolysis of bacopasaponin B and C yielded bacogenin A1 which is known as an artifact of pseudojujubogenin. Hence, the aglycon moieties of bacopasaponin A, B & C were confirmed as jujubogenin and pseudojujubogenin. The glycon moieties were identified as arabinose for saponin A and B and arabinose and glucose for Saponin C. The glycosylation shifts were studied to ascertain the point of attachment of sugar units to the aglycon. On the basis of spectral analysis, the structures of bacopasaponin A, B and C were assigned as 3-*O*-α-L-arabinopyranosyl-20-*O*-α-L- arabinopyranosyl-jujubogenin,3-*O*-[α-L-arabinofuranosyl(1→2)α-L-arabinopyranosyl]pseudojuju bogeninand3-*O*-[β-D-glucopyranosyl(1→3){α-L-arabinofuranosyl(1→2)}α-L-arabinofuranosyl]pseudojujubogenin, respectively [26].

Three other saponins named Bacopasaponin D, E and F (**19-21**) were also identified from the butanol fraction of the leaves. Bacopasaponin D is a sugar derivative of pseudojujubogenin, having two sugar units attached to C-3. Bacopasponin E is a jujubogenin derivative with three arabinose units attached to C-3, while in Bacopasaponin F, one glucose and two arabinoses are attached to C-3. As earlier, the identities of the sugar molecules were confirmed by hydrolysis and attachment patterns by comparing the $^{13}$C-NMR chemical shifts. The structures of saponins were established as 3-O-[α-L-arabinofuranosyl- (1→2)- β-D-glucopyranosyl]pseudojujubogenin,3-O-[β-D-glucopyranosyl-(1→3){α-    L-arabinofuranosyl-(1→2)}-α-Larabinopyranosyl]-20-O-(α-L-arabinopyranosyl) jujubogeninand3-O-[β-D-glucopyranosyl(1→3){α-L-arabinofuranosyl(1→2)} β-d-glucopyranosyl]-20-O-α-L-arabinopyranosyl) jujubogenin for Bacopasa ponin D, E and F, respectively [27 - 28].

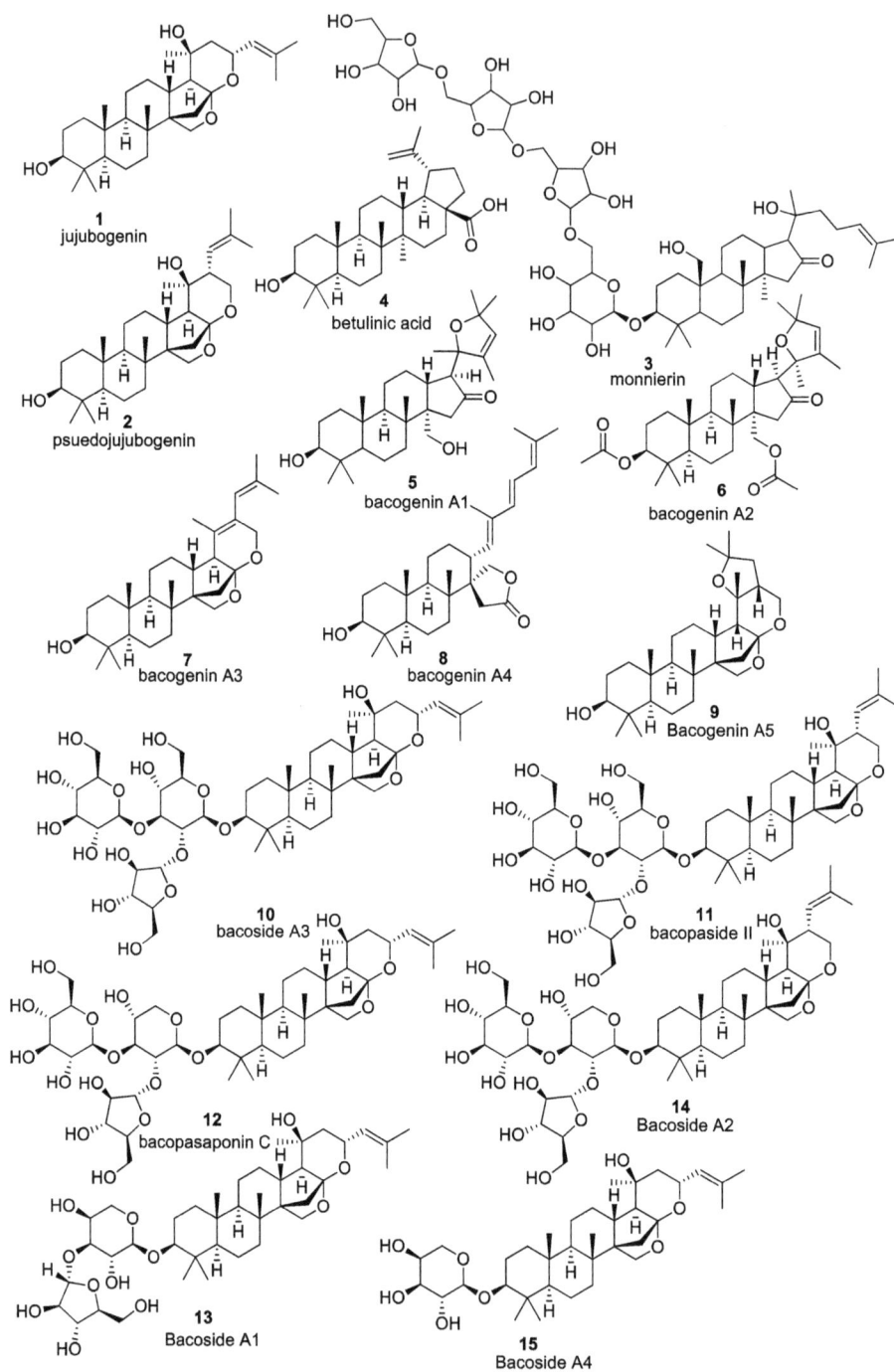

**Fig. (2).** Structure of isolated compounds **1-15**.

The *n*-butanol fraction of methanolic extract of the fresh whole plant was chromatographed over Sephadex LH-20, yielding two saponins as bacopasaponin G (**22**) and bacopaside III (**23**) (Fig. **3**). The aglycon part of bacopasaponin G was identified as pseudojujubogenin with adiglyceride attached to the C-3 position. Bacopaside III was sulphonylated at theC-6 position of glucose attached to C-3. The structure of the aglycon part of both the compounds was established on the basis of hydrolysis products and spectral analysis [29]. Another saponin identified as arabinose derivative of pseudojujubogenin has been isolated from the plant, and the structure was confirmed by chemical and spectral data. The compound was named bacopasaponin H (**24**) and characterized as 3-O-α-L-arabinopyranosyl pseudojujubojenin [30] (Mandal and Mukhopadhyay, 2004). Dang *et al.* [31] reported the isolation and identification of bacopaspon in I (**25**) Fig. (**3**) from the whole plant. The sugar units are attached to C-3 of aglycon confirmed by comparing the NMR signals with reported data of bacoside A3, A6 and bacopaside III. The sapogenin of the molecule was assigned by comparing the literature data of bacopasaponin G. Hence, the structure of the molecule was found to be 3-O-[β-D-glucopyranosyl-(1→3)-O-{α-L-arabinofuranosyl- (1→2)}-O-β-D-glucopyranosyl]-20-deoxypsedojujubogenin [31]. In 2001, Chakravarty *et al.* [9] identified bacopaside I and II (**26 & 27**) and their structures were established as 3-*O*-α-L-arabinofuranosyl-(1→2)-[6-*O*-sulphonyl-β-D- glucopyranosyl-(1→3)]-α-L-arabinopyranosyl pseudojujubogenin and 3-*O*-α- L-arabinofuranosyl-(1→2)-[β-D-glucopyranosyl (1→3)]-β-D-glucopyranosyl pseudojujubogenin by analysis of 2D NMR and other spectral data [32]. In continuation of the search for novel saponins from *B. monnieri*, the group further reported the structures of Bacoside III-V (**28-30**). A literature survey revealed that the asulphonylated saponin previously reported by Hou *et al.* was already named Bacoside III, but the structures of both compounds are different. To avoid the ambiguity, in this chapter, we will address this newly isolated compound as Bacopaside IIIa. A combination of liquid partitioning, normal phase conventional column chromatography and automated reverse phase prep HPLC afforded Bacopaside III-V. High resolution FAB MS and 22D NMR data were examined to interpret the structures. The aglycon moieties of the compounds were ascertained by comparing 13C chemical shifts with jujubogenin and psedojujubogenin while the sugar linkages by 2DNMR data principally, heteronuclear multiple bond correlations. In conclusion, Bacopaside III-V were represented as 3-O-α- L-arabinofuranosyl-(1→2)-O-β-D-glucopyranosyljujubogenin,3-O-β-D-gluco pyra-nosyl-(1→3)-O-α-L-arabinopyranosyljujubogenin and 3-O-β-D-glucopyra nosyl-(1→3)-O-α-L-arabinopyranosylpseudojujubogenin respectively [33]. In continuation of searching for plant-based antidepressants, bacopasides VI-VIII (**31-33**) (Fig. **4**), along with bacopa saponin C, bacopaside I and II, were reported

[10]. Considering earlier described saponins from the plant species, it was speculated that the sapogenin of the compounds was pseudojujubogenin [34].

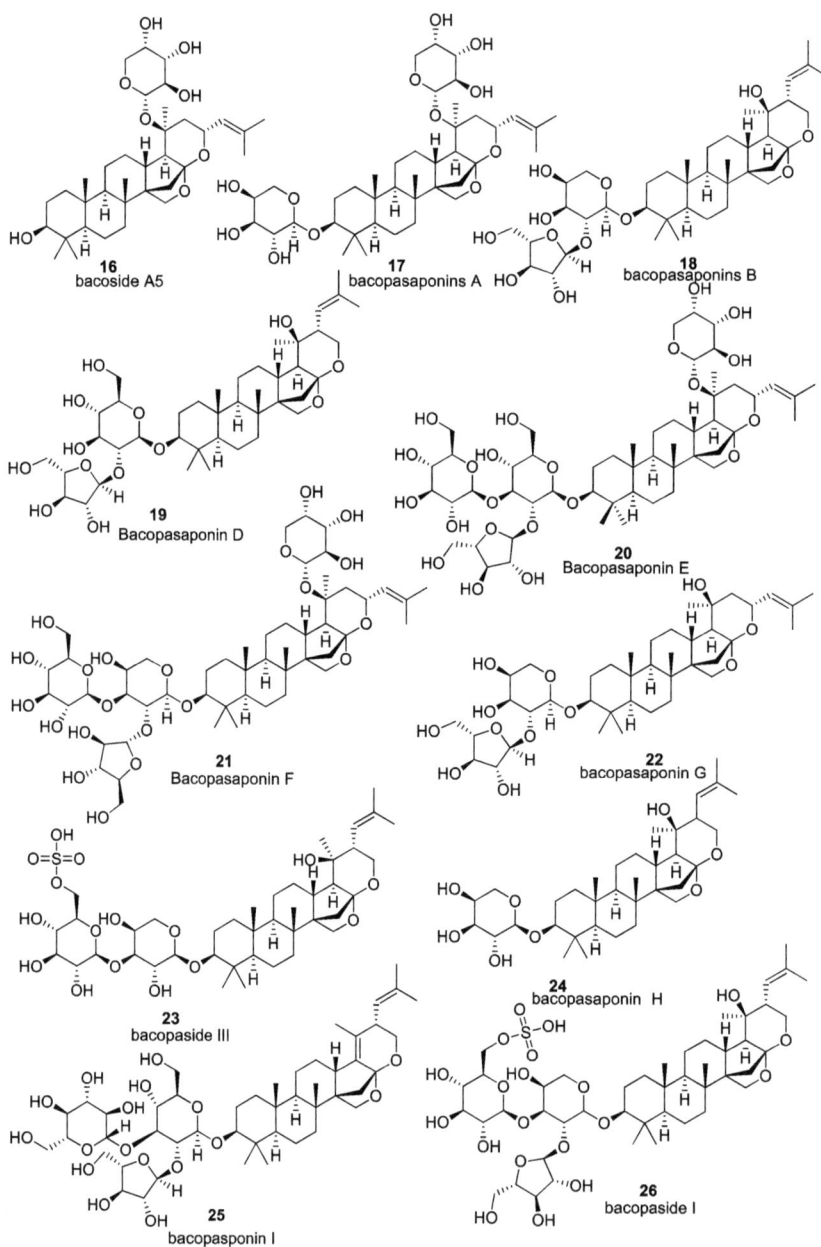

**Fig. (3).** Structure of isolated compounds **16-26**.

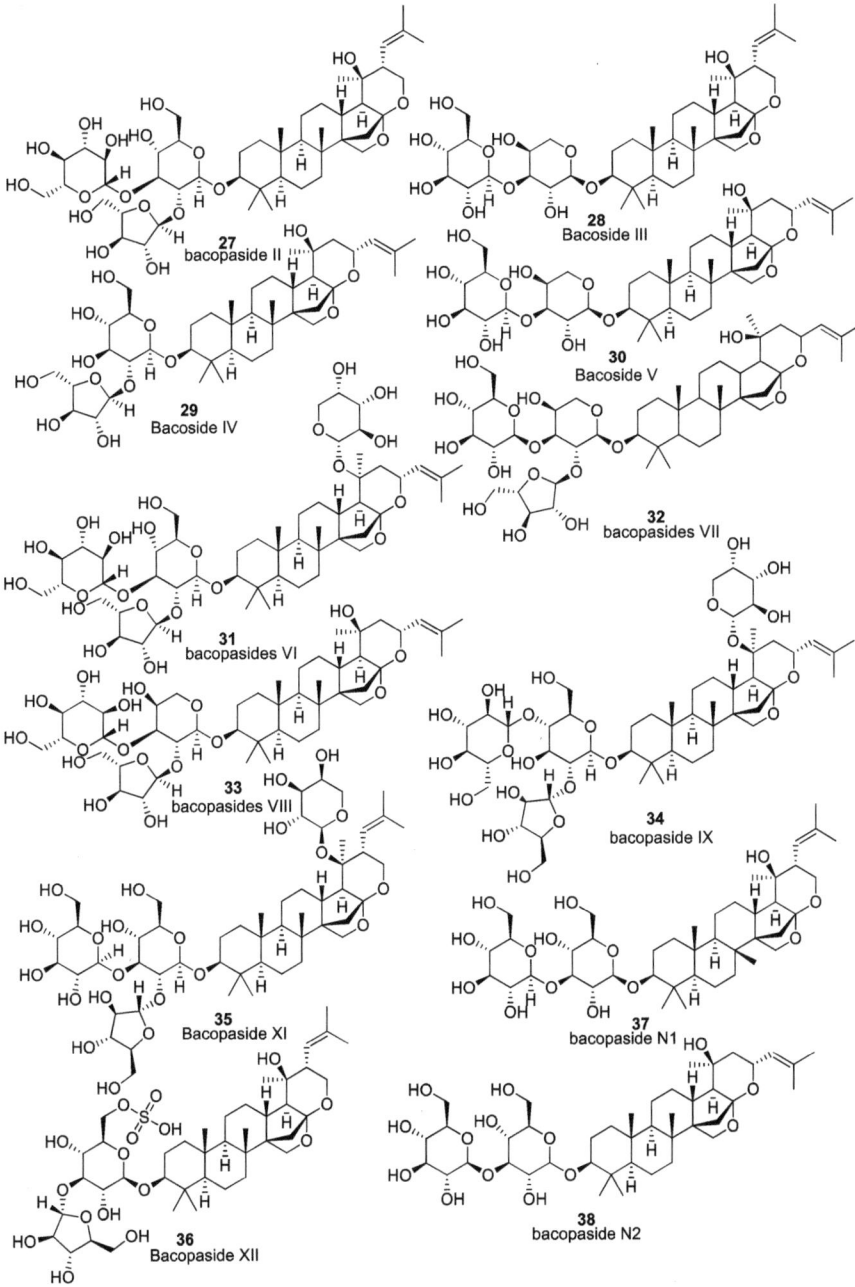

**Fig. (4).** Structure of isolated compounds **27-38**.

Aside from the 13C data of aglycone, eleven oxymethines corroborated the existence of a hexose and a pentose sugar. Acid hydrolysate of the compounds was subjected to GC analysis to identify sugar derivatives revealing the existence of D-glucose and L-arabinose. The loss of 180 amu in ESIMS spectra indicates the loss of a sulfate group. NMR data were compared with those of the known bacopaside V; the two compounds were found to be very similar except for an additional terminal glucose moiety in VI. Hence, these dammarane glycosides, bacopasides VI-VIII, were identified to be 3-O-{β-D-glucopyranosyl-(1→3)- [α-L-arabinofuranosyl-(1→2)]-O-α-L-arabinopyranosyl}jujubogenin, 3-O-[6-O-sulfonyl-β-D-glucopyranosyl-(1→3)]-O-α-L-arabinopyranosyl pseudojuju bogenin and 3-O-{β-D-glucopyranosyl-(1→3)[α-L-arabinofuranosyl-(1→2)]-β - D-gluco pyranosyl}-20-O-α-L-arabinopyranosyljujubogenin along with previously established homologues, *i.e.*, bacopasaponin C, bacopaside I & II, from the whole plant of *Bacopa monnieri*. The structures were elucidated by 2D NMR and other spectral analyses. Sugar molecules were assigned on the basis of hydrolysis products [10]. Later, Zhou *et al.* [10] described bacopaside IX (**34**) was identified as 3-O-{β-D-glucopyranosyl(1 → 4)[α-l-arabinofuranosyl-(1→2)]-β-D-glucopyranosyl}-20-O-α-l-arabinopyranosyljujubogenin through chemical and spectral data [35].Chromatography of the ethylacetate extract of aerial parts of the plant over diaion HP20 resin afforded two triterpenoids. Isolated triterpenoids were elucidated as 3-O-[α-L-arabinofuranosyl (1→3)]-6-O-sulfonyl-β-D-glu copyranosyl pseudojujubogenin and 3-O-{β-D-glucopyranosyl (1→3)[α-L-arabinofuranosyl(1→2)]-O-β-D-glucopyranosyl}-20-O-α-L-arabinopyranosyl pseudojujubogenin. The compounds were trivially named as Bacopaside XI (**35**) and Bacopaside XII (**36**), respectively. Both the compounds were obtained as white amorphous powder. Bacoside XI was a diglyceride with a 6-sulphonylated glucopyranosyl, linked to arabinofuranosyl at C-3 of pseudojujubogenin aglycon. Bacoside XII was a tetraglyceride with two glucose and two arabinose sugars. Linkages were established through spectroscopic evidence [35].

In the quest of delineating the spectrum of pure bacopasaponins and unequivocal identification of bacoside A & B, Sivaramakrishna *et al.* [36] isolated twelve saponins from the plant. Among these twelve saponins, two molecules bacopaside N1 and bacopaside N1 were first report in nature. Besides isolation and identification, the report reveals the identity of bacoside B which was described as the mixture of bacopaside N1(**37**), bacopaside N2 (**38**) (Fig. **4**), Bacopaside IV and bacopasideV with bacoside IV being the major constituent of the saponin mixture [36].

Two acylated dammarane triterpene oligoglycosides, bacomosaponins A and B (**39 &40**), were identified from the whole plant of *B. monnieri*. The identification of the compounds was done on the basis of physicochemical as well as spectral data analysis. It was the first report on acylated dammarane-type triterpene oligo glycosides from *B. monnieri*. Spectral data analysis suggested that the structure of bacomosaponin A was 3-O-{$\beta$-D-glucopyranosyl(1→3)[α-L-arabino furan osyl(1→2)]-$\beta$-D-glucopyranosyl}-20-O-(3,4-diacetyl-α-L-arabinopyranosyl) jujubogenin and bacomosaponins B as 3-O-{$\beta$-D-glucopyranosyl(1→3)[α-L-arabinofuranosyl(1→2)]-α-L-arabinopyranosyl}-20-O-(3,4-diacetyl-α-L-arabino pyranosyl) jujubogenin [37].

Apart from dammaranes, the plant exhibits a wide variety of phytochemicals, including alkaloids, steroids, phenylethanoids, chalcones and cucurbitacins. A literature survey revealed the first report of an alkaloid named brahmine from the plant [38]. After that, nicotine and herpestine were also reported [30]. Subsequent extraction of the plant with petroleum ether and chloroform yielded a triterpene acid. Later this acid was identified as betulinic acid by its acetyl and methyl derivative. Ephenylethanoids and monnierasides I-III (**41-43**), with known analogue plant ainoside B (**44**), were reported from the ethylacetate soluble fraction of defatted methanolic extract of *B. monnieri* [39]. A combination of conventional normal phase chromatography, size exclusion chromatography and reverse phase preparative HPLC was used to separate the chemical entities from the complex mixture. The high resolution FAB-MS and 2D-NMR spectral data, which includes COSY, HMQC and HMBC, led to the structural identification of the eisolates [40]. Four compounds from a different class of triterpenoids, namely cucurbitacins were also isolated and characterized. The compounds were named as bacobitacin A-D (**45-48**) (Fig. **5**). Apart from these novel compounds, a known cytotoxic, cucurbitacin, *i.e.,* cucurbitacin E, was identified through spectral exploration and ESI-QTOF-MS/MS evaluation [41].

The phytochemical examination of aerial parts of *B. monnieri* led to the isolation of an ewsterol 13,14-seco-stigma-9(11),14(15)-diene-3β-ol which was named as bacosterol (**49**). A lupane triterpenoid bacosine was also isolated from the aerial part. The compounds were subjected to NMR, mass, IR and UV analysis and chemical transformation to corroborate the structure as lup-20(29)-ene-3α-ol- 27-oicacid [42]. A 13-14 secosteroid, bacosterol-3-O-$\beta$-D-glucopyranoside (**50**), was isolated as an amorphous powder after chromatography and crystallization of ethyl acetate partitioned fraction. A flavonoid luteolin-7-O-$\beta$-glucopyranoside (**51**) has also been isolated from the same fraction. IR, 1D & 2D NMR, mass and other physical data were investigated to establish the structure of compound **51** [43]. Another report revealed the structure of glucuronyl flavonoids from the stem and leaves of the *B. monnieri*. In glucuronyl flavonoids, the methylene group of glucose oxidizes to carboxyl. Identified flavones were characterized as glucuronyl-7-apigenin and glucuronyl-7-luteolin (**52 & 53**) by chromatographic and spectroscopic analyses [44]. A feruloyl derived phenyl ethylglycoside, 3,4-

dihydroxyphenylethylalcohol(2-*O*-feruloyl)-*β*-D-glucopyran oside (**54**) and a new glycoside, phenylethyl alcohol[5-O-*p*-hydroxybenzoyl-α- D-apiofuranosy- -(1→2)]-α-D-glucopyranoside (**55**), were isolated and identified by chromatographic and spectral analyses [29]. A chalcone was isolated and identified as 2,4,6-trihydroxy-5-(3,3-dimethylpropenyl)-3-(4-hydroxyphenyl) propiophenone (**56**) (Fig. **6**) from ethyl acetate extract and identified through chemical and spectral methods [45]. For comprehensive metabolic profiling, the ethanolic extract of *B. monnieri* was subjected to LC-ESI-QTOF-MS in both positive and negative ionization modes [46].

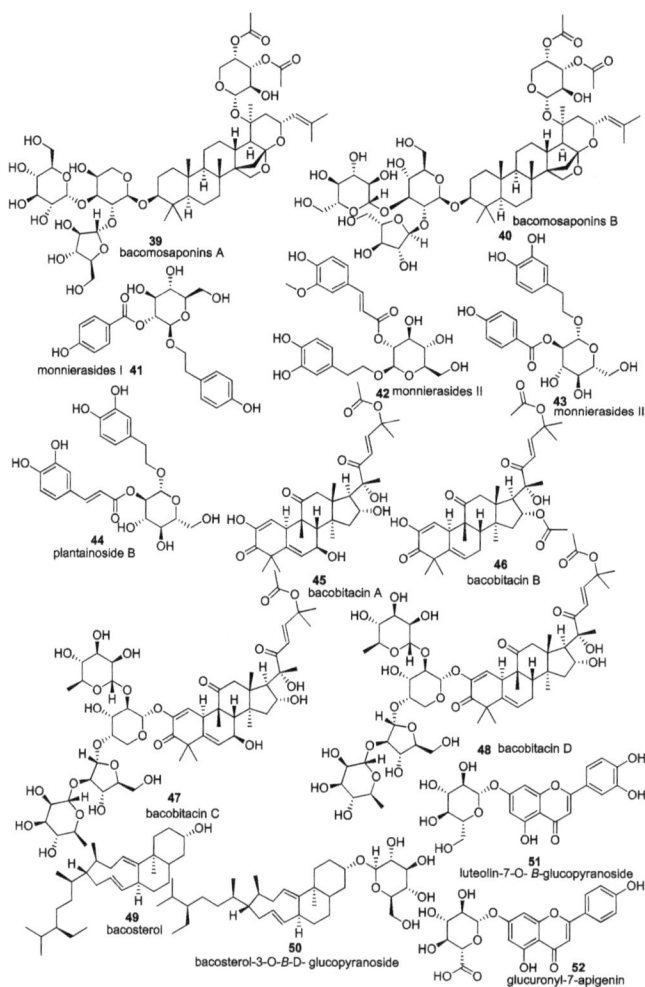

**Fig. (5).** Structure of isolated compounds **39-52.**

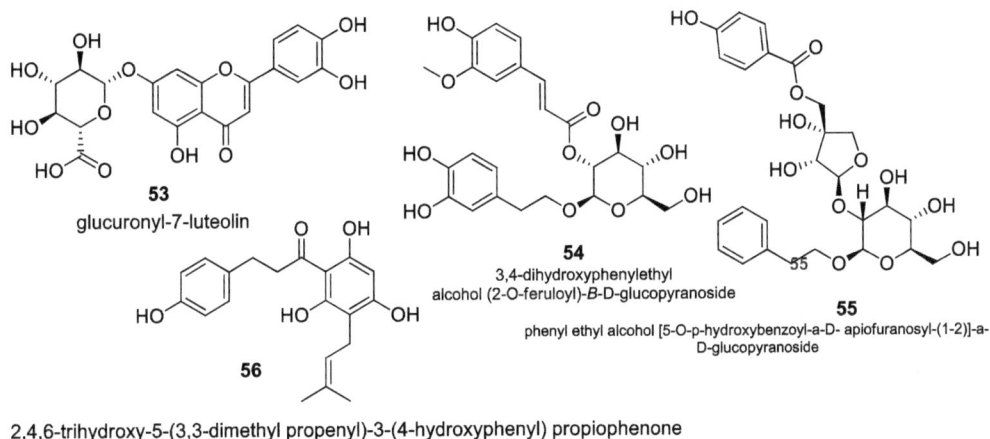

**53**
glucuronyl-7-luteolin

**54**
3,4-dihydroxyphenylethyl
alcohol (2-O-feruloyl)-*B*-D-glucopyranoside

**55**
phenyl ethyl alcohol [5-O-p-hydroxybenzoyl-a-D- apiofuranosyl-(1-2)]-a-D-glucopyranoside

**56**
2,4,6-trihydroxy-5-(3,3-dimethyl propenyl)-3-(4-hydroxyphenyl) propiophenone

**Fig. (6).** Structure of isolated compounds **53-56.**

**Table 1. Extraction and Isolation of Bacopasides.**

| Sl. No | Name | Extraction | PurificationProcedure | Reference |
|---|---|---|---|---|
| 1. | BacopasideN1 | Extracted with 70% methanol under reflux f6r four hours | The extract was dissolved in *n*-butanol and further extracted with EtOAc. The insoluble part was subjected to chromatography over silica gel and reversed phase polymer resin. | [36] |
| 2. | BacopasideN2 | | | |
| 3. | BacopasideIV | | | |
| 4. | BacopasideV | | | |
| 5. | BacopasideA3 | | | |
| 6. | BacopasideII | | | |
| 7. | BacopasideX | Extracted with 70% methanol under reflux f6r four hours | The extract was dissolved in *n*-butanol and further extracted with EtOAc. The insoluble part was subjected to chromatography over silica gel and reversed phase polymer resin. | [36] |
| 8. | Bacopasaponin | | | |
| - | C | - | - | - |
| 9. | BacopasideI | | | |
| 10. | BacopasideIII | | | |
| 11. | BacopasaponinE | | | |
| 12. | BacopasaponinF | | | |
| 13. | BacopasideIII | MeOH Extract by cold percolation | The extract was partitioned by n-BuOH. The n-BuOH part was adsorbed on silica gel, extracted with acetone using Soxhletapparatus. The extract was purified over silica gel and then reverse phase prep HPLC. | [33] |
| 14. | BacopasideIV | | | |
| 15. | BacopasideV | | | |
| 16. | BacopasaponinA | | | |
| 17. | BacopasaponinA | | | |

(Table 1) cont.....

| Sl. No | Name | Extraction | PurificationProcedure | Reference |
|---|---|---|---|---|
| 18. | BacosideA2 | Ethanolicextract | Silica gel and reverse phase C-18 flash chromatography. | [23] |
| 19. | BacogeninA5 | | | [20] |
| 20. | BacopasideI | MeOH extract | The extract was chromatographed over silica gel and eluted with CHCl$_3$–MeOH mixtures. The fractions were subjected to preparative HPLC. | [32] |
| 21. | BacopasideII | | | |
| 22. | BacopasaponinsA | MeOH extract by cold percolation | The extract was partitioned between n-BuOH and H$_2$O. The n-BuOH fraction was adsorbed on silica gel and extracted with EtOAc, Me$_2$CO and CHCl$_3$-MeOH (4:1). | [26, 27] |
| 23. | BacopasaponinsB | | | |
| 24. | BacopasaponinsC | | | |
| 25. | BacopasaponinsC | - | These fractions were subjected to column chromatography on silica gel and similar fractions were further purified by prep TLC followed by crystallization. | - |
| 26. | BacopasideIII | MeOH extract | The extract was suspended in water and partitioned with n-BuOH. The n-BuOH fraction was concentrated and chromatographed over Sephadex LH-20, Diaion HP-20 column, MCI-gel CHP 20P and silica gel. | [29] |
| 27. | BacopasaponinG | | | |
| 28. | BacopasideA | | | |
| 29. | BacopasideB | | | |
| 30. | BacopasideC | | | |
| 31. | BacopasaponinE | MeOH Extract by cold percolation | The n-butanol partitioned fraction of methanol extract was adsorbed on silica gel and extracted with 20% methanol in chloroform. This extraction purification was done by column chromatography reverse phase prep HPLC. | [28] |
| 32. | BacopasaponinF | | | |
| 33. | BacopasideA3 | Ethanolicextract | The ethanolic extract was purified over normal silica gel and flash chromatography. | [24] |
| 34. | Bacopaside-XI | 50% Methanolicextract | The MeOH extract was diluted with MeOH (250mL), kept overnight to precipitate a deep green residue. The residue was filtered and the filtrate was partitioned with EtOA c, and the fraction was subjected to column chromatography on Diaion HP-20. | [35] |

# 3. NEUROLOGICAL PROPERTIES OF *BACOPA MONNEIRI*

Neurological disorders are defined as disorders that affect the brain as well as the nerves found throughout the human body and the spinal cord, including neuronal deterioration, cognitive decline, depression, and anxiety, and have been considered one of the greatest risks to human health. Slow and progressive loss of neuronal cells in specified regions of the brain is the main pathologic feature of Alzheimer's disease, Parkinson's disease, *etc.* [47]. In addition to environmental factors, genetic mutations and brain aging, several cellular and molecular events are also responsible, such as an increase in oxidative stress, impaired mitochondrial functions, deposition of aggregated proteins, inflammatory response, activation of neuronal apoptosis, altered cell signaling and gene expression [48].

*Bacopa monneiri* is an important herb in the management of neurological disorders (Fig. 7). The protective effect of BM over neuronal loss is well documented.

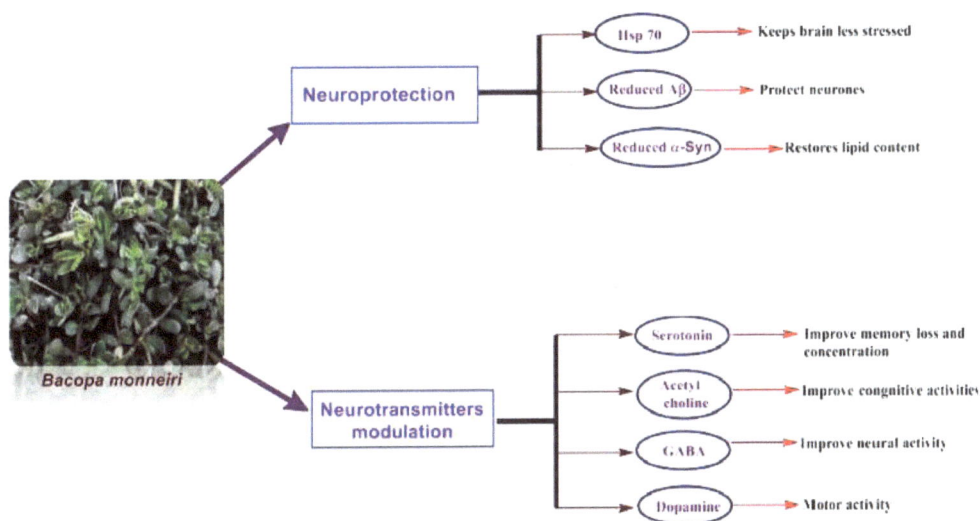

**Fig. (7).** Various neurological properties of *B. monneiri.*

A study was conducted on *in vivo* model; transient 2 vessels occlusion (T2VO)-induced cognitive deficits in mice using oxygen- and glucose-deprivation (OGD)-induced hippocampal cell damage and *in vitro* model for ischemia. In the *in vivo* experiments, mice were treated and administered with a standardized BM extract either orally or intraperitoneally, and in case of *in vitro* experiments, the organotypic hippocampal slice cultures (OHSCs) were incubated with triterpenoid saponins (bacosides) from isolated *Bacopa monneiri*. The BM treatment significantly improved T2VO-induced damages and *in vitro* experiments bacopasideI (25μM) exhibited potent neuroprotective effects against OGD-induced neuronal cell damage. These findings indicate that BM played a role in the neuroprotective effects in the mouse model and in *in vitro* studies [49]. The effect of methanolic extract of BM on toxicity induced by the nitric oxide donor, S-nitroso-N-acetyl-penicillamine (SNAP), in culture of purified rat astrocytes was studied. The extract suppressed the production of reactive species and DNA damage in a dose-dependent manner, thus suggesting its therapeutic potential in cure or prevention of neurological diseases [50].

## 3.1. Anti-Alzheimer's Activity

Alzheimer's disease (AD) is a progressive and irreversible neurodegenerative disorder, which leads to deterioration of memory, disorientation, increased confusion, and other psychological manifestations. The appearance of extracellular amyloid-beta (Aβ) deposits in senile plaques and the development of intracellular neurofibrillary tangles, reactive micro gliosis, and astrogliosis are the significant histopathological characteristics of AD. Crude Brahmi extract and other dammarane triterpene components, bacoside A, bacoside B, baco saponins, were found to be responsible for attenuating the tau mediated toxicity in neurons. Tau is a microtubule-associated protein known to be involved in the progression of Alzheimer's disease [51]. Bacoside A and B repair neurons by promoting kinases activity, synaptic activity restoration and nerve transmission enhancement. U87MG cells were treated with bacoside-A3 before stimulation with $\beta$-amyloid ($10\mu M$) to induce characteristics of Alzheimer's disease *in vitro*. The study suggested that bacoside-A3 prevented $\beta$-amyloid-mediated suppression of U87MG cell viability, and inhibited the generation of oxidative radicals, PGE2, and synthesis of iNOS. Therefore, bacoside-A3 has therapeutic potential for Alzheimer's disease [52].

## 3.2. Anti-Parkinson Activity

Parkinson's disease (PD) is characterized by progressive loss of dopaminergic neurons. It is the second most common neurodegenerative disorder, which affects approx. 1% of the population over the age of 60 years. Since the neurotransmitter dopamine is associated with motor activity, therefore, loss of dopaminergic neurons leads to tremors, muscle rigidity, and bradykinesia. Moreover, PD also affects cognition, mental state, sleep, personality, and behavior leading to depression and anxiety.

*Bacopa monnieri* (L.) Wettst extract (BM) was used to assess the neuroprotective and neurorescue properties in a mice model of 1-methyl-4-phenyl-1,2-3,6-tetrahydropyridine (MPTP)-induced PD. The animals were administered with BM extract at doses of 40mg/kg body weight orally before and after MPTP administration in the neuroprotective (BM+MPTP) and neurorescue (MPTP +BM) experiments, respectively. Neurobehavioral parameters and levels of dopamine, glutathione, lipid peroxide, and nitrites were monitored. BM treatment group leads to a significant decrease in glial fibrillary acidic protein (GFAP) immunostaining and expression of inducible nitric oxide synthase (iNOS) in the substantia nigra region, however, results were more effective in mice receiving BM treatment before MPTP administration. Thus, BM plays both neuroprotective and neurorescue roles against MPTP-induced degeneration of the nigrostriatal dopaminergic neurons [53]. Dopaminergic anti-parkinsonian medications cause complications in the majority of patients with PD. Rotenone (RT) induced rat model of PD was used for testing the cholinergic system. Rats were divided into four groups.

Group 1 received saline water (1ml/kg), Group 2 received RT (2.5mg/kg) through *i.p.* route of administration for 60 days to induce PD. Group 3 received BM extract (180mg/kg/day) for 20 days orally before induction of PD and Group 4 received Levodopa (LD)(10mg/kg/day) orally as reference control. Acetylcholine was decreased and Acetyl cholinesterase was increased in LD and BM treated rats. Thus it is concluded that BM can modulate the cholinergic system; offering an effective treatment against PD [54].

### 3.3. Anti-stroke Activity

Brain stroke is one of the leading geneses of brain injury, and a leading cause of disability and the second leading cause of death in India. In every 40 seconds, one person has a stroke in India, out of which one-fourth of the patients are under the age of 50s. *Bacopa monniera* is a cognitive tonic. It is reported that a surge of free radicals is produced in the course of cerebral ischemia and, at the inception of reperfusion, later cerebral ischemia. Hence, some investigations have been conducted to appraise the role of Brahmi against ischemia and reperfusion induced brain injury. It was demonstrated that aqueous extracts of *Bacopa monnieri* exert neuroprotection against ischemia and reperfusion-induced cerebral injury in mice [55]. Ischemic-reperfusion stimulation leads to increased infarct size and diminished short-term memory and motor balance. Application of Brahmi at the dosage of 120 mg/kg, 160 mg/kg and 240 mg/kg reduced the infarct size and ameliorated primary memory and motor balance in mice. The biochemical screening of this experiment has shown that Brahmi diminishes total nitrite and lipid peroxidation, which corroborates neuro protection through free radical scavenging activity of the plant. Furthermore, Brahmi improved the coordination of muscles and catalase activity in rats [56]. To extend these studies, Kamkaew *et al.* [57] investigated the impact of ethanolic extract of *B. monnieri* on cerebral blood flow. Cognitive deterioration is associated with the cerebral cortex and the hippocampus, which are susceptible to vascular affliction [58]. The study revealed that *B. monnieri* extract increases neocortical blood flow. Although *B. monnieri* causes more effective vaso-relaxation in basilar and mesenteric arteries, the effect is poor on femoral and renal arteries, corroborating that the action is tissue specific favoring the brain [59]. The rats were administered with a dose of 40mg/Kg of Brahmi extract for 8 weeks, and subsequently, the cerebral blood flow was measured. The herb-treated group augmented the cerebral blood flow (CBF) by 25% in rats without affecting the blood pressure. These outcomes ratified the potency of Brahmi in the treatment of neurological disorders [57].

### 3.4. Anticonvulsant Activity

Epilepsy is a sporadic brain dysfunction accompanied by intermittent capricious seizures. Temporal lobe epilepsy (TLE) is a cardinal form of epilepsy. A number of evidences indicate to the sclerotic hippocampus, as the place of origination of chronic seizures in patients with TLE through glutamate excite toxicity. Additionally, glutamate acts as a primary excitatory neurotransmitter in the brain. Many experimental data support that at the seizure focus, the release of glutamate is the mechanism of initiation and regulation of seizures. Pathophysiology of TLE is the imbalance in excitatory and inhibitory synaptic neurotransmission in key brain parts such as the hippocampus, in which fast excitatory transmission is arbitrated by the activation of glutamate receptors like NMD A receptors. Recently, interest has been drawn to herbal drugs and formulations for the treatment of epilepsy. Brahmi is one of the important herbal drugs that alleviate nervous dysfunction, convulsions and inflammation, as well as boosts memory. Hence, to examine the neuroprotective effect of Brahmi, epileptic rats were administered with herbal medication. The results showed that treatment of Brahmi reversed the alterations in binding of glutamate receptor and NMDA R1 gene expression, which is a common feature of epilepsy. Thus, resulting in diminished glutamate-mediated excite toxicity in the over induced hippocampal neurons. These experimental outcomes substantiate the anticonvulsant property of *B. monnieri* at the molecular level. The study established the therapeutic significance of *B. monnieri*, alone as well as an adjuvant, in the management of epilepsy [39].

### 3.5. Anti-depressant Activity

Brahmi accomplishes a surplus of actions in the central nervous system. Besides the treatment of brain dysfunctions, Brahmi shows anti-depressant activity. Shen *et al.* studied the anti-depressant activity of methanolic extract and chloroform, ethyl acetate and butanol partitioned fractions of methanol extract. The activity was evaluated through tail suspension test (TST) and forced swimming test (FST) in mice. The mice were supplemented with 50, 100, and 200mg/kg for 5 consecutive days, and it was observed that methanol extract, ethyl acetate and *n*-butanol fractions reduced the immobility in FST and TST [60].

Brain derived neurotrophic factor (BDNF) is an important nerve growth factor family that is vital to the growth, repairs, and persistence of nerve cells and works *via* axon specific receptor tyrosine kinase (Trk). Lower levels of BDNF are observed in patients with severe depression. Banerjee *et al.*, studied the antidepressant effect of extract of BM having total bacosides at the level of 40.0-50.0%. The molecular mechanism of antidepressant action was investigated by measuring BDNF protein and mRNA levels in the brain tissues of rats. This study revealed that 80 mg/kg is the most effective dosage to produce anti-depressant effects in chronic unpredictable stress (CUS) induced depression in rats [61]. Another study revealed the activity of *Bacopa monnieri* methanolic extract on morphine withdrawal induced depression in mice. Firstly, the phytochemical constituents of the extract were analyzed by using HPLC-UV. The analysis showed the highest content of bacoside $A_3$ in the extract. Mice were introduced to chronic morphine treatments for eight days to induce opioid withdrawal related depression. The mice were dosed at the level of 10, 20, and 30 mg/kg body weight (b.w).The study revealed the impending role of Brahmi in the treatment of depression, which may be attributed to bacoside $A_3$, due to its abundance in the extract [62].

## 3.6. Anxiolytic Activity

Sathyanarayanan *et al.* [63] carried out a preclinical study on a healthy adult human population to test the long-term effect of Brahmi on learning performance, recollection capacity, and anxiety. The study was designed as a randomized, double-blind, placebo-controlled parallel trial. Seventy-two healthy participants between the age of 35–60 years were given a single dose of 450 mg daily. State and trait anxiety were considered as result variables to study the effect. Results revealed that although there was no substantial difference between the administered and placebo groups, the participants who took the dosage of Brahmi showed lower anxiety scores [63]. Another study was performed to evaluate the anxiolytic effect of a standardized extract of *B. monnieri* (BM) with bacoside A content of 25.5 ± 0.8%. The animal model of anxiety was claimed to be an extensively validated model, which includes elevated plus maze, social interaction, novelty-suppressed feeding latency and open-field performances in rats. The rats were given a dose of 5, 10 and 20 mg/kg, p.o. and the outcomes were compared with the effect of lorazepam, which is an established benzodiazepine anxiolytic drug. Lorazepam was used at a dose of 0.5 mg/kg, *i.p.*The results deduced that standardized BM extract produced a dose-dependent anxiolytic effect, comparable to that of lorazepam. However, comparable results were shown by higher two doses of BM, *i.e.*,10 and 20 mg/kg. The findings give firm evidence for the clinical use of the plant as medhya rasayana in Ayurveda. The usage of *B. monnieri* was shown more beneficial than Lorazepam and other benzodiazepine anxiolytics as it possesses additional nootropic action contrary to the amnesic effect of benzodiazepine [64].

## 4. TOXICOLOGICAL STUDIES

*B. monnieri*is an Ayurvedic medicine used for brain health promotion for centuries and considered as safe for therapeutic applications. There are some scientific investigations that have been carried out to investigatethe safety profile of the herb. The study was conducted in rats to assess the safety profile of aqueous and alcoholic extracts of *B. monnieri* in rats given through the intraperitoneal route and found the LD50 of aqueous and alcoholic extracts at 1 g and 15 g/kg, respectively, whereas the aqueous extract given orally did not show any toxicity up to a dose of 5 g/kg [65]. The recommended daily dose of *B. monnieri* is 5-10 g of powder, or 30 ml of syrup or 8-16ml of infusion. In a study of safety evaluation of *B. monnieri* performed on 23 healthy volunteers with 350 mg daily did not show any annoying symptoms in the treated volunteers during pre and post-treatment period [66]. A single dose of this herb at 5000 mg/kg to female rats did not show any severe side effects and toxicity [67]. In healthy old persons, the plant has shown digestive side effects such as nausea, abdominal cramps, *etc.* [68, 69].

## 5. CLINICAL STUDIES

Several clinical studies have been carried out to ascertain the clinical efficiency of *B. monnieri* to improve learning capacity and other cognitive functions. A study was conducted to examine the chronic effects of the extract of *B. monnieri* [70] Stough *et al.*, 2001) *via* the double-blind placebo-controlled method. In a study, 76 adults aged between 40 and 65 years volunteered to investigate the effect of *B. monnieri* on the retention of new information and improvement of memory, and tests showed that the retention rate of newly acquired information was significantly increased as compared to placebo, however, the learning rate and anxiety level were found to be unaffected [71]. A randomized double blind placebo controlled study of the standardized *B. monnieri* extract (CDRI 08) supplementation for the first 16 weeks over male children (6-14 years of age) significantly improved the symptoms of hyperactivity or Attention Deficit Hyperactivity Disorder (ADHD) and also mended cognitive functions [72]. The literature survey evidenced the anti-anxiolytic activity of *B. monnieri* through human clinical trials [73].

## CONCLUSION AND FUTURE PROSPECTS

*B. monnieri* is a highly reputed herb of Ayurveda, and it has been widely explored for its bioactive constituents and pharmacological activities with special emphasis on neuroprotection. The chapter comprises a brief discussion of bioactive chemical constituents, methods of extractions and isolation and their neurological activities. *B. monnieri* contains mainly two types of bacopa saponin, *i.e.*, jujubogenin and pseudojujubogenin. These saponins have a typical glycosylation pattern with $\beta$-D-glucopyranosyl or $\alpha$-L-arabinofuranosyl glycone units directly attached to the C-3 center of the dammarane triterpene units in most of the cases. However, in some cases, the sulphated glucopyranosyl sugar units are also present. The interesting neuroprotective effect of the plant opens up enthralling prospects for future research like formulation development and may offer innovative perceptions in the treatment of different neurodiseases. New formulation development is required to increase the bioavailability of the active constituents of the Brahmi in the brain to improve cognitive functions. Further clinical studies should be conducted to evaluate the synergistic effect of different compounds of the herb rather than considering only bacoside A and B. The structure activity relationships (SAR) should also be developed to generate new leads or formulations for further translational research. This herb possesses huge pharmacological potential and interesting metabolites, which open new dimensions in neurological research.

## ACKNOWLEDGMENTS

The authors are thankful to Director, CSIR-CIMAP, for encouragement and support. We also acknowledge CSIR for financial support in the form of an in-house MLP (DU1/MLP-10) project.

## ABBREVIATIONS

| | |
|---|---|
| **BM** | *Bacopa monnieri* |
| **CNS** | Central Nervous System |
| **HPLC** | High Performance Liquid Chromatography |
| **FAB-MS** | Fast Atom Bombardment Mass Spectrometry |
| **2D-NMR** | Two Dimensional Nuclear Magnetic Resonance |
| **IR** | Infrared Spectroscopy |
| **UV** | Ultraviolet |
| **MeOH** | Methanol |
| **BuOH** | Butanol |
| **T2VO** | Transient 2 vessels occlusion |
| **OGD** | Oxygen- and glucose-deprivation |
| **OHSCs** | Organotypic Hippocampal Slice Cultures |
| **Aβ** | Amyloidalβ-proteinorbeta-amyloid |
| **SNAP** | S-nitroso-N-acetyl-penicillamine |

**AD** Alzheimer's disease

**I.P.** Intra parenteral

**PD** Parkinson's Disease

**iNOS** Inducible Nitric Oxide Synthase

**PGFAPD** Glial Fibrillary Acidic Protein

**CBF** Cerebral Blood Flow

**TLE** Temporal lobe epilepsy

**ADHD** Attention Deficit Hyperactivity Disorder

# REFERENCES

[1]    Russo, A.; Borrelli, F. *Bacopa monniera*, a reputed nootropic plant: An overview. *Phytomedicine,* **2005**, *12*(4), 305-317.
       [http://dx.doi.org/10.1016/j.phymed.2003.12.008] [PMID: 15898709]

[2]    Sharma, P.V.. *Dravyagunavijñāna,Chaukhambha Bhārati Academi.,* **1988**.

[3]    Sharma, P., Yelne, M., Dennis, T., Joshi, A. & Billore, K.. *Database on medicinal plants used in Ayurveda,* **2000**.

[4]    Aguiar, S.; Borowski, T. Neuropharmacological review of the nootropic herb *Bacopa monnieri*. *Rejuvenation Res.,* **2013**, *16*(4), 313-326.
       [http://dx.doi.org/10.1089/rej.2013.1431] [PMID: 23772955]

[5]    Channa, S.; Dar, A.; Anjum, S.; Yaqoob, M.; Atta-ur-Rahman, Anti-inflammatory activity of *Bacopa monniera* in rodents. *J. Ethnopharmacol.,* **2006**, *104*(1-2), 286-289.
       [http://dx.doi.org/10.1016/j.jep.2005.10.009] [PMID: 16343831]

[6]    Kongkeaw, C.; Dilokthornsakul, P.; Thanarangsarit, P.; Limpeanchob, N.; Norman Scholfield, C. Meta-analysis of randomized controlled trials on cognitive effects of *Bacopa monnieri* extract. *J. Ethnopharmacol.,* **2014**, *151*(1), 528-535.
       [http://dx.doi.org/10.1016/j.jep.2013.11.008] [PMID: 24252493]

[7]    Pase, M.P.; Kean, J.; Sarris, J.; Neale, C.; Scholey, A.B.; Stough, C. The cognitive-enhancing effects of *Bacopa monnieri*: A systematic review of randomized, controlled human clinical trials. *J. Altern. Complement. Med.,* **2012**, *18*(7), 647-652.
       [http://dx.doi.org/10.1089/acm.2011.0367] [PMID: 22747190]

[8]    Stough, C.; Scholey, A.; Cropley, V.; Wesnes, K.; Zangara, A.; Pase, M.; Savage, K.; Nolidin, K.; Downey, L.; Downey, L. Examining the cognitive effects of a special extract of Bacopa monniera (CDRI08: Keenmnd): A review of ten years of research at Swinburne University. *J. Pharm. Pharm. Sci.,* **2013**, *16*(2), 254-258.
       [http://dx.doi.org/10.18433/J35G6M] [PMID: 23958194]

[9]    Chakravarty, A.K.; Sarkar, T.; Masuda, K.; Shiojima, K.; Nakane, T.; Kawahara, N. Bacopaside I and II: Two pseudojujubogenin glycosides from *Bacopa monniera*. *Phytochemistry,* **2001**, *58*(4), 553-556. a
       [http://dx.doi.org/10.1016/S0031-9422(01)00275-8] [PMID: 11576596]

[10]   Zhou, Y.; Shen, Y.H.; Zhang, C.; Su, J.; Liu, R.H.; Zhang, W.D. Triterpene saponins from Bacopa monnieri and their antidepressant effects in two mice models. *J. Nat. Prod.,* **2007**, *70*(4), 652-655.
       [http://dx.doi.org/10.1021/np060470s] [PMID: 17343408]

[11]   Dutta, T.; Basu, U.P. Terpenoids: Part II-Isolation of new triterpene saponin, monnierin,from *Bacopa monniera* Wettst. *Indian J. Chem.,* **1963**, *1*, 400-408.

[12] TAPAN. Triterpenoids.II.Isolation of a new triterpenesaponin,monnierin,from *Bacopa monniera.* *Indian J. Chem.,* **1963**, *1*, 408-409.

[13] CHATTERJEE. Chemical examination of *Bacopa monniera* Wettst.PartII: The Constitution of Bacoside A. *Indian J. Chem.,* **1965**, *3*, 24-29.

[14] RASTOGI,R.P.&MEHROTRA,B. *Compendium of Indian medicinal plants,Central Drug Research Institute.,* **1990**.

[15] BASU. Chemical examination of *Bacopa monniera*,Wettst: PartIII BacosideB. *Indian J. Chem.,* **1967**, *5*, 84-86.

[16] Kulshreshtha, D.K.; Rastogi, R. Bacogenin A2: A new sapogenin from bacosides. *Phytochemistry,* **1974**, *13*(7), 1205-1206.
[http://dx.doi.org/10.1016/0031-9422(74)80101-9]

[17] Chandel, R.S.; Kulshreshtha, D.K.; Rastogi, R.P. Bacogenin-A3: A new sapogenin from *Bacopa monniera.* *Phytochemistry,* **1977**, *16*(1), 141-143.
[http://dx.doi.org/10.1016/0031-9422(77)83039-2]

[18] Kulshreshtha, D.K.; Rastogi, R.P. Identification of ebelin lactone from bacoside A and the nature of its genuine sapogenin. *Phytochemistry,* **1973**, *12*(8), 2074-2076. b
[http://dx.doi.org/10.1016/S0031-9422(00)91552-8]

[19] Kulshreshtha, D.K.; Rastogi, R.P. Bacogenin-A1: A novel dammarane triterpene sapogenin from *Bacopa monniera. Phytochemistry,* **1973**, *12*(4), 887-892. a
[http://dx.doi.org/10.1016/0031-9422(73)80697-1]

[20] Rastogi. Bacogenin-A5: Arearranged sapogenin from the saponins of *Bacopa monnieri. Indian J. Heterocycl. Chem.,* **1993**, *2*, 149-150.

[21] Deepak, M.; Sangli, G.K.; Arun, P.C.; Amit, A. Quantitative determination of the major saponin mixture bacoside A in*Bacopa monnieri* by HPLC. *Phytochem. Anal.,* **2005**, *16*(1), 24-29.
[http://dx.doi.org/10.1002/pca.805] [PMID: 15688952]

[22] Jain, P.; Kulshreshtha, D.K. Bacoside A1, A minor saponin from *Bacopa monniera. Phytochemistry,* **1993**, *33*(2), 449-451.
[http://dx.doi.org/10.1016/0031-9422(93)85537-2]

[23] Rastogi. Bacoside A2: A triterpenoid saponin from *Bacopa monniera. Indian J. Chem.,* **1999**, *38B*, 353-356.

[24] Rastogi, S.; Pal, R.; Kulshreshtha, D.K. Bacoside A3-A triterpenoid saponin from Bacopa monniera. *Phytochemistry,* **1994**, *36*(1), 133-137.
[http://dx.doi.org/10.1016/S0031-9422(00)97026-2] [PMID: 7764837]

[25] PAWAR. R.&Bhutani.k.2006.New dammarane triterpenoidal saponins from *Bacopa monniera. Indian J. Chem. Sect. B,* **1511-1514**, *45B*(6)

[26] Garai, S.; Mahato, S.B.; Ohtani, K.; Yamasaki, K. Dammarane-type triterpenoid saponins from *Bacopa monniera. Phytochemistry,* **1996**, *42*(3), 815-820. b
[http://dx.doi.org/10.1016/0031-9422(95)00936-1] [PMID: 8768327]

[27] Garai, S.; Mahato, S.B.; Ohtani, K.; Yamasaki, K. Bacopasaponin D-A pseudojujubogenin glycoside from *Bacopa monniera. Phytochemistry,* **1996**, *43*(2), 447-449. a
[http://dx.doi.org/10.1016/0031-9422(96)00250-6] [PMID: 8862037]

[28] Mahato, S.B.; Garai, S.; Chakravarty, A.K. Bacopasaponins E and F: Two jujubogenin bisdesmosides from *Bacopa monniera. Phytochemistry,* **2000**, *53*(6), 711-714.
[http://dx.doi.org/10.1016/S0031-9422(99)00384-2] [PMID: 10746885]

[29] Hou, C.C.; Lin, S.J.; Cheng, J.T.; Hsu, F.L. BacopasideIII, bacopasaponinG, and bacopasides A,B,and C from *Bacopa monniera. J. Nat. Prod.,* **2002**, *65*(12), 1759-1763.

[http://dx.doi.org/10.1021/np020238w] [PMID: 12502309]

[30] MANDAL. S.&Mukhopadhyay.s.2004.Bacopa saponin H:A pseudojujubogenin glycoside from *Bacopa monniera. Indian J. Chem.,* **1802-1804**, *43B*, 201.

[31] Dang, P.H.; Pham, H.K.T.; Phan, T.H.N.; Nguyen, K.D.H.; Nguyen, M.T.T.; Nguyen, N.T. A New 20-Deoxypseudojujubogenin Glycoside from *Bacopa monniera. Chem. Nat. Compd.,* **2018**, *54*(1), 124-126.
[http://dx.doi.org/10.1007/s10600-018-2273-7]

[32] Chakravarty, A.K.; Sarkar, T.; Masuda, K.; Shiojima, K.; Nakane, T.; Kawahara, N. Bacopaside I and II: Two pseudojujubogenin glycosides from *Bacopa monniera. Phytochemistry,* **2001**, *58*(4), 553-556. b
[http://dx.doi.org/10.1016/S0031-9422(01)00275-8] [PMID: 11576596]

[33] Chakravarty, A.K.; Garai, S.; Masuda, K.; Nakane, T.; Kawahara, N. Bacopasides III-V: Three new triterpenoid glycosides from *Bacopa monniera. Chem. Pharm. Bull.,* **2003**, *51*(2), 215-217.
[http://dx.doi.org/10.1248/cpb.51.215] [PMID: 12576661]

[34] Zhou, Y.; Kong, D.Y.; Peng, L.; Zhang, W.D. A new triterpenoid saponin from Bacopa monniera. *Chin. Chem. Lett.,* **2009**, *20*(5), 569-571.
[http://dx.doi.org/10.1016/j.cclet.2009.01.004]

[35] BHANDARI. Dammaranetriterpenoidsaponinsfrom *Bacopa monnieri. Can. J. Chem.,* **2009**, *87*, 1230-1234.

[36] Sivaramakrishna, C.; Rao, C.V.; Trimurtulu, G.; Vanisree, M.; Subbaraju, G.V. Triterpenoid glycosides from *Bacopa monnieri. Phytochemistry,* **2005**, *66*(23), 2719-2728.
[http://dx.doi.org/10.1016/j.phytochem.2005.09.016] [PMID: 16293276]

[37] Ohta, T.; Nakamura, S.; Nakashima, S.; Oda, Y.; Matsumoto, T.; Fukaya, M.; Yano, M.; Yoshikawa, M.; Matsuda, H. Chemical structures of constituents from the whole plant of *Bacopa monniera. J. Nat. Med.,* **2016**, *70*(3), 404-411.
[http://dx.doi.org/10.1007/s11418-016-0986-0] [PMID: 27010932]

[38] CHOPRA,R.N.N.,S.I.;CHOPRA,I.C. *Glossary of Indian Medicinal Plants*; , **1956**.

[39] Rastogi, R. P. D. Chemical examination of *Bacopa monnieri. J. Sci. Ind. Res.,* **1960**, *19B*, 455-456.

[40] Chakravarty, A.K.; Sarkar, T.; Nakane, T.; Kawahara, N.; Masuda, K. New phenylethanoid glycosides from *Bacopa monniera. Chem. Pharm. Bull.,* **2002**, *50*(12), 1616-1618.
[http://dx.doi.org/10.1248/cpb.50.1616] [PMID: 12499603]

[41] Bhandari, P.; Kumar, N.; Singh, B.; Kaul, V.K. Cucurbitacins from *Bacopa monnieri. Phytochemistry,* **2007**, *68*(9), 1248-1254.
[http://dx.doi.org/10.1016/j.phytochem.2007.03.013] [PMID: 17442350]

[42] AHMED. Bacosterol,a new 13,14-seco-steroid and bacosine, a new triterpene from *Bacopa monnieri. Indian J. Chem.,* **2000**, *39B*, 620-625.

[43] Bhandari, P.; Kumar, N.; Singh, B.; Kaul, V.K. Bacosterol glycoside, a new 13,14-seco-steroid glycoside from *Bacopa monnieri. Chem. Pharm. Bull.,* **2006**, *54*(2), 240-241.
[http://dx.doi.org/10.1248/cpb.54.240] [PMID: 16462073]

[44] PROLIAC. TwoO-glucuronyl flavones in the stems and leaves of *Bacopa monnieri* L.(Scrofulariaceae). *Pharm. Acta Helv.,* **1991**, *66*, 153-154.

[45] Suresh, A.; Sheela, X.Q.R.; Kanmani, R.; Mani, C.; Lalith, E.; Stanley, A.L.; Ramani, V.A.J.A.J.O.C. Isolation and identification of a chalcone from *Baccopa monnieri. Asian J. Chem.,* **2010**, *22*, 965-970.

[47] Available from: https://www.who.int/news-room/questions-and-answers/item/mental-he-lth-neurological-disorders

[48] Solanki, I.; Parihar, P.; Parihar, M.S. Neurodegenerative diseases: From available treatments to

prospective herbal therapy. *Neurochem. Int.,* **2016**, *95*, 100-108.
[http://dx.doi.org/10.1016/j.neuint.2015.11.001] [PMID: 26550708]

[49]    Le, X.T.; Nguyet Pham, H.T.; Van Nguyen, T.; Minh Nguyen, K.; Tanaka, K.; Fujiwara, H.; Matsumoto, K. Protective effects of *Bacopa monnieri* on ischemia-induced cognitive deficits in mice: The possible contribution of bacopaside I and underlying mechanism. *J. Ethnopharmacol.,* **2015**, *164*, 37-45.
[http://dx.doi.org/10.1016/j.jep.2015.01.041] [PMID: 25660331]

[50]    Russo, A.; Borrelli, F.; Campisi, A.; Acquaviva, R.; Raciti, G.; Vanella, A. J. L. S. *Nitric oxide-related toxicity in cultured astrocytes: Effect of Bacopa monniera,* **2003**, *73*, 1517-1526.

[51]    Dubey, T.; Chinnathambi, S. Brahmi (*Bacopa monnieri*): An ayurvedic herb against the Alzheimer's disease. *Arch. Biochem. Biophys.,* **2019**, *676*, 108153.
[http://dx.doi.org/10.1016/j.abb.2019.108153] [PMID: 31622587]

[52]    Bai, Q.K.; Zhao, Z.G.J.B.; Biochemistry, A. Isolation and neuronal apoptosis inhibitory property of bacoside-A3 *via* downregulation of β-amyloid induced inflammatory response. *Biotechnol. Appl. Biochem.,* **2021**, 1-9.
[PMID: 33687113]

[53]    Singh, B.; Pandey, S.; Rumman, M.; Kumar, S.; Kushwaha, P.P.; Verma, R.; Mahdi, A.A. Neuroprotective and neurorescue mode of action of *Bacopa monnieri*(L.)Wettst in 1-methyl-4-phe-yl-1, 2, 3, 6-tetrahydropyridine-induced Parkinson's disease: an *in silico* and *in vivo* study. *Front. Pharmacol.,* **2021**, *12*, 616413.
[http://dx.doi.org/10.3389/fphar.2021.616413] [PMID: 33796021]

[54]    Swathi, G.; Bhuvaneswar, C; Rajendra, W.J.I.J.P.B.S. Alterations of cholinergic neurotransmission inrotenone induced parkinson's disease: protective role of Bacopa, **2013**.

[55]    Rehni, A.K.; Pantlya, H.S.; Shri, R.; Singh, M. Effect of chlorophyll and aqueous extracts of *Bacopa monniera* and *Valeriana wallichii* on ischaemia and reperfusion-induced cerebral injury in mice. *Indian J. Exp. Biol.,* **2007**, *45*(9), 764-769.
[PMID: 17907741]

[56]    Saraf, M.K.; Prabhakar, S.; Anand, A. Neuroprotective effect of *Bacopa monniera* on ischemia induced brain injury. *Pharmacol. Biochem. Behav.,* **2010**, *97*(2), 192-197.
[http://dx.doi.org/10.1016/j.pbb.2010.07.017] [PMID: 20678517]

[57]    Kamkaew, N.; Norman Scholfield, C.; Ingkaninan, K.; Taepavarapruk, N.; Chootip, K. *Bacopa monnieri* increases cerebral blood flow in rat independent of blood pressure. *Phytother. Res.,* **2013**, *27*(1), 135-138.
[http://dx.doi.org/10.1002/ptr.4685] [PMID: 22447676]

[58]    Brown, W.R.; Thore, C.R. Review: Cerebral microvascular pathology in ageing and neurodegeneration. *Neuropathol. Appl. Neurobiol.,* **2011**, *37*(1), 56-74.
[http://dx.doi.org/10.1111/j.1365-2990.2010.01139.x] [PMID: 20946471]

[59]    Kamkaew, N.; Scholfield, C.N.; Ingkaninan, K.; Maneesai, P.; Parkington, H.C.; Tare, M.; Chootip, K. *Bacopa monnieri* and its constituents is hypotensive in anaesthetized rats and vasodilator in various artery types. *J. Ethnopharmacol.,* **2011**, *137*(1), 790-795.
[http://dx.doi.org/10.1016/j.jep.2011.06.045] [PMID: 21762768]

[60]    Shen, Y.H.; Zhou, Y.; Zhang, C.; Liu, R.H.; Su, J.; Liu, X.H.; Zhang, W.D. Antidepressant effects of methanol extract and fractions of *Bacopa monnieri*. *Pharm. Biol.,* **2009**, *47*(4), 340-343.
[http://dx.doi.org/10.1080/13880200902752694]

[61]    Banerjee, R.; Hazra, S.; Ghosh, A.K.; Mondal, A.C. Chronic administration of *bacopa monniera* increases BDNF protein and mRNA expressions: A study in chronic unpredictable stress induced animal model of depression. *Psychiatry Investig.,* **2014**, *11*(3), 297-306.
[http://dx.doi.org/10.4306/pi.2014.11.3.297] [PMID: 25110503]

[62] Rauf, K.; Subhan, F.; Abbas, M.; Ali, S.M.; Ali, G.; Ashfaq, M.; Abbas, G. Inhibitory effect of bacopasides on spontaneous morphine withdrawal induced depression in mice. *Phytother. Res.,* **2014,** *28*(6), 937-939.
[http://dx.doi.org/10.1002/ptr.5081] [PMID: 24243728]

[63] Sathyanarayanan, V.; Thomas, T.; Einöther, S.J.L.; Dobriyal, R.; Joshi, M.K.; Krishnamachari, S. Brahmi for the better? New findings challenging cognition and anti-anxiety effects of Brahmi (*Bacopa monniera*) in healthy adults. *Psychopharmacology (Berl.),* **2013,** *227*(2), 299-306.
[http://dx.doi.org/10.1007/s00213-013-2978-z] [PMID: 23354535]

[64] Bhattacharya, S.K.; Ghosal, S. Anxiolytic activity of a standardized extract of *Bacopa monniera*: An experimental study. *Phytomedicine,* **1998,** *5*(2), 77-82.
[http://dx.doi.org/10.1016/S0944-7113(98)80001-9] [PMID: 23195757]

[65] Joshua Allan, J.; Damodaran, A.; Deshmukh, N.S.; Goudar, K.S.; Amit, A. Safety evaluation of a standardized phytochemical composition extracted from *Bacopa monnieri* in Sprague–Dawley rats. *Food Chem. Toxicol.,* **2007,** *45*(10), 1928-1937.
[http://dx.doi.org/10.1016/j.fct.2007.04.010] [PMID: 17560704]

[66] Pravina, K.; Ravindra, K.R.; Goudar, K.S.; Vinod, D.R.; Joshua, A.J.; Wasim, P.; Venkateshwarlu, K.; Saxena, V.S.; Amit, A. Safety evaluation of BacoMind™ in healthy volunteers: A phase I study. *Phytomedicine,* **2007,** *14*(5), 301-308.
[http://dx.doi.org/10.1016/j.phymed.2007.03.010] [PMID: 17442556]

[67] Sireeratawong, S.; Jaijoy, K.; Khonsung, P.; Lertprasertsuk, N.; Ingkaninan, K. Acute and chronic toxicities of *Bacopa monnieri* extract in Sprague-Dawley rats. *BMC Complement. Altern. Med.,* **2016,** *16*(1), 249.
[http://dx.doi.org/10.1186/s12906-016-1236-4] [PMID: 27460904]

[68] Morgan, A.; Stevens, J. Does *Bacopa monnieri* improve memory performance in older persons? Results of a randomized, placebo-controlled, double-blind trial. *J. Altern. Complement. Med.,* **2010,** *16*(7), 753-759.
[http://dx.doi.org/10.1089/acm.2009.0342] [PMID: 20590480]

[69] Singh, H.; Dhawan, B. Neuropsychopharmacological effects of the ayurvedic nootropic bacopa monniera linn.(Brahmi). *Indian J. Pharmacol.,* **1997,** *29*, 259.

[70] C, S.; P, N.; J, L.; J, C.; C, H.; L, D.; T, R. The chronic effects of an extract of *Bacopa monniera(Brahmi)* on cognitive function in healthy human subjects. *Psychopharmacology (Berl.),* **2001,** *156*(4), 481-484.
[http://dx.doi.org/10.1007/s002130100815] [PMID: 11498727]

[71] Roodenrys, S.; Booth, D.; Bulzomi, S.; Phipps, A.; Micallef, C.; Smoker, J. Chronic effects of Brahmi (*Bacopa monnieri*) on human memory. *Neuropsychopharmacology,* **2002,** *27*(2), 279-281.
[http://dx.doi.org/10.1016/S0893-133X(01)00419-5] [PMID: 12093601]

[72] Kean, J.; Kaufman, J.; Lomas, J.; Goh, A.; White, D.; Simpson, D.; Scholey, A.; Singh, H.; Sarris, J.; Zangara, A.; Stough, C. A randomized controlled trial investigating the effects of a special extract of bacopa monnieri *(CDRI 08)* on hyperactivity and inattention in male children and adolescents: BACHI Study Protocol (ANZCTRN12612000827831). *Nutrients,* **2015,** *7*(12), 9931-9945.
[http://dx.doi.org/10.3390/nu7125507] [PMID: 26633481]

[73] Sarris, J.; McIntyre, E.; Camfield, D.A. Plant-based medicines for anxiety disorders, part 2: A review of clinical studies with supporting preclinical evidence. *CNS Drugs,* **2013,** *27*(4), 301-319.
[http://dx.doi.org/10.1007/s40263-013-0059-9] [PMID: 23653088]

# CHAPTER 6

# Carcinogenicity of Hexavalent Chromium and Its Effects

**Sachin Verma**[1], **Pallavi Kumari**[1], **Shailesh Kumar**[1] and **Ashok Kumar Jha**[1,*]

[1] *University Department of Chemistry, Tilka Manjhi Bhagalpur University, Bhagalpur-812007, Bihar, India*

**Abstract:** Hexavalent chromium has been a potential threat to human beings due to its toxicity and carcinogenesis. The pathway of entry of hexavalent chromium in an aqueous medium is both anthropogenic and natural through ores of chromium. Prolonged exposure to hexavalent chromium may cause DNA mismatch and gene mutation, resulting in cancer. Cr(VI)- induced malignant cell and its study has become very important towards the possible mechanism of Cr(VI) binding. When a cell of the human lungs adsorbs hexavalent chromium due to prolonged ingestion of Cr(VI) contaminated water or inhalation, oxidative DNA damage is caused in the specific gene. This causes mutations in adenine and guanine bases of DNA in cases of lung cancer.

**Keywords:** Cr(VI), Carcinogenicity, DNA, Mutation.

## 1. BACKGROUND

People working in industrial processes of chromium suffer from lung and nasal cancers. The saliva, gastric juice and liver have been associated with the elimination of Cr(VI) from the body. First time people of Hinkley faced cancer of liver, heart, brain, kidney, uterus and gastrointestinal system. A suit against Pacific gas and Electric Company has also been filed for claim. Since then the use of Cr(VI) in the industry was curbed. A few groundwater samples of Naugachia, Koshi region in Bhagalpur district of Bihar, India, have also been found to be contaminated with hexavalent chromium, resulting in cases of liver cancer.

## 2. INTRODUCTION

The aquatic kingdom is very susceptible to the adverse health effects of Cr(VI). Chromium has three oxidation states 0, 3+ and 6+, out of which Cr(VI) is very toxic and carcinogenic [1 - 4]. Hexavalent chromium migrates in an aqueous med-

---

* **Corresponding author Ashok Kumar Jha:** University Department of Chemistry, Tilka Manjhi Bhagalpur University, Bhagalpur-812007, Bihar, India; E-mail: ashokjha39@gmail.com

**Ashok Kumar Jha & Ravi S. Singh (Eds.)**

ium and is reduced to trivalent chromium, which gets precipitated or adsorbed. Cr(VI) is obtained by extraction of chromite ore and finds its way into water bodies through geological and anthropogenic activities, *i.e.,* leather tanning, anticorrosive agent, paints and other industrial activities [5, 6].

Chromium is a d block of 3d series having atomic number 24. Extraction of chromium is done from chromite mineral which is found in large amounts in South Africa, out of a total reserve of 11 billion tons. The use of chromium in stainless steel is very common as an anticorrosive agent. India is also one of the important countries producing Cr from the ore deposit. The processes of mining, grinding, smelting, and refining add chromium concentration to the water. In addition to this, geological factors also increase the concentration of Chromium (III) and Chromium (VI) in groundwater [7, 8]. In the Ferro alloy industry, chromites are also used, thus increasing hexavalent chromium. A comparison of the toxicity of chromium (III) and (VI) shows that chromium (III) is the more common but inert.

The cases of acute chromium carcinogenicity first came to light in 1987 and were published as —Hexavalent chromium – one Town's Story on 7 December 1987. Hexavalent chromium has been detected at a level of 580 micrograms per liter. Pacific gas and Electric company used Cr(VI) as an anticorrosive agent in the cooling towers of the compressor station in the Mojave Desert town of Hinkley. Until 1972, PG and E had knowingly released 370 million gallons of wastewater contaminated with Cr(VI) into the water bodies, which finally polluted the groundwater. Hinkley plaintiffs filed suit for compensation of settlement, and finally, a compensation of 333 million was settled, followed by restrictions on the use of Cr(VI) and cleaning up the contamination. People of Hinkley town have been facing liver, heart, respiratory, cancer of the brain and uterus-related health problems for a long time due to the use of Cr(VI) by PG and E company.

Project on case studies regarding Cr(VI) contamination and the latest remediation techniques have been started in my laboratory since 2008 which is still ongoing. Some liver cancer cases have been detected in place where people use Cr(VI) contaminated water in a particular region.

Almost all compounds having oxidation state of +6 are carcinogenic [9, 10]. Lung cancer has been detected in workers due to prolonged inhaling of Cr(VI) [11]. Prolonged use of Cr(VI) contaminated drinking water causes liver cancer and nasal epithelia [12, 13]. It has been observed that the effect of hexavalent chromium on the stress response plays an important role in carcinogenesis [14, 15]. This may be one of the probable mechanisms. Lung tissues and biopsies of patients having prolonged exposure to Cr(VI) in industries revealed particulate deposits at the bronchial bifurcations [16]. Prolonged exposure of lung epithetical cells to chromate causes an increased risk of lung cancer. The inhalation of particulate Cr(VI) in the air is a potential source of cancer. This is why industries related to chrome plating, leather tanning and extraction of chromium from its ores have become a potential threat to the workers engaged in such industries. A large portion of Cr(VI) gets converted to Cr(III) in the stomach. Chromium may be measured in the urine, serum red blood cells and whole blood. Secondary uses of chemicals having chromium refractory brick industry, steel grinding and welding also increase the contamination of chromium in water, and air workers of these industries have exposure to chromium and face an increased risk of lung cancer, liver cancer and genetic disorders. In many countries, workers in chromate industries have been found to be associated with respiratory tract and gastrointestinal tract problems [17, 18].

The physico-chemical properties of chromium decide the toxicity. Hexavalent chromium generally occurs as $HCrO_4^-$, $CrO_4^{2-}$ and $Cr_2O_7^{2-}$.

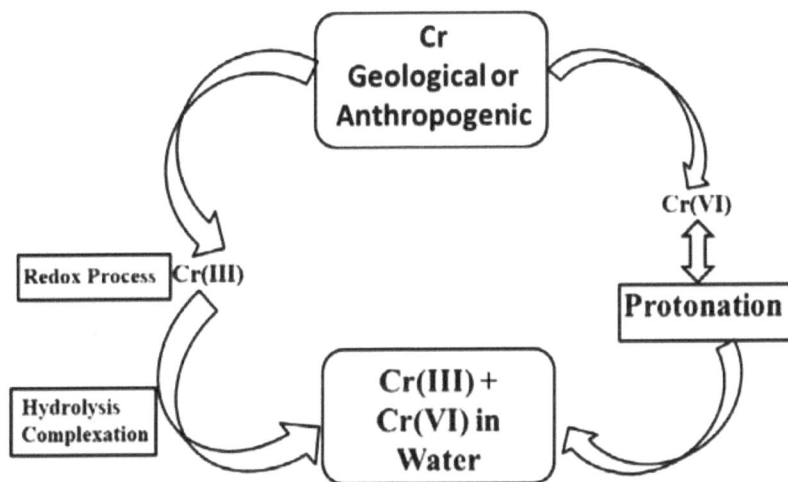

**Fig. (1).** Geochemistry of Cr.

Hexavalent chromium is reduced to trivalent chromium and thus precipitated. If the aqueous medium has a greater content of ferrous ion, the reduction of Cr(VI) to Cr(III) is facilitated.

But $CrO_4^{2-}$ anion is isostructural with sulphate and phosphate ions. Due to structural similarity, they easily move through the cellular membrane, whereas large-sized Cr(III) do not enter the cellular membrane, and consequently, Cr(III) remains inert [19, 20]. If there is an organic matter or ferrous ion, the reduction of hexavalent chromium to trivalent chromium is increased [21]. The hexavalent chromium in an aqueous medium depends on complex formation, redox reactions and adsorption. In an aqueous solution, Cr(III) forms coordination complexes and even chelates with suitable ligands. Cr(III) also forms complexes with niacin, and the common ligands are sulphates, organic acids and halides. The hexavalent form is carcinogenic and changes to a trivalent form when it comes in contact with organic matter. Thus hexavalent chromium moves fast in an aqueous medium [22]. The trivalent chromium migrates only in acidic conditions and remains more or less inert. Thus the migration of chromium ions in water and soil can be understood with geochemistry. Migration in an aqueous medium can also decide the greater toxicity of hexavalent chromium.

## 3. CASE STUDIES OF CANCER CAUSED BY CR(VI)

As per data in the state of Maryland lung cancer death in different age groups under a range of cumulative exposure (mg $CrO_3/$ m$^3$-years), it has become clear that the observed lung cancer deaths in the age group 50-59 and 60-69 are 10 each under the range of cumulative exposure (mg $CrO_3/$ m$^3$-years) 0.00150- 0.0089). The model has been used to examine the cases of lung cancer due to Cr(VI) exposure. The signs of irritation, exposure and working hours have also been taken into account. The ratio of inhalation of Cr(III) and Cr(VI) from air and consumption from an aqueous medium becomes important in view of lung and liver cancer. As per the report of the International Agency for Research on Cancer 1987, causes of lung cancer have increased among workers in chromate production, chrome plating and other related industries.

When biopsy of samples of chromate industry workers was done, deposition of Cr(VI) compounds was found at the bronchial bifurcation [23, 24]. It has been supposed that inhalation of Cr(VI) compounds as particulates are very dangerous because of exposure of lung epithelial cells to chromates [25]. Now it has been established completely that Cr(VI) compounds are highly carcinogenic.

The first suspicion of lung cancer due to hexavalent chromium exposure has been observed in Scotland among chrome pigment workers. In 1980's it has been established beyond any doubt that hexavalent chromium is a strong human lung carcinogen [26].

## 4. DNA REPAIR AND CANCER

In carcinogenesis, genetic mutations take place stepwise and uncontrolled cell proliferation is a cause of DNA damage which in due course converts to malignant cancer cells.

DNA structure may also be altered by environmental factors. Such alterations may also induce permanent changes in the genetic information called mutations. Mutations accumulate in an individual and may lead to carcinogenesis.

It has been established that DNA damage is caused due to the presence of reactive chemicals in the environment by industries, *e.g.,* hexavalent chromium in the environment. These carcinogens in water or air modify bases in DNA and produce cancer. Thus the permanent change or mutations replace one base pair with another. Consequently, abnormal growth of cells takes place and a tumor is formed. The genes which control cell division may get damaged by mutations. Changes in DNA-repair genes increase the rate of mutation, which leads to greater chances of cancer [26]. DNA mismatch repair, defects in gene encoding and recombinational repair are all related somehow to human cancer. In addition, a large number of protons are required for nucleotide-excision repair.

This repair works with DNA polymerase η in normal human cells. When polymerase η activity is lost, the cells become more mutagenic. If other DNA repair systems are absent, mutations increase, leading to cancer.

The effect of Cr(VI) on the lung causes lung carcinogenesis. It has also been reported that Zinc chromate nanoparticles cause interstitial pneumonitis. Inflammatory cytokines such as IL-6 and TNF-α were involved. Cr(VI) may damage DNA as it generates oxidative stress. Cr(VI) undergoes reduction in multi-steps leading to intermediate products and finally Cr(III). Thus Cr(III)-DNA complexes are formed along DNA protein crosslinks. Hexavalent chromium causes damage to DNA by loss of thiol redox control, and this antioxidant defense system is somehow disturbed [27]. During the study of the effect of Cr(VI) on rat lungs, the formation of 8-hydroxy-2-deoxyguanosine has been observed, which shows that DNA is damaged by hexavalent chromium exposure due to the production of oxidative stress [28]. DNA damage also takes place through the interaction of these molecules with Cr(III), giving rise to Cr(III) –DNA adducts. These adducts influence several cellular DNA repair systems through impediments to normal DNA replication and transcription. Mutations in key proteins involved in DNA repair systems have been observed [29, 30].

## 5. PROTEOTOXIC STRESS

A stress response is also one of the important factors in carcinogenesis. Hexavalent chromium on inhalation promotes proteotoxic stress, which activates the cell death pathways. In all cellular processes, proteins regulate accurate folding and assembling. Cells use proteostasis networks to monitor protein homeostasis. Proteostasis networks help synthesis, folding and even start degradation of proteins. Cell deaths due to proteotoxic stress have been proposed to take place through different routes. Activating transcription factor 4 (ATF4) has a very short half-life. This ATF4 is a binding protein of DNA but interacts with many partners. As a result of this, ATF4 controls the expression of many genes which play important roles in resolving proteotoxic stress [31]. ATF4 may promote cell death in an independent manner. These ATF4 proteins may bind to block caspase activities [32, 33].

ATF4 regulates TF, *e.g.,* CCAAT enhancer binding protein is responsible for apoptotic response [34]. Oxidative stress has also been observed during proteotoxic stress [35]. During proteotoxic stress, alternate forms of death can be explained due to the enhanced levels of ROS and calcium [36]. Thus every cell is involved in proteostasis. Proteotoxic stress also enhances neurodegenerative diseases, *e.g.,* Parkinson's and Alzheimer's diseases [37]. Reactive oxygen species (ROS) has been established to be one of the important cellular stresses which damage proteins and start mutations in DNA. In the initial state, a large number of DNA mutations are present, which produce a higher level of mutant protein, finally giving rise to proteotoxic stress. Finally, malignant progression is attained through chromosomal instability and genotoxic stress. There is no doubt that oxidative, proteotoxic and genotoxic stress all are important in the propagation of cancer due to hexavalent chromium [38]. Normal cells cannot survive in such stress situations.

Heat shock proteins (HSP) explain stress response. It has been known that heat shock factor 1 (HSF1) is one of the important transcriptional regulators of the stress response [39]. When HSF1 activity is increased, the HSP level also increases, which results in the loss of the tumor suppressor protein P53 [40].

In eukaryotic cells, unfolded protein response (UPR) functions in the endoplasmic reticulum (ER), which acts as a site for the folding and transport of trans membrane proteins. In the tumor cases, increased ROS levels aggravate the situation. In the case of B cell-derived malignancy, a high amount of immunoglobulins is produced, giving rise to ER stress [41]. When the ER stress becomes chronic, apoptotic pathways are activated due to abnormal calcium signaling from ER to mitochondria [42]. It may be concluded that one of the pathways of carcinogenesis may be due to resistance to mitochondrial and ER stresses [43].

Specific HSP has been found to be instrumental in cancer invasiveness [44]. Due to proteotoxic stress, many proteins mismatch or misfold, and tumor suppressor proteins can prevent such misfolding. The stress response has become important as it protects cells on the one hand, and on the other hand, it has a great role to play in cancer. More study is required to understand well the link between stress response and carcinogenesis.

## CONCLUSION

Due to proteotoxic stress, many proteins mismatch or misfold, and tumor suppressor proteins can prevent such misfolding. Stress response has become important as it protects cells on the one hand, and on the other hand, it has a great role to play in cancer. More study is required to understand well the link between stress response and carcinogenesis.

## REFERENCES

[1]     Jha, A.K.; Kumar, U. Studies on removal of heavy metals by cymbopogon *flexuosus*. *Int. J. Agric. Environ. Biotechnol.,* **2017**, *10*(1), 89-92.
        [http://dx.doi.org/10.5958/2230-732X.2017.00017.1]

[2]     Jha, A.K.; Kumar, U.; Gupta, Y.C. Biosorption of heavy metals by aquatic weeds. *Chemical Science Review Letters,* **2015**, *4*, 827-834.

[3]     Jha, A.K. Adsorption of cr(vi) and arsenic onto bentonite. *Chemical Science Review and Letters,* **2014**, *3*(12), 1182-1189.

[4]     Kumari, K.; Jha, A.K. Studies on concentration of arsenic(iii) and chromium(vi) in ground water resources of naugachia region. *J. Emerg. Technol. Innov. Res.,* **2019**, *6*(2).

[5]     Jha, A.K.; Majumder, S. Removal of cr and mn from aqueous medium using bentonites and their derivatives. *J. Chem. Sci.,* **2020**, 132-135.

[6]     Jha, A.K.; Kumar, U. Estimation of arsenic(iii) and chromium(vi) contamination in gangetic plains of bhagalpur. *IJIRSET,* **2020**, *12*(4), 9-13.

[7]     Jha, A.K.; Dubey, R.K. A modern approach to water pollution. MeenakashiPrakashan: Delhi, **2012**; pp. 44-45.

[8]     Cheryl, P.; Susan, M.B. Environ. health perspect. **2000**, 108.

[9]     Tor, N. The carcinogenicity of chromium. Environmental Health Perspective, **1981**; 40, pp. 121-130.

[10]    Langard, S.; Norseth, T. Chromium In: *Handbook on the toxicology of metals*; Friberg, L.; Nordberg, G.F.; Vouk, V.B., Eds.; Amsterdam: Elsevier, **1979**; pp. 383-410.

[11]    Occupational exposure to chromium(VI). National Institute of Occupational Safety and Health: Washington, D.C., **1975**.

[12]    William Sunderman, F., Jr A review of the carcinogenicities of nickel, chromium and arsenic compounds in man and animals. *Prev. Med.,* **1976**, *5*(2), 279-294.
        [http://dx.doi.org/10.1016/0091-7435(76)90045-1] [PMID: 778825]

[13]    Hong, S; Yuanliang, G; Xin, S; Jinshun, Z; Wang, Y. Carcinogenicity of chromium and chemoprevention: A brief update. *Onco Targets Ther.,* **2017**, *10*, 4065-4079.
        [http://dx.doi.org/10.2147/OTT.S139262]

[14]    Alexander, J.; Aaseth, J. Uptake of chromate in human red blood cells and isolated rat liver cells: The role of the anion carrier. *Analyst ,* **1995**, *120*(3), 931-933.
        [http://dx.doi.org/10.1039/an9952000931] [PMID: 7741257]

[15]    O'Brien, T.; Ceryak, S.; Patierno, S.R. Complexities of chromium carcinogenesis: Role of cellular response, repair and recovery mechanisms. *Mutat. Res.,* **2003**, *533*(1-2), 3-36.
        [http://dx.doi.org/10.1016/j.mrfmmm.2003.09.006] [PMID: 14643411]

[16]  Fearon, E.R.; Vogelstein, B. A genetic model for colorectal tumorigenesis. *Cell,* **1990**, *61*(5), 759-767.
[http://dx.doi.org/10.1016/0092-8674(90)90186-I] [PMID: 2188735]

[17]  Pitot, H.C. The molecular biology of carcinogenesis. *Cancer,* **1993**, *72*(S3) Suppl., 962-970.
[http://dx.doi.org/10.1002/1097-0142(19930801)72:3+<962::AID-CNCR2820721303>3.0.CO;2-H]
[PMID: 8334671]

[18]  Ferreira, L.M.R. Cancer metabolism: The warburg effect today. *Exp. Mol. Pathol.,* **2010**, *89*(3), 372-
380.
[http://dx.doi.org/10.1016/j.yexmp.2010.08.006] [PMID: 20804748]

[19]  Acharya, A.; Das, I.; Chandhok, D.; Saha, T. Redox regulation in cancer: A double-edged sword with
therapeutic potential. *Oxid. Med. Cell. Longev.,* **2010**, *3*(1), 23-34.
[http://dx.doi.org/10.4161/oxim.3.1.10095] [PMID: 20716925]

[20]  Ferreira, L.M.R.; Cunha-Oliveira, T.; Sobral, M.C.; Abreu, P.L.; Alpoim, M.C.; Urbano, A.M. Impact
of carcinogenic chromium on the cellular response to proteotoxic stress. *Int. J. Mol. Sci.,* **2019**, *20*(19),
4901.
[http://dx.doi.org/10.3390/ijms20194901] [PMID: 31623305]

[21]  IARC. Monographs on the evaluation of carcinogenic risks to humans. Lyons, France.International
Agency for Research on Cancer,, **1987**.

[22]  Ishikawa, Y.; Nakagawa, K.; Satoh, Y.; Kitagawa, T.; Sugano, H.; Hirano, T.; Tsuchiya, E.
Characteristics of chromate workers' cancers, chromium lung deposition and precancerous bronchial
lesions: An autopsy study. *Br. J. Cancer,* **1994**, *70*(1), 160-166.
[http://dx.doi.org/10.1038/bjc.1994.268] [PMID: 8018529]

[23]  Ishikawa, Y.; Nakagawa, K.; Satoh, Y.; Kitagawa, T.; Sugano, H.; Hirano, T.; Tsuchiya, E. *Hot spots*
of chromium accumulation at bifurcations of chromate workers' bronchi. *Cancer Res.,* **1994**, *54*(9),
2342-2346.
[PMID: 8162579]

[24]  Yatera, K.; Morimoto, Y.; Ueno, S.; Noguchi, S.; Kawaguchi, T.; Tanaka, F.; Suzuki, H.; Higashi, T.
Cancer risks of hexavalent chromium in the respiratory tract. *J. UOEH,* **2018**, *40*(2), 157-172.
[http://dx.doi.org/10.7888/juoeh.40.157] [PMID: 29925735]

[25]  Kondo, K.; Takahashi, Y.; Ishikawa, S.; Uchihara, H.; Hirose, Y.; Yoshizawa, K.; Tsuyuguchi, M.;
Takizawa, H.; Miyoshi, T.; Sakiyama, S.; Monden, Y. Microscopic analysis of chromium
accumulation in the bronchi and lung of chromate workers. *Cancer,* **2003**, *98*(11), 2420-2429.
[http://dx.doi.org/10.1002/cncr.11818] [PMID: 14635077]

[26]  Gibb, H.J.; Lees, P.S.J.; Pinsky, P.F.; Rooney, B.C. Lung cancer among workers in chromium
chemical production. *Am. J. Ind. Med.,* **2000**, *38*(2), 115-126.
[http://dx.doi.org/10.1002/1097-0274(200008)38:2<115::AID-AJIM1>3.0.CO;2-Y]              [PMID:
10893504]

[27]  Abreu, P.L.; Ferreira, L.M.R.; Alpoim, M.C.; Urbano, A.M. Impact of hexavalent chromium on
mammalian cell bioenergetics: Phenotypic changes, molecular basis and potential relevance to
chromate-induced lung cancer. *Biometals,* **2014**, *27*(3), 409-443.
[http://dx.doi.org/10.1007/s10534-014-9726-7] [PMID: 24664226]

[28]  Dubrovskaya, V.; Wetterhahn, K.E. Effects of Cr(VI) on the expression of the oxidative stress genes in
human lung cells. *Carcinogenesis,* **1998**, *19*(8), 1401-1407.
[http://dx.doi.org/10.1093/carcin/19.8.1401] [PMID: 9744536]

[29]  O'Brien, T.J.; Brooks, B.R.; Patierno, S.R. Nucleotide excision repair functions in the removal of
chromium-induced DNA damage in mammalian cells. *Mol. Cell. Biochem.,* **2005**, *279*(1-2), 85-95.
[http://dx.doi.org/10.1007/s11010-005-8225-0] [PMID: 16283517]

[30]  Xie, H.; Wise, S.S.; Holmes, A.L.; Xu, B.; Wakeman, T.P.; Pelsue, S.C.; Singh, N.P.; Wise, J.P., Sr
Carcinogenic lead chromate induces DNA double-strand breaks in human lung cells. *Mutat. Res.*

*Genet. Toxicol. Environ. Mutagen.,* **2005**, *586*(2), 160-172.
[http://dx.doi.org/10.1016/j.mrgentox.2005.06.002] [PMID: 16112599]

[31]    Pitale, P.M.; Gorbatyuk, O.; Gorbatyuk, M. Neurodegeneration: Keeping ATF4 on a tight leash. *Front. Cell. Neurosci.,* **2017**, *11*, 410.
[http://dx.doi.org/10.3389/fncel.2017.00410] [PMID: 29326555]

[32]    Rzymski, T.; Milani, M.; Singleton, D.C.; Harris, A.L. Role of ATF4 in regulation of autophagy and resistance to drugs and hypoxia. *Cell Cycle,* **2009**, *8*(23), 3838-3847.
[http://dx.doi.org/10.4161/cc.8.23.10086] [PMID: 19887912]

[33]    Wang, Q.; Mora-Jensen, H.; Weniger, M.A.; Perez-Galan, P.; Wolford, C.; Hai, T.; Ron, D.; Chen, W.; Trenkle, W.; Wiestner, A.; Ye, Y. ERAD inhibitors integrate ER stress with an epigenetic mechanism to activate BH3-only protein NOXA in cancer cells. *Proc. Natl. Acad. Sci.,* **2009**, *106*(7), 2200-2205.
[http://dx.doi.org/10.1073/pnas.0807611106] [PMID: 19164757]

[34]    Cnop, M; Toivonen, S; Igoillo-Esteve, M; Salpea, P. Endoplasmic reticulum stress and eIF2α phosphorylation: The Achilles heel of pancreatic β cells. *Mol Metab,* **2017**, *6*(9), 1024-1039.
[http://dx.doi.org/10.1016/j.molmet.2017.06.001]

[35]    Ciotti, S.; Iuliano, L.; Cefalù, S.; Comelli, M.; Mavelli, I.; Di Giorgio, E.; Brancolini, C. GSK3β is a key regulator of the ROS-dependent necrotic death induced by the quinone DMNQ. *Cell Death Dis.,* **2020**, *11*(1), 2.
[http://dx.doi.org/10.1038/s41419-019-2202-0] [PMID: 31919413]

[36]    Vanlangenakker, N.; Berghe, T.; Krysko, D.; Festjens, N.; Vandenabeele, P. Molecular mechanisms and pathophysiology of necrotic cell death. *Curr. Mol. Med.,* **2008**, *8*(3), 207-220.
[http://dx.doi.org/10.2174/156652408784221306] [PMID: 18473820]

[37]    Jones, C.L.; Tepe, J.J. Proteosome activation to combat proteotoxicity. *Molecules,* **2019**, *24*(15), 2841.
[http://dx.doi.org/10.3390/molecules24152841] [PMID: 31387243]

[38]    Csermely, P.; Schnaider, T.; Soti, C.; Prohászka, Z.; Nardai, G. The 90-kDa molecular chaperone family: Structure, function, and clinical applications. A comprehensive review. *Pharmacol. Ther.,* **1998**, *79*(2), 129-168.
[http://dx.doi.org/10.1016/S0163-7258(98)00013-8] [PMID: 9749880]

[39]    Lindquist, S. The heat-shock response. *Annu. Rev. Biochem.,* **1986**, *55*(1), 1151-1191.
[http://dx.doi.org/10.1146/annurev.bi.55.070186.005443] [PMID: 2427013]

[40]    Whitesell, L.; Lindquist, S. Inhibiting the transcription factor HSF1 as an anticancer strategy. *Expert Opin. Ther. Targets,* **2009**, *13*(4), 469-478.
[http://dx.doi.org/10.1517/14728220902832697] [PMID: 19335068]

[41]    Obeng, E.A.; Carlson, L.M.; Gutman, D.M.; Harrington, W.J., Jr; Lee, K.P.; Boise, L.H. Proteasome inhibitors induce a terminal unfolded protein response in multiple myeloma cells. *Blood,* **2006**, *107*(12), 4907-4916.
[http://dx.doi.org/10.1182/blood-2005-08-3531] [PMID: 16507771]

[42]    Carreras-Sureda, A.; Pihán, P.; Hetz, C. The unfolded protein response: At the intersection between endoplasmic reticulum function and mitochondrial bioenergetics. *Front. Oncol.,* **2017**, *7*, 55.
[http://dx.doi.org/10.3389/fonc.2017.00055] [PMID: 28421160]

[43]    Hsu, C.C.; Tseng, L.M.; Lee, H.C. Role of mitochondrial dysfunction in cancer progression. *Exp. Biol. Med. ,* **2016**, *241*(12), 1281-1295.
[http://dx.doi.org/10.1177/1535370216641787] [PMID: 27022139]

[44]    Oesterreich, S.; Weng, C.N.; Qiu, M.; Hilsenbeck, S.G.; Osborne, C.K.; Fuqua, S.A. The small heat shock protein hsp27 is correlated with growth and drug resistance in human breast cancer cell lines. *Cancer Res.,* **1993**, *53*(19), 4443-4448.
[PMID: 8402609]

# CHAPTER 7

# Medicinal Plants: A Future of Modern Medical System

**Aakansha Singh**[1] and **Anjani Kumar**[2,*]

[1] *Department of Bioengineering and Biotechnology, Birla Institute of Technology, Mesra, Ranchi-835215, Jharkhand, India*

[2] *ICAR-RCER, Farming System Research Centre for Hill & Plateau Region, Ranchi-834010, Jharkhand, India*

**Abstract:** Humans, since their evolution, have always been in close contact with mother nature. Early life has been dependent solely on environmental resources for their livelihood. The trial-and-error approach in utilizing different resources came up with incorporating plants as a whole or their parts for food and survival. Gradually, the knowledge of medicinal plants was gained by our ancestors, and there started the Indian medical history of Ayurveda. In the current scenario, a huge number of medicinal herbs are being consumed in day-to-day life, which imparts tremendous benefits to human health. Our interest in gaining knowledge of medicinal components present in these herbs has led to many important discoveries in the area of drug development. Nowadays, numerous plants derived compounds are being used in modern medicines. In view of utilizing these natural resources efficiently, we need to understand their components in a better way. This chapter is towards gaining a deeper knowledge about medicinal plants, their role in different diseases, and insights into drug discovery.

**Keywords:** Bioactive compound, Medicinal plants.

## 1. INTRODUCTION

The co-existence of humans and plants has established ages ago, and plants have always played a pivotal role in human life. From consuming plants as a food source to utilizing them in curing several diseases, we have evolved our knowledge at an accelerating pace. Primitive man, in search of sustenance and to alleviate human misery, began to identify plants that were suitable for medicinal purposes, having some pharmacological qualities. This relationship between humans and plants bloomed, and a plethora of medicinal plants came into use. In

* **Corresponding author Anjani kumar:** IICAR-RCER, Farming System Research Centre for Hill & Plateau Region, Ranchi-834010, Jharkhand, India; E-mail: anjani0039@gmail.com

**Ashok Kumar Jha & Ravi S. Singh (Eds.)**

terms of therapeutic herbs, Mother Nature has blessed our land abundantly. In the Eastern Himalayan areas, the Western Ghats, and the Andaman and Nicobar Islands, India has a concentrated hotspot of medicinal plants [1]. This is the reason why India is often regarded as a hub for medicinal plants. The clinical use of a huge number of medicinal plants has been reported in Indian Vedas and was used by our ancestors in treating diseases. Several herbs and plants, including species, are consumed by us regularly to enhance our immunity. Scientists are keenly interested in understanding the pharmacology of the biologically active compounds of these herbs. In the 21$^{st}$ century, we have many herbal-compound-based medicines in treating a large spectrum of diseases, and the discoveries are still on. From treating most common disorders like diabetes to treating deadly diseases like cancer, medicinal plants are contributing a major portion all over the world. With evolving knowledge of science and technology, researchers are trying to set a benchmark for the use of medicinal plants and their bioactive compounds. Concepts like herbal drug designing and chemo-informatics have become more common in the field of drug discovery.

## 2. TRADITIONAL MEDICAL SYSTEM

Ayurveda, or "Science of Life," is an ancient Indian medical system that dates back around 5000 years. Ayurveda was practiced in India's medical system during the Vedic period. During the first millennium BC, the CharakaSamhita and SushrutaSamhita list roughly 700 plant species. This medicinal system is widely used as a supplemental medicine in many parts of the world. India's Ayurveda attempts to preserve, promote and sustain human health and wellbeing. Studies report the use of over 7500 different plant species as medicine in tribal and rural areas of India [2]. Herbal products account for nearly half of all medications that are in clinical use in the 21$^{st}$ century, either directly or as purified components. Through its global network, India's ancient medical system AYUSH (Ayurveda, Yoga, Unani, Siddha, and Homeopathy) is moving forward to revolutionize the healthcare sector [1].

## 3. WHAT ARE MEDICINAL PLANTS?

Medicinal plants are plants containing chemicals in different organs which can be utilized for therapeutic reasons or are precursors to manufacture valuable pharmaceuticals. Information about their constituents makes it simpler to distinguish between medicinal plants whose therapeutic and chemical functions have been scientifically established and those that are considered medicinal but have not been exposed to scientific study. Numerous plants have been used in traditional medicines, some of them are effective against diseases but do not have any scientific reporting [3]. These plant or their extract need to qualify as medical plants. According to Sofowora & Evans (2008), for categorizing plants as medicinal ones, they should fall under the following categories:

• Microscopic plants, like fungi, actinomycetes, *etc.,* used in drug formulations, mostly antibiotics. For example, *Streptomyces griseus* and ergot.

• Plants or their extracts that have direct medicinal use or their Hemi- synthetic formulations as medicinal compounds. For example, diosgenin, used for the hemi synthesis of sex hormones.

• Spices, food, and perfumery plants used for medical purposes like ginger.

## 4. ENVIRONMENTAL FACTORS AND SECONDARY METABOLITE PRODUCTION

Plants are thought to be a living chemical factory that creates a wide range of secondary metabolites (SMs), which are the foundation for many commercial pharmaceutical medications and herbal therapies derived from medicinal plants. Various compounds found in these plants have biological activities that benefit human health. Metabolites like alkaloids, terpenes, polyphenols, *etc.,* are some of the vital chemicals that are considered well for drug development [4]. Before going deep into how plants regulate secondary metabolite production, we need to get a brief of some terms used in advanced science these days. The first is the metabolome, which is used to define all of a cell's tiny components and is the fourth most important term in the "systems" approach to biology. Genomic (DNA), transcriptomics (RNA), and proteomics (protein) are the other three. In this context, secondary metabolites are a subgroup of the metabolome produced by plants, distinct from primary metabolites such as glycolysis intermediates and TCA cycle intermediates, which are vital in development and growth. A technique called mass spectroscopy has emerged to be the workhouse of recent studies that aim to identify and quantify metabolome [5].

Thousands of SMs exist in the plant kingdom; however, they are confined to specific taxonomic levels. SM synthesis is usually tightly controlled and restricted to specific tissues, organs, or developmental phases. The production of SMEs, which are important for adaptive responses, mediates the chemical interaction between the environment and plants. Abiotic and biotic stresses influence how plants interact with their environment to survive, which leads to the production of a variety of SMs. These stresses redirect the plant's primary metabolism and help in increased enzymatic activity and SMs production (Fig. **1**).

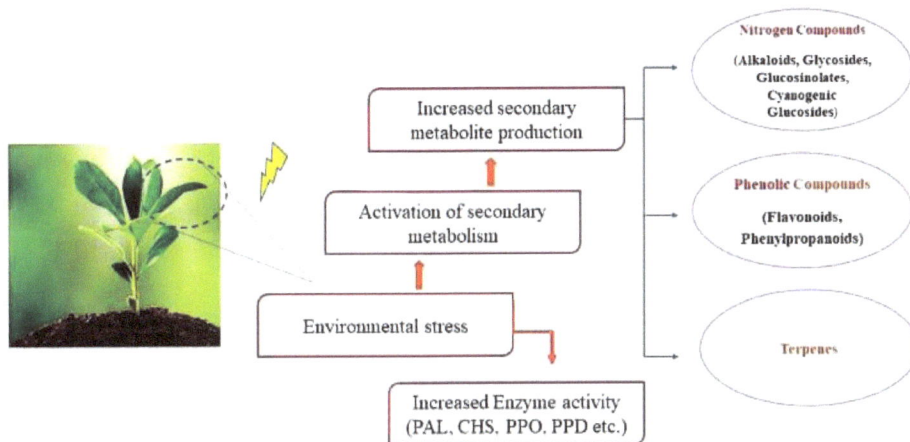

**Fig. (1).** Representation of the mechanism plant during environmental stresses (Adopted and modified from Ghorbunpour *et al.* 2017).

Nitrogen compounds (alkaloids, glycosides, glucosinolates, and cyanogenic glycosides), phenolic compounds (phenylpropanoids and flavonoids), and terpenes are the three primary types of SMs based on their metabolic pathways. Although the precursor molecules in SMs vary in structure, they all come from basic metabolic processes. The Calvin cycle and the pentose phosphate pathway, for example, give carbon skeleton for erythrose-5-phosphate, which is then converted to shikimate. The shikimic acid, mevalonate, and non-mevalonate pathways produce a variety of compounds that are classified as terpenes, flavonoids, alkaloids, and anthocyanins. In plants, amino acids are the precursor molecules for a range of SMs. The aliphatic SMs are produced from amino acids, like leucine, isoleucine, alanine, methionine, and valine. While the aromatic SMs are produced from precursor-like tyrosine, phenylalanine, and tryptophan (Fig. **2**). Aromatic amino acids are most likely the primary precursor for the production of SMs in plants. Alkaloids, glycosides, phytoalexins, and indole glucosinolates are all made up of tryptophan. Alkaloids, quinones, and isoquinoline are all precursors to tyrosine, while flavonoids, phenylpropanoids, and condensed tannins are all precursors to phenylalanine. We will go through some of the most important plant metabolites here [6].

## 4.1. Alkaloids

Alkaloids are organic compounds with heterocyclic rings and at least one nitrogen atom in them [7]. These are primarily found in plants and notably flowering plants and medicinal plants. The most common alkaloids found in plants are morphine, nicotine, strychnine, quinine, ephedrine, *etc.* In their pure form, these compounds are crystalline, colourless, and non-volatile solids. They have a diverse medicinal property, morphine is considered a strong narcotic and helps relieve pain. A drug like lobeline is clinically used in the treatment of respiratory disorders. Ergonovine, another alkaloid is used in reducing uterine hemorrhage during childbirth.

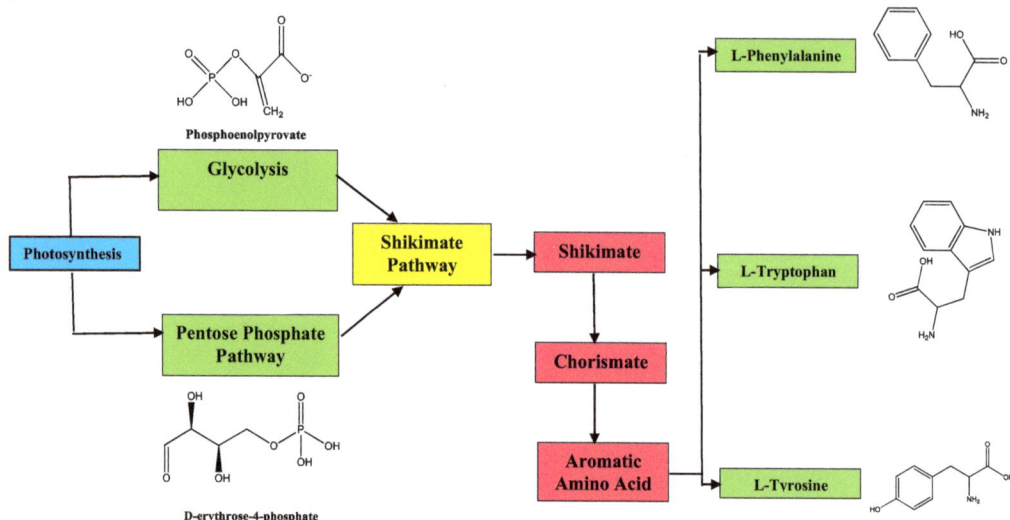

**Fig. (2).** Schematic representation of aromatic amino acid derived SMs in plants (Adopted & modified from Borges *et al.* 2017).

## 4.2. Flavonoids

Flavonoids are plant metabolites that have a wide range of health advantages and are effective antioxidants. These are water-soluble polyphenolic compounds with 15 carbon atoms. Flavones, chalcones, isoflavonoids, flavanones, anthocyanins, and anthoxanthins are the six major subgroups of these metabolites. Pigmentation in plant parts is mainly caused by anthocyanins and anthoxanthins. Flavonoids are plant metabolites with immense health benefits and are potent anti-oxidants. These flavonoids are found in abundance in plants and perform several functions like nitrogen fixation, UV fixation, and cell cycle inhibition and act as chemical messengers [8]. Flavonoids have relatively low toxicity in comparison to any other plant compounds and hence can be consumed in large quantities. Taking about their health benefits, these compounds show antiviral, antioxidant, anti-inflammatory and anti-cancer properties. Studies suggest flavonoids help in decreasing the risk of cardiac disease and act as a chemopreventive agent against cancer. Quercetin is a flavonoid that is useful in the treatment of asthma, sinusitis, and eczema. Flavonoids are prominently present in fruits, vegetables, dried beans, red wine, black coffee, green tea, *etc.* It is said that the more colourful a food item is, the higher the flavonoid content is.

## 4.3. Terpenes

Terpenes are aromatic compounds present in plants and show a characteristic aroma. The concentration of terpenes is found to be abundant in cannabis. Plants show certain fragrances because of a combination of different terpenes. These terpenes protect plants against grazers and infectious organisms. Because of their high concentration in cannabis, research is focused on their possible benefits. Terpenes are mainly categorized as limonene, pinene, linalool, myrcene, humulene, *etc.* Terpenes show some notable therapeutic properties like anticancer, antiviral, antidiabetic, antianxiety, neuroprotective, and antidepressant [9]. The common plant source for terpenes is cannabis, spinach sages, tea, thyme, citrus fruits, and many more. Curcumin, a terpene, generally holds antiplasmodial, antiseptic, astringent, and antiviral properties. Terpenes have also been found to act as an antimalarial agent, and their mode of action is similar to the drug chloroquine.

## 5. BIOACTIVE COMPOUNDS

Bioactive components are usually referred to as the chemical components present in plants or their products and have a direct or indirect impact on human health. Usually, these chemical compounds are present in a small quantities and confer various therapeutic benefits, including antimicrobial, antiviral, anticancer, and antiparasitic activities. Traditionally, plant extracts were used to cure many diseases. The modern medical system is moving ahead to include these biologically active components in their healthcare and biomedical sectors. Natural products from medicinal plants or their crude extract possess enormous diversity and many provide an unlimited opportunity in new drug discoveries [10]. Studies suggest the presence of numerous organic compounds in medicinal plants, like alkaloids, flavonoids, tannins, terpenoids, saponins, glycosides, *etc.* These are wide range of chemically and taxonomically diverse compounds. A large number of these chemicals belong to different classes and are important in different areas like medical science, veterinary, and agriculture [11]. Table **1** describes bioactive phytochemicals, their major classification, compounds, and biological functions [12].

## 6. HERBAL DRUGS AND THEIR IMPORTANCE IN MODERN MEDICINE

Herbal drugs or medicines are those that are obtained from natural extracts, like stem, leaf bark, and roots. These plant parts are thought to have comparatively more bioactive components and are used in diseases or as immunity boosters. The modern medical sectors are now inclining towards the usage of herbal drugs in the treatment of several diseases. This is because the present allopathy-based medications have a range of side effects. For decades, we have been considering natural remedies in treating common ailments like cough, cold, fever, headache, *etc.,* and the trend has been steadily increasing. With the shift from synthetic to natural alternates of medications, we can say —we are going back to our roots‖ in treating the disease, and this can prove to be a prominent option in the near future. WHO has reported that around 80% of the total world's population uses herbal formulations in primary treatment [13]. In recent advancements, a plethora of bioactive compounds have been identified and incorporated into the treatment of diseases, including diabetes, cardiac disease, and cancer. Table **2** summarizes some of the most frequently used plants and their extracts as herbal medicine [14]. Different methods like combinatorial chemistry, synthetic biology, and advanced bioinformatics approaches are employed for the isolation, extraction, and purification and natural extracts for developing drugs. Although plentiful research is ongoing in the area of synthetic medicines, the interest is inclining more toward finding medical solutions using natural extracts and herbal formulations. WHO has emphasized the use of herbal medicines in developing as well as developed countries [15]. In developed countries, people are shifting towards traditional approaches for acute as well as chronic diseases with a belief of effectiveness in herbal medications, fewer side effects than synthetic medicines, and pocket-friendly to society.

**Table 1. Bioactive Phytochemicals in Medicinal Plants.**

| S. No. | Classification | Major Group of Compounds | Biological Functions |
|---|---|---|---|
| 1. | Non-starch polysaccharides (NSA) | Cellulose, Hemicellulose, Pectin, Lignin, Mucilage | Binding toxins and bile acids. Water holding capacity. |
| 2. | Anti-fungals & Anti-bacterials | Terpenoids, Alkaloids, Phenolics | Reduce the risk of fungal infection. Inhibit micro-organisms. |
| 3. | Anti-oxidants | Polyphenolic compounds, Flavonoids, Tocopherols | Inhibit lipid peroxidation. Help in free radicle scavenging. |
| 4. | Anti-cancerous | Carotenoids, Curcumin, Flavonoids | Inhibit cancer development. Inhibit metastasis. |
| 5. | Detoxifying agents | Aromatic isothiocyanates, Retinoids, Reductive acids | Induce drug binding of carcinogens. Inhibit tumorigenesis. |
| 6. | Others | Volatile flavor compounds, Alkaloids, Biogenic amines | Cancer chemoprevention,.Neuropharmacological agents. |

**Table 2. Some most common medicinal plants and their properties.**

| S. No. | Plant Species | Common Name | Bioactive Agents | Medicinal Use | Ref. |
|---|---|---|---|---|---|
| 1. | *Catharant hus roseus* | Sadabahar | Alkaloids (Vincristine, Vinblastine) | Anti-cancer. | [16] |
| 2. | *Curcuma longa* | Turmeric | Flavonoid (Curcumin) | Anti-cancerous, anti-inflammatory. | [17] |
| 3. | *Terminali a chebula* | Harra | Tannin, Triterpenoid, | Anti-diabetic, renoprotective. | [18] |
| 4. | *Withania s omnifera* | Ashwagan dha | Steroidal lactones | Chemoprotective, immunomodulator, memory enhancer. | [19] |
| 5. | *Zingiber of ficinale* | Ginger | Mono & Sesquiterpenes | Anti-oxidant, anti-atherosclerosis. | [20] |
| 6. | *Azadirach ta indica* | Neem | Limonoids | Blood purifier, anti- allergic. Inhibit carcinoma. | [21] |
| 7. | *Tinospora cordifolia* | Geloy | Diterpenoidsfura nolactones | Cardioprotective, immunomodulator. | [22] |
| 8. | *Silybum marianum* | Milk thistle | Flavonoids silymarin (Silibinin) | Liver tonic, anti- inflammatory. | [23] |
| 9. | *Aloe vera* | Ghreetku mari | Aloin, Campesterol | Healing property, antiviral, antiseptic effect. | [24] |
| 10. | *Berberis vulgaris* | Barberry | Berberine | Antimicrobial, hepatoprotective. | [25] |
| 11. | *Digitalis lanata* | Tilapushpi | Digoxin | In heart disease. | [26] |

# 7. PLANT SECONDARY METABOLITES IN CANCER PREVENTION

Cancer prevention talks about the use of specific synthetic, natural or hemi-synthetic compounds to suppress or reverse the cancer progression. Due to the presence of numerous SMs, the plant explicit some anti-cancer properties. Several herbal compounds are in clinical use for cancer treatment, and every year so many cytotoxic SMs are identified, explored and incorporated into the list. In the last few decades, a range of plant SMs were discovered, but a very few of them managed to reach clinical trials after successfully passing different screenings. Each of the SMs that passed the selection has their own history of success and shortcomings [27]. From the historical, clinical and therapeutic point of view, several plant-based drugs have been incorporated into cancer treatment, Vincristine, being one of them. Vincristine, isolated from Catharanthus roseus is one of the earliest plant-derived anti-cancer drugs. Food and Drug Administration (FDA), in 1963, approved this drug for its clinical use to treat cancer. Its incorporation into the treatment has been very effective and has shown around 80% increase in survival of cancer patients [27]. Some other FDA-approved plant-based drugs for cancer are Paclitaxel, Homoharringtonine, Vinblastine, Topotecan, Etoposide, Cannabidiol, *etc.* (Fig. **3**). For industrial production of these plant-derived compounds, a new technology called Synthetic Biology has recently been introduced. Synthetic biology implies the use of different microbial strains in the same way that industry uses *E. coli* for the production of insulin.

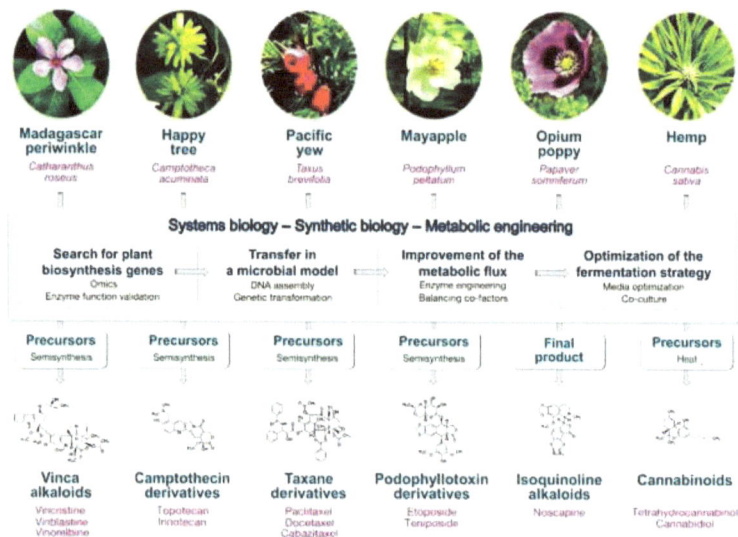

**Fig. (3).** Schematic representation of plant-derived drugs and incorporation of synthetic biology towards the development of plant-based medications.

Centre for Drug Evaluation and Research (CDER) is a U.S. based governing body that performs essential health tasks to ensure the safe effective use of drugs by people. CDER is part of the U.S. FDA and works over the counter and prescription-based drugs, including generic and therapeutic drugs. In the year 2020, CDER has approved some novel drugs for the treatment of different ailments. Table **3** discusses some of the novel drugs approved by CDER in 2020 for treating cancer.

**Table 3. CDER approved novel anti-cancer drugs.**

| Active agent | Approval | Trade | Summary of | Mode of |
|---|---|---|---|---|
| - | Date | Name | Approval | Intake |
| Avapritinib | 09/01/20 | Ayvakit | In treating metastatic gastrointestinal stromal cancer. | Tablet |

*(Table 3) cont.....*

| Active agent | Approval | Trade | Summary of | Mode of |
|---|---|---|---|---|
| - | Date | Name | Approval | Intake |
| Belantamab mafodotin blmf | 0508/20 | Blenrep | In treating recurrent multiple myeloma. | Injection |
| Fluoroestradiol F18 | 20/05/20 | Cerianna | As a diagnostic imaging agent in breast cancer. | Injection |
| Naxitamab-gqgk | 25/11/20 | Danyelza | To treat relapsed neuroblastoma. | Injection |
| Pralsetinib | 04/09/20 | Gavreto | In treating non-small lung cancer. | Capsule |
| Margetuximab-cmkb | 16/12/20 | Margenza | In metastatic breast cancer (Her-2 positive). | Injection |

# 8. COMPLEMENTARY AND ALTERNATIVE (CAM) APPROACHES TO HERBAL MEDICINE

In developing countries, 80 percent or more of the population cannot afford basic medications, immunizations, or treatments [28]. Complementary and alternative approaches are becoming increasingly popular among the affluent populations of both developing and developed countries. However, there is currently modest evidence of their safety and efficacy. Ayurveda, which is based on scientific evidence, is gaining popularity in India and around the world. The United States Federal Government established the National Centre for Complementary and Alternative Medicine as the primary agency for scientific research in this branch of medicine. Its mission is to examine complementary and alternative therapies in the context of rigorous science, fund advanced research, train researchers, inform the public about beneficial modalities, and explain the scientific basis for findings. It is considered that those who employ these methods do so because they are less expensive than traditional therapies or systems. Although, they are more or less the same when compared to conventional medication. However, convenience and traditional healing are the major factors that draw people to the CAM approach. Nowadays, people are inkling more towards this approach as they believe there are lesser side effects than conventional medications. Table **4** illustrates various herbal compositions commonly utilized in the Indian Ayurvedic system [29]. It will also highlight the plant parts that are considered for medication, their ratio, and the appropriate doses required.

**Table 4. Some frequently used herbal formulations in the Indian Ayurvedic System.**

| S. No. | Disease | Herbal Formulations | Plant Parts Used | Ratio | Dosage |
|---|---|---|---|---|---|
| 1. | Anemia | *Asparagus racemosus* | Roots | 20% | 4gm of mixed powder twice a day with water |
| | | *Withania somnifera* | Roots | 20% | |
| | | *Glycyrrhiza glabra* | Roots | 15% | |
| | | *Piper longum* | Fruits | 5% | |
| | | *Phyllanthus emblica* | Fruits | 15% | |
| | | *Plumbago zeylanica* | Roots | 5% | |
| | | *P. amarus* | Leaves | 10% | |
| | | *Tephrosia purpurea* | Leaves | 10% | |
| 2. | Cancer | *Azadirachta indica* | Bark | 20% | 4 gm of mixed powder twice a day (morning & night) with lukewarm honey |
| | | *Bauhinia variegate* | Bark | 15% | |
| | | *Terminalia chebula* | Fruits | 15% | |
| | | *Tinospora cordifolia* | Stem | 15% | |
| | | *T. bellerica* | Fruits | 10% | |
| | | *Crataeva nurvala* | Bark | 15% | |
| | | *Holarrhena antidysenterica* | Bark | 10% | |
| 3. | Dislocation | *Asparagus racemosus* | Roots | 15% | 3 gm of mixed powder twice a day with water |
| | | *Withania somnifera* | Roots | 15% | |
| | | *Azadirachta arabica* | Bark | 20% | |
| | | *Terminalia arjuna* | Bark | 20% | |
| | | *T. chebula* | Fruits | 10% | |
| | | *T. bellerica* | Fruits | 10% | |
| | | *Phyllanthus emblica* | Fruits | 10% | |
| 4. | Diabetes | *Gymnema sylvestre* | Leaves | 30% | 4gm of mixed powder twice a day with water |
| | | *Tinospora cordifolia* | Stem | 15% | |
| | | *Azadirachta indica* | Leaves | 10% | |
| | | *Curcuma longa* | Roots | 10% | |
| | | *Phyllanthus emblica* | Fruits | 20% | |
| | | *Aegle marmelos* | Leaves | 15% | |

*(Table 4) cont.....*

| S. No. | Disease | Herbal Formulations | Plant Parts Used | Ratio | Dosage |
|---|---|---|---|---|---|
| 5. | Female sterility | *Asparagus racemosus* | Roots | 20% | 3 gm of mixed powder twice a day before a meal, with milk |
| | | *Withania somnifera* | Roots | 20% | |
| | | *Glycyrrhiza glabra* | Roots | 20% | |
| | | *Phyllanthus emblica* | Fruits | 10% | |
| | | *Ficus glomerata* | Bark | 10% | |
| | | *F. religiosa* | Bark | 10% | |
| 6. | High blood pressure | *Terminalia arjuna* | Bark | 35% | 4 gm of mixed powder twice a day (morning & night) with honey |
| | | *T. chebula* | Fruits | 15% | |
| | | *Asparagus racemosus* | Roots | 15% | |
| | | *Zingiber officinale* | Roots | 10% | |
| | | *Withania somnifera* | Roots | 25% | |
| 7. | Heart tonic | *Withania somnifera* | Roots | 10% | 3 gm of mixed powder twice a day with water |
| | | *Terminalia arjuna* | Bark | 30% | |
| | | *T. bellerica* | Fruits | 10% | |
| | | *T. chebula* | Fruits | 10% | |
| | | *Cyperus rotundus* | Roots | 10% | |
| | | *Phyllanthus emblica* | Fruits | 10% | |
| | | *Ocimum sanctum* | Leaves | 10% | |
| 8. | Migraine | *Curcuma longa* | Roots | 15% | 4 gm of mixed powder twice a day with honey |
| | | *Glycyrrhiza glabra* | Roots | 15% | |
| | | *Azadirachta indica* | Bark | 15% | |
| | | *Tinospora cordifolia* | Stem | 15% | |
| | | *Terminalia chebula* | Fruits | 10% | |
| | | *Ocimum sanctum* | Leaves | 15% | |
| | | *Eclipta alba* | Leaves | 15% | |
| 9. | Paralysis | *Curcuma zedoaria* | Roots | 20% | 3 gm of mixed powder thrice a day with honey |
| | | *Withania somnifera* | Roots | 20% | |
| | | *Tribulus terrestris* | Fruits | 20% | |
| | | *Zingiber officinale* | Roots | 20% | |
| | | *Piper longum* | Fruits | 5% | |
| | | *Crataeva nurvala* | Leaves | 10% | |
| | | *Plumbago zeylanica* | Roots | 5% | |

*(Table 4) cont.....*

| S. No. | Disease | Herbal Formulations | Plant Parts Used | Ratio | Dosage |
|---|---|---|---|---|---|
| 10. | Sleeplessness | *Withania somnifera* | Roots | 20% | 3 gm of mixed powder at night with milk, before going to bed |
| | | *Centella asiatica* | Leaves | 30% | |
| | | *Piper longum* | Roots | 20% | |
| | | *Glycyrrhiza glabra* | Roots | 10% | |
| | | *Terminalia bellerica* | Fruits | 10% | |
| 11. | Urinary tract infection | *Tribulus terrestris* | Fruits | 25% | 4 gm of mixed powder twice a day with water |
| | | *Zingiber officinale* | Roots | 10% | |
| | | *Solanum xanthocarpum* | Whole plant | 10% | |
| | | *Crataeva nurvala* | Bark | 25% | |
| | | *Tinospora cordifolia* | Stem | 10% | |
| | | *Asparagus racemosus* | Roots | 10% | |
| | | *Tephrosia purpurea* | Leaves | 10% | |
| 12. | Thyroid problems | *Crataeva nurvala* | Bark | 20% | 3 gm of mixed powder twice a day with lukewarm water |
| | | *Bauhinia variegata* | Bark | 20% | |
| | | *Sida cordifolia* | Leaves | 15% | |
| | | *Terminalia chebula* | Fruits | 15% | |
| | | *T. bellerica* | Fruits | 10% | |
| | | *Glycyrrhiza glabra* | Roots | 15% | |
| | | *Zingiber officinale* | Roots | 10% | |
| 13. | Arthritis | *Piper longum* | Fruits | 10% | 4 gm of mixed powder with ginger juice, twice a day, before one hour of meal |
| | | *S. xanthocarpum* | Whole plant | 15% | |
| | | *Terminalia chebula* | Fruits | 10% | |
| | | *Withania somnifera* | Roots | 10% | |
| | | *Terminalia bellerica* | Fruits | 10% | |
| | | *Curcuma zedoaria* | Roots | 15% | |
| | | *Phyllanthus emblica* | Fruits | 15% | |
| | | *Ricinus communis* | Roots | 15% | |

# 9. ETHNOPHARMACOLOGICAL STUDY OF MEDICINAL PLANTS

There is no doubt that medicinal plants possess many biologically active chemicals that help in numerous disease treatments. As these chemicals are produced in small quantities, their efficacy needs to be enhanced. The ethnopharmacology approach proves to be a prominent option in this regard. This is the interdisciplinary scientific exploration of bioactive compounds that are traditionally being used. This field utilizes the amalgamation of disciplines like botany, chemistry, and pharmacology. The emphasis of this study is on field observation, utilizing folk medicines, their botanical identification, and pharmacological research.

Drug discovery from natural extracts in the light of ethnopharmacological study has a pivotal role in current therapeutics [30]. Much attention has been recently gained by pharmaceutical companies towards phytochemical and pharmacological studies of traditional plants and introducing them to clinical trials. Fig. (4) shows the schematic representation of the work plan followed in the ethnopharmacological study of the natural extracts.

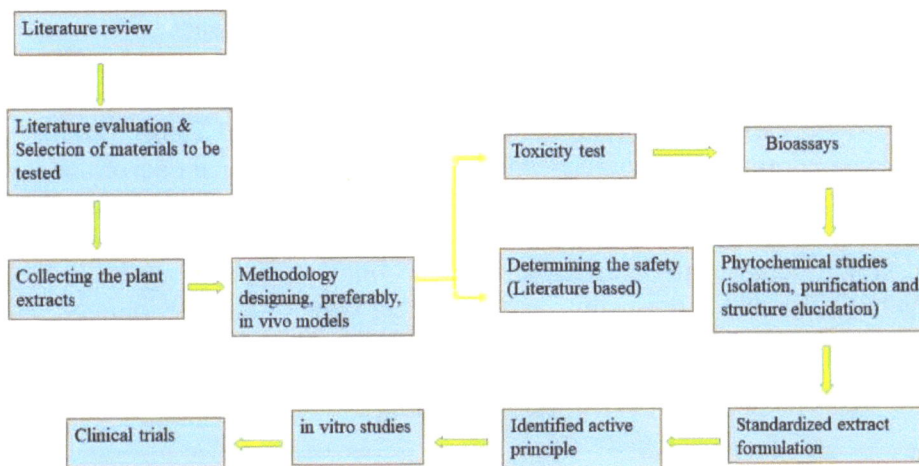

**Fig. (4).** Illustration of ethnopharmacological study of natural extracts.

## 10. MEDICINAL PLANTS AND DRUG DISCOVERY

Many structural features, like aromatic rings, chiral centres, *etc.,* that are common to a different natural product have been reported to show relevance towards drug discovery. Human genome sequencing has led to the identification of thousands of new molecular targets essential in disease progression. Drugs focusing on these molecular targets can help in the treatment of diseases in different ways. Even if new structures are not discovered, medicinal plants having different biological activities can provide new drug leads. Numerous known compounds from traditional mediational plants are effective against the new molecular targets, for example, Indirubin, which binds to cyclin-dependent kinases (CDKs) and interferes with cell division [31]. Medicinal plants and their derivatives are being efficiently explored in the field of oncology. Recent chemotherapies in cancer patients lead to a range of side effects. Therefore, the advancement in research is towards developing plant-based formulations to minimize the adverse effect of medicines.

## 10.1. Anti-cancer Drug Discovery

Globally, large cases of deaths are due to cancer these days. Different categories of cancer contribute to mortality at different levels. There has been a 22% increase in the incidence and mortality rate since the 1990s, and the most frequently occurring cancers are, Breast cancer, Lung cancer, Gastrointestinal cancer, and colorectal cancer. Evolving lifestyle increased food adulterations, and preservatives have led to a steady increase in cancer cases in India. Drug discovery has played an important role in the treatment of cancer. From the 1940s to 2002, around 40% of all the available drugs are natural derivatives [32]. Plant-derived formulations that are currently in clinical use are majorly classified as alkaloids, taxanes, epidophyllotoxins, and camptothecins. Table **5**, emphasizes some most commonly used anti-cancerous drugs and their mode of action [33]. Cancer drug discovery using medicinal plants imparts a vital role in therapeutics. Plant-derived medicines and drugs have been incorporated in the treatment over the past half-century and have witnessed a decline in cancer mortality [34]. These drugs basically target the pathways that cancer cells utilize for their growth and development, thus limiting their growth.

**Table 5. Some medicinal plants and their use in cancer drugs.**

| S. No. | Natural Extract | Source | Activity |
|---|---|---|---|
| 1. | Yondelis | Sea squirt | Interferes with cell division. Blocks transcription. |
| 2. | Halichondrin B (Eisai) | South Pacific Sea sponge | Blocks tubulin formation. |
| 3. | Paclitaxel | Pacific yew tree | Stabilizes microtubule formation. |
| 4. | Vincristine & Vinblastine | Madagascar periwinkle plant | Inhibits tubulin formation. |
| 5. | Etoposide | Mayapple | Inhibits topoisomerase II. |
| 6. | Camptothecin | Chinese *Camptotheca accum inata* tree | Inhibits DNA topoisomerase II. |
| 7. | Thapsigargin | Ibizan*Thapsiagarg anica* plant | Induces apoptosis |

## 11. DRUG DISCOVERY FOR CHEMOPREVENTION

Chemoprevention is defined as the strategy of controlling cancer by introducing natural or synthetic formulations that may help in the suppression or reversion of cancer. Cancer is a multistage disease where normal cells transform into cancerous ones because of several mutations. This transformation involves changes in DNA repair genes, protooncogenes, and tumor suppressor genes and further accelerates cellular growth and invasion. The chemopreventive drugs target these stages and help in controlling tumor growth. The drug action includes anti-initiation and anti-proliferative mechanisms like interfering with replication, increased free radical scavenging, *etc* [35]. The incorporation of herbal medicines, dietary fibres, and traditional herbs regularly is highly recommended and serves as a chemopreventive agent without any adverse effects, as these sources have been incorporated in human consumption for a long time.

## 12. CHALLENGES IN DRUG DISCOVERY FROM NATURAL EXTRACTS

Despite the success of herbal drug discovery, numerous challenges are faced by future endeavors. As bioactive compounds are produced in small quantities, pharmacologists and phytochemists are trying hard to enhance their quality, quantity, and efficacy. In the current scenario, herbal formulations are majorly used in combination with chemotherapy or other therapeutic options [36]. The *de-novo* process of drug discovery takes around 10 years or more and a huge capital. There is a strong need to direct the research to modifying and enhancing the already known herbal compounds so that these may bind to different new molecular targets. Fig. (**5**) illustrates the major steps involved in the process of drug discovery.

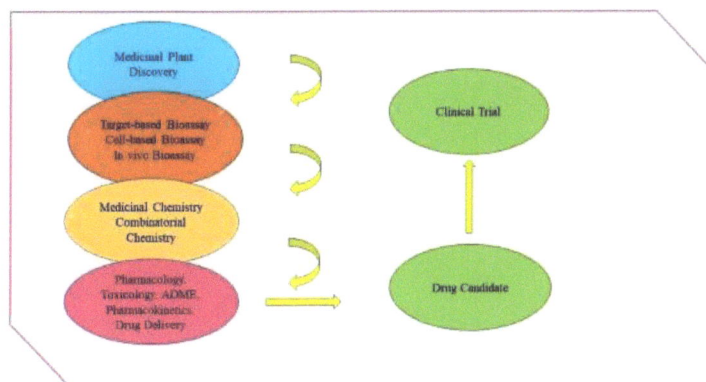

**Fig. (5).** Flowchart showing medicinal plant-based drug discovery.

Drug discovery from natural products has been considered more complicated than any other source. Therefore, faster and better methods are to be employed for plant identification, collection, bioassays, compound isolation, and drug lead development.

## 13. FUTURE PROSPECT OF MEDICINAL PLANTS

There is a promising future for medicinal plants in healthcare, as there are a plethora of plant species that are yet to be identified for their different medicinal properties. In today's modern market of medicines, many plants derived compounds are being used directly or indirectly, for example, aspirin. Many herbs that we consume on a regular basis contain several antimicrobial and antiviral activities, that help us boost our immunity. Keeping this view in mind, there is accelerating growth of research in this field, and many compounds are being incorporated as medicines either directly or as adjuvants. The research is leading to the discovery of novel medicines. In the coming decades, we may see herbal drugs replacing the current synthetic medicines.

## CONCLUSION

In the coming decades, herbal medicines may revolutionize the medical system and establish a new era in disease management. A large portion of the world's population relies on traditional remedies for different ailments. Over the past decades, there has been a resurgence of interest in introducing natural compounds as herbal medicines. There is much research needed in this field for developing a sound medication in terms of herbal drugs. The recent pandemic has witnessed an accelerating demand for herbal products and their incorporation into day-to-day life. AYUSH and PATANJALI are emerging to modernize traditional compounds with advanced medical science.

## REFERENCES

[1]   Dar, R.A.; Shahnawaz, M.; Qazi, P.H. General overview of medicinal plants: A review. *J. Phyto.*, **2017**, *6*(6), 349-351.
      [http://dx.doi.org/10.31254/phyto.2017.6608]

[2]   Arora, S.; Kaur, K.; Kaur, S. Indian medicinal plants as a reservoir of protective phytochemicals. *Teratog. Carcinog. Mutagen.*, **2003**, *23*(S1) 1, 295-300.
      [http://dx.doi.org/10.1002/tcm.10055] [PMID: 12616620]

[3]   Sofowora, A.; Ogunbodede, E.; Onayade, A. The role and place of medicinal plants in the strategies for disease prevention. *Afr. J. Tradit. Complement. Altern. Med.*, **2013**, *10*(5), 210-229.
      [http://dx.doi.org/10.4314/ajtcam.v10i5.2] [PMID: 24311829]

[4]   Li, Y.; Kong, D.; Fu, Y.; Sussman, M.R.; Wu, H. The effect of developmental and environmental factors on secondary metabolites in medicinal plants. *Plant Physiol. Biochem.*, **2020**, *148*, 80-89.
      [http://dx.doi.org/10.1016/j.plaphy.2020.01.006] [PMID: 31951944]

[5]   Borges, C. V.; Minatel, I.O.; Gomez-Gomez, H. O.; Lima, G. P. P. Medicinal plants: Influence of

environmental factors on the content of secondary metabolites. In: *Medi. Plants Envir. Challen*; , **2017**.

[6]   Chakraborty, P. Herbal genomics as tools for dissecting new metabolic pathways of unexplored medicinal plants and drug discovery. *Biochim. Open,* **2018**, *6*, 9-16.
      [http://dx.doi.org/10.1016/j.biopen.2017.12.003] [PMID: 29892557]

[7]   Mueller-Haevey, I. Tannins: their nature and biological significance in secondary plants products. Antinutritional and beneficial actions in animal feeding. *Nottingham Univ Press,* **1999**, 17-70.

[8]   Pridham, J.B. Phenolics in plants, in health and disease. Pergamon Press: NewYork, **1960**; pp. 34-35.

[9]   Halliwell, B.; Gutteridge, J.M.C. Role of free radicals and catalytic metal ions in human disease: An overview. *Methods Enzymol.,* **1990**, *186*, 1-85.
      [http://dx.doi.org/10.1016/0076-6879(90)86093-B] [PMID: 2172697]

[10]  Mustafa, G.; Arif, R.; Atta, A.; Sharif, S.; Jamil, A. Bioactive compounds from medicinal plants and their importance in drug discovery in Pakistan. *Matrix Science Pharma,* **2017**, *1*(1), 17-26.
      [http://dx.doi.org/10.26480/msp.01.2017.17.26]

[11]  Saxena, M.; Saxena, J.; Neema, R.; Singh, D.; Gupta, A. Phytochemistry of medicinal plants. *J. Pharmacogn. Phytochem.,* **2013**, *1*(6).

[12]  Ravishankar, B.; Shukla, V.J. Indian systems of medicine: A brief profile. *Afr. J. Tradit. Complement. Altern. Med.,* **2008**, *4*(3), 319-337.
      [http://dx.doi.org/10.4314/ajtcam.v4i3.31226] [PMID: 20161896]

[13]  Gurib-Fakim, A. Medicinal plants: Traditions of yesterday and drugs of tomorrow. *Mol. Aspects Med.,* **2006**, *27*(1), 1-93.
      [http://dx.doi.org/10.1016/j.mam.2005.07.008] [PMID: 16105678]

[14]  Pandey, M.M.; Rastogi, S.; Rawat, A.K.S. Indian traditional ayurvedic system of medicine and nutritional supplementation. *Evid. Based Complement. Alternat. Med.,* **2013**, *2013*, 1-12.
      [http://dx.doi.org/10.1155/2013/376327] [PMID: 23864888]

[15]  WHO. The regulatory situation of herbal medicines. a worldwide review. Geneva, SwitzerlandWHO, **2017**; pp. 1-5.

[16]  Priyadarshini, K Paclitaxel against cancer: A short review. *Med. Chem.,* **2012**, *2*, 139-141.

[17]  Sharma, V. Part based hplc-pda quantification of podophyllotoxin in populations of podophyllumhexandrumroyle indian mayapple from higher altitude himalayas. *Journal of Medicinal Plants Studies,* **2013**, *1*(3), 176-183.

[18]  Jena, J.; Gupta, A.K. RicinusCommunis linn: A phyto pharmacological review. *Int. J. Pharm. Pharm. Sci.,* **2012**, *4*(4), 25-29.

[19]  Rathinamoorthy, R.; Thilagavathi, G. TerminaliaChebula : Review on pharmacological and biochemical studies. *Int. J. Pharm. Tech. Res.,* **2014**, *6*(1), 97-116.

[20]  Umadevi, M.; Rajeswari, R. Traditional and medicinal use of withaniasomnifera. *Pharma Innov.,* **2012**, *1*(9), 102-110.

[21]  Gupta, S.; Sharma, A. Medicinal properties of zingiber officinale roscoe : A review. *IOSR J. Pharm. Biol. Sci.,* **2014**, *9*(5), 124-129.
      [http://dx.doi.org/10.9790/3008-0955124129]

[22]  Ahmad, N.; Fazal, H.; Abbasi, B.H.; Farooq, S.; Ali, M.; Khan, M.A. Biological role of Piper nigrum L. (Black pepper): *A review. Asian Pac. J. Trop. Biomed.,* **2012**, *2*(3), S1945-S1953.
      [http://dx.doi.org/10.1016/S2221-1691(12)60524-3]

[23]  Akram, M.; Shahab-Uddin, A.A.; Usmanghani, K.H.A.N.; Hannan, A.B.D.U.L.; Mohiuddin, E.; Asif, M. Curcuma longa and curcumin: A review article. *Rom J Biol Plant Biol,* **2010**, *55*(2), 65-70.

[24]  Mittal, J.; Sharma, M.M.; Batra, A. Tinosporacordifolia: A multipurpose medicinal plant-A.

*Faslnamah-i Giyahan-i Daruyi,* **2014**, *2*(2).

[25]   Jain, S.; Mohan, R.; Rai, R. Ocimum sanctum as an herbal medicine: A review. *I. J. Maxillofacial Res.,* **2015**, *1*(1), 1-12.

[26]   Chauhan, R.; Km, R.; Dwivedi, J. Bergenia ciliata mine of medicinal properties: A review *IJPSR,* **2012**, *15*(2), 20-23.

[27]   Courdavault, V.; O'Connor, S.E.; Oudin, A.; Besseau, S.; Papon, N. Towards the microbial production of plant-derived anticancer drugs. *Trends Cancer,* **2020**, *6*(6), 444-448.
       [http://dx.doi.org/10.1016/j.trecan.2020.02.004] [PMID: 32459998]

[28]   Debas, T.H.; Laxminarayan, R.; Straus, S.E. Complementary and alternative medicine. In: *Dis. Con. Prior. Devel. Coun,* 2nd ed; Jamison, D.T.; Breman, J.G.; Measham,, A.R., Eds.; Oxford University Press: New York, NY, USA, **2006**.

[29]   Narayana, A.; Subhose, V. Standardization of ayurvĕdic formulations : A scientific review *Bull Indian Inst. Hist. Med.,* **2005**, *35*(1), 21-32.

[30]   Süntar, I. Importance of ethnopharmacological studies in drug discovery: Role of medicinal plants. *Phytochem. Rev.,* **2019**.

[31]   Shakya, A.K. Medicinal plants: Future source of new drugs. *Int. J. Herb. Med.,* **2016**, *4*(4), 59-64.

[32]   Parkin, D.M.; Bray, F.; Ferlay, J.; Pisani, P. Estimating the world cancer burden: Globocan 2000. *Int. J. Cancer,* **2001**, *94*(2), 153-156.
       [http://dx.doi.org/10.1002/ijc.1440] [PMID: 11668491]

[33]   Seca, A.; Pinto, D. Plant secondary metabolites as anticancer agents: Successes in clinical trials and therapeutic application. *Int. J. Mol. Sci.,* **2018**, *19*(1), 263.
       [http://dx.doi.org/10.3390/ijms19010263] [PMID: 29337925]

[34]   Newman, D.J.; Cragg, G.M.; Snader, K.M. Natural products as sources of new drugs over the period 1981-2002. *J. Nat. Prod.,* **2003**, *66*(7), 1022-1037.
       [http://dx.doi.org/10.1021/np030096l] [PMID: 12880330]

[35]   Roy, A.; Jauhari, N.; Bharadvaja, N. Medicinal plants as a potential source of chemopreventive agents. In: *Anti. Plan.: Nat. Prod. Biotech. Imple*; , **2018**; pp. 109-139.

[36]   Balunas, M.J.; Kinghorn, A.D. Drug discovery from medicinal plants. *Life Sci.,* **2005**, *78*(5), 431-441.
       [http://dx.doi.org/10.1016/j.lfs.2005.09.012] [PMID: 16198377]

# CHAPTER 8

# Shikonin, a Naphthaquinone of Commercial Importance: its Biosynthesis and Prospect for Use as Drugs

**Ravi S. Singh**[1,*] and **Sanjay Kumar**[2]

[1] *Department of Plant Breeding and Genetics, Bihar Agricultural University, Sabour, Bhagalpur, Bihar-813 210, India*

[2] *CSIR-Institutes of Himalyan Bioresource Technology, Palampur, Himachal Pradesh-176 061, India*

**Abstract:** Shikonin is a red naphthaquinone pigment present in the roots of plants of the Boraginaceae family. This pigment is an as active ingredient in several pharmaceutical and cosmetics preparations, and as a dye for fabrics and food items. It shows many bioactivities such as stimulation of peroxidase, protection against UV-radiation, inhibition of microsomal monooxygenase and induction and secretion of nerve growth factor. In this book chapter, we have provided detailed information on its biosynthesis and prospects for pharmaceutical use.

**Keywords:** Biosynthesis, Naphthaquinone, Secondary metabolites, Shikonin.

## 1. INTRODUCTION

Shikonin is a monoterpenoid with IUPAC name 5, 8-dihydroxy-2-[(1R)-1-hydroxy-4-methylpent-3-enyl] naphthalene-1,4-dione (Fig. **1**; redrawn [1]). Various derivatives of shikonin are formed by variation in the "–R" group attached to the naphthazarin (5,8-dihydroxy-1,4-naphthoquinone). The history of the importance of shikonins to mankind, notably as medicines and dyestuff for silk and food products, was known since ancient times [1, 2]. The use of shikonins in traditional Chinese medicine might have originated with the great surgeon Hua To (born ca. 136 ± 141 AD). Records of the use of shikonin in Chinese medicine can be found in Pen Ts'ao Kang Mu, the classic compilation of traditional Chinese medicine, which was written in 1596 AD 1[]. This molecule

* Corresponding author **Ravi S. Singh:** Department of Plant Breeding and Genetics, Bihar Agricultural University, Sabour, Bhagalpur, Bihar- 813 210, India; E-mail: ravissingh0202@gmail.com

**Ashok Kumar Jha & Ravi S. Singh (Eds.)**

was the major constituent of the red pigment extract of the roots of *Lithospermum erythrorhizon* Sieb. et Zucc., and is known in Chinese by name as tzu tsao, tzu-ken, and hung-tzu ken and other boraginacae plants, including *Arnebia euchroma* (Royle) Johnston.

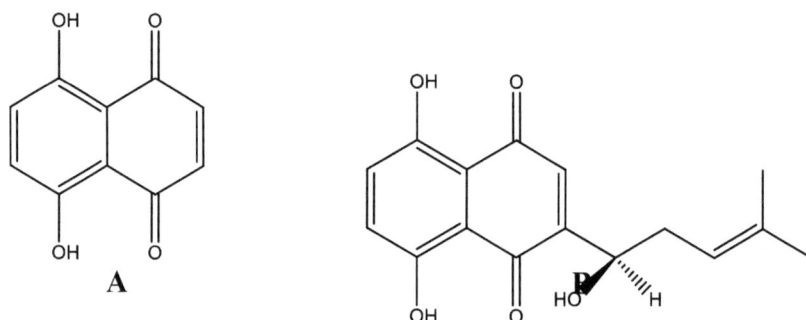

**Fig. (1).** All shikonin and its derivatives are derived from the basic structure of naphthazarin (**A**), wherein the variation in "–R" group attached to the naphthazarin moiety determines the structures of shikonin and its derivative (**B**).

Shikonins have wider uses in phytoceuticals, andcosmetics products, and are also used as a colorant for fabrics and food products [1 - 3]. Other bioactivities of shikonins include stimulation of peroxidase, antimicrobial properties, protection against UV-radiation, inhibition of microsomal monooxygenase and induction and secretion of nerve growth factor [4]. Shikonins are also present in *Onosma paniculatum, Arnebia hispidissima, Arnebia guttata, Arnebia tibetiana, Cynoglossum officinale*, and *Echium lycopsis*.

## 2. BIOSYNTHESIS OF SHIKONIN

### 2.1. Routes for The Biosynthesis of Secondary Metabolites

Most of the secondary metabolites are derived from three basic biosynthetic pathways, the shikimate pathway, the isoprenoid/terpenoid pathway, and the polyketide pathway. After the synthesis of the major basic skeletons, further modification by hydroxyl, methoxy, aldehyde, carboxyl groups, and carbon atoms creates a large variety of compounds [5]. Analysis of *Arabidopsis thaliana* and other plant genomes suggested that nearly 15-25% of the genes encode for enzymes involved in secondary metabolism [6]. Since the majority of secondary metabolites are plant or species specific, and the biosynthetic enzymes are substrate-exclusive, it is likely that thousands of enzymes and hence are genes involved in secondary metabolite biosynthesis, and most of these remain to be elucidated [7].

The biosynthesis of secondary metabolites and their accumulation, storage and release occurs in specialized organs or tissues. Flowers, fruits and seeds are usually rich in secondary metabolites, especially in annual plants. While in perennial species, a high amount of secondary metabolites is found in bulbs, roots and stems [7]. In many cases, the site of biosynthesis, processing and accumulation are different [8]. The corresponding product could be detected in several other tissues *via* transport routes, such as the xylem or phloem for the translocation of secondary metabolites [9]. For example, nicotine synthesized in the roots of tobacco is transported upwards *via* the xylem to the leaves, where it is accumulated as well as transformed into a wide array of products. Vacuoles occupy the most part of the inner volume of plant cells (40-90%) and play a critical role in the accumulation of secondary metabolites [10]. Water soluble compounds are usually stored in the vacuole [7, 11], whereas lipophilic substances are sequestered in resin ducts, lactifers, glandular hairs, trichomes, thylakoid membranes or the cuticle [12]. Two major mechanisms were proposed for the vacuolar transport of secondary metabolites: $H^+$-gradient-dependent secondary transport *via* $H^+$-antiport and directly energized primary transport by ABC transporters [13].

## 2.2. IPP Biosynthesis Pathways

IPP is the central intermediate in the biosynthesis of isoprenoids. Two routes of IPP biosynthesis have been established in cells [14]: the mevalonate (MVA) pathway and the methylerythritol 4-phosphate (MEP) pathway [15, 16]. The evolutionary history of the enzymes of these pathways and the phylogenetic distribution of their genes suggested an archaebacterial link to the MVA pathway and an eubacterial link to the MEP pathway [17]. This implies the prokaryotic origin of IPP biosynthesis and eukaryotes have inherited genes of these pathways.

### 2.2.1. MVA Pathway

In the MVA pathway (Fig. **2**), HMG-CoA results from the coupling of three molecules of acetyl-CoA, which is reduced by the enzyme HMGR to yield MVA. In the next two steps, MVK and PMVK catalyse conversion of MVA to form MVD, which in turn is decarboxylated to yield IPP. IPP is converted into GPP using the enzyme GDPS. The MVA pathway provides IPP for the synthesis of various isoprenoids/metabolites, for example, natural rubber, linalool, dolichol, and ubiquinone [16, 18, 19, 20]. This pathway (Fig. **2**) was first discovered in yeasts and animals in the 1950s [21, 22]. HMGR is a major enzyme of the pathway that has been studied extensively. It is considered to be the major point of regulation of substrate flux through the pathway [23, 24]. MVA pathway involves a range of enzyme, namely, ACTH, HMGS, HMGR, MVK, PMVK, MVDD, IPPI and GDPS which are described in the following section.

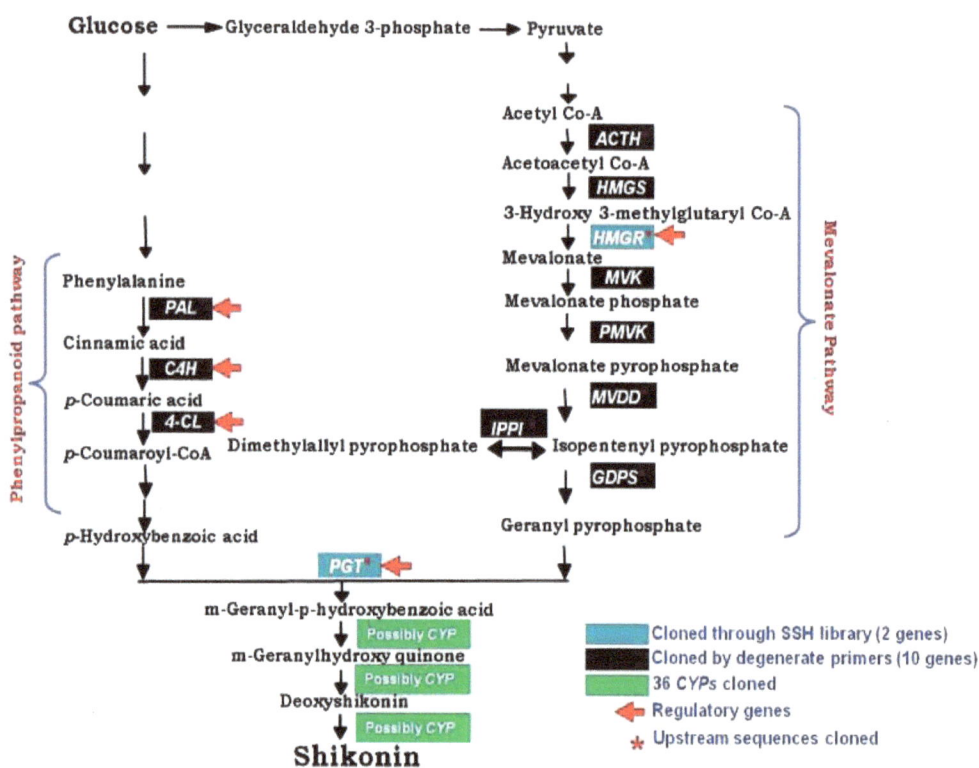

**Fig. (2).** Status of cloned genes and upstream sequences of shikonins biosynthesis pathway in *A. euchroma* [14]. The figure shows a total of 12 genes cloned in the present work, upstream putative promoter sequences of the genes, and the *cytochrome P450* (*CYP*) genes as putative genes associated with terminal steps of the shikonins biosynthesis pathway. Arrows indicate the regulatory genes of the pathway, as evidenced by expression analysis.

## 2.2.2. MEP Pathway

The reassessment of the isoprenoid biosynthesis in plants and microorganisms was initiated in the late 1980s by studies performed independently by Rohmer, Sahm, Arigoni and co-workers [25]. Experiments [26] incorporating $^{13}$C-labeled acetate into bacterial hopanoids, such as aminobacteriohopanetriol, had revealed unexpected labelling patterns in the terpenoid moiety of the molecules under study. The existence of distinct acetyl CoA pools was proposed to explain how anomalous labeling patterns could arise *via* the MVA pathway [26], but other possibilities were also considered. Reinterpretation of these data s hinted the existence of a new pathway, the MEP pathway [26]. Independently, Arigoni and co-workers studied the incorporation of $^{13}$C-labeled glucose into the isoprenoid side chain of ubiquinone in *E. coli* and the same into ginkgolides in seedlings of *Ginkgo bilolia* [27]. The detailed analysis of specimens of ginkgolides generated from various specifically labeled $^{13}$C isotopomers of glucose established that the synthesis of the isoprenoid monomers proceeded by the contribution of a three-carbon and a two-carbon fragment from glucose. Clearly, this could not be explained *via* the MVA pathway, which had been shown long ago to utilize exclusively a two-carbon building block (acetyl CoA).

MEP pathway has been reported in many eubacteria, apicomplexa parasites, and photosynthetic eukaryotes, but *Homo sapiens* lack this pathway [17]. The genes and enzymes of this pathway are attractive targets for the development of new antibacterial and antiparasitic drugs and herbicides [28, 29]. A number of compounds produced by this pathway also have nutritional or medicinal value, and are important targets for biotechnological manipulation. For example, carotenoids, tocopherols and anti-oncogenic drugs [30, 31]. Several major plant hormones are produced through this pathway either from direct biosynthesis (gibberellins) or as cleavage derivatives, such as abscisic acid and the recently discovered hormone strigolactone [32, 33]. MEP pathway is involved in the synthesis of some notable monoterpenes, for example, borneol (*Conocephalum conicum* [34], cineole (*Eucalyptus globules* [35], geraniol (*Pelargonium graveolens* [25], *Vitis vinifera* [36], linalyl acetate (*Mentha citrate* [37], menthol (*Mentha piperita* [25], pulegone (*Mentha* pulegium [25], and thymol (*Thymus vulgaris* [25]. MEP pathway involves seven enzymes namely DXS, DXR, MCT, CMK, MDS, HDS and HDR which are discussed in the following section.

Shikonins consist of an isoprenoid moiety derived from GPP and PHB. PHB is formed through the PP pathway, whereas GPP could be through MVA [16] and MEP [15] pathways. GPP flow is essential for the yield of isoprenoids [38], therefore, a study on the regulation of gene expression in GPP biosynthesis is of immense significance. Depending upon the metabolite and species under consideration, the preference for the route to GPP biosynthesis might differ. For example, natural rubber and stevioside rely on the MVA pathway and MEP pathway, respectively [20, 39]. Comparative analysis of MVA and MEP pathways plays a role in shikonins biosynthesis using inhibitors such as mevinolin and fosmidomycin, respective inhibitors of HMGR (of MVA pathway) and DXR (of MEP pathway) [40, 41]. A cell suspension culture system was used for this study that showed an increase in shikonins content from negligible quantity by 82.8 fold from day zero to day 10 of transferring the suspension cultures from low shikonin production system (LSPS) to high shikonin production system (HSPS) [42]. Mevinolin severely inhibited (92.82%) shikonins accumulation, whereas the fosmidomycin effect was milder (49.97%). Thus, implying a major role of the MVA pathway in shikonins biosynthesis in comparison to the MEP pathway. Similar observation was reported in *L. erythrorhizon* in which mevinolin inhibited the shikonins biosynthesis by 98% [43]. Twelve genes of shikonin biosynthesis, including the different pathways involved, *i.e., AeHMGR* (of MVA pathway), *AePGT* (involved in the coupling of GPP and PHB) and PP pathway were up-regulated in HSPS as compared to the LSPS. HMGR is known to play a key role in the regulation of IPP biosynthesis in plants [44, 45].

HMGR, as an early enzyme in isoprenoid biosynthesis, was proposed to control the metabolic flux into the MVA pathway by Lange *et al.* [46], while the downstream enzymes of the pathway are involved in the synthesis of specialized end products. We also reported *AeHMGR* could be a key regulatory gene in shikonins biosynthesis [42].

Increased activity of the PP pathway appeared to be a general feature for shikonins biosynthesis in *A. euchroma* [42]. The PP pathway supplies one of the substrates, PHB, for shikonins biosynthesis [47, 48]. While contrasting results were reported in *L. erythrorhizon* of expression of genes of the PP pathway [49], and similar findings as in *A. euchroma* were reported on tea [50, 51]. *AePGT* encodes for PGT, which showed up-regulation in HSPS and was positively correlated with shikonins content. A study [52] reported higher (thirty five times) activity of PGT in *L. erythrorhizon* shikonin producing culture than in the non-shikonins producing culture. These results suggest PGT has an important regulatory role in the biosynthesis of shikonins.

## 3. COMPARTMENTATION AND CROSS-TALK AMONG PATHWAYS FOR THE ISOPRENOID BIOSYNTHESIS

Compartmentation was found to be important in isoprenoid biosynthesis [53, 54]. Several isoprenoids are synthesized in the cytosol from the MVA pathway, such as steroids, some sesquiterpenes, and triterpenes [55]. Whereas MEP pathway derived metabolites are synthesized in the plastids, for example, isoprene, monoterpenes, certain sesquiterpenes, diterpenes, tetraterpenes and carotenoids [15]. This separation in different organelles and parts of the cell involves the synthesis of some of the diterpenoids and tetraterpenoid compounds for various biological processes, including photosynthesis, for the constitution of plant membranes [56]. Further, evidences also suggest the movement of intermediates across these compartments. Cross-talk between the plastidial and the cytosolic pathways was evident from the previous studies of feeding experiments using stable isotopes in the biosynthesis of the dieter pene ginkgolide in *Ginkgo biloba* [57]. The study revealed that in the presence of $^{13}C$ glucose, three isoprene units were incorporated according to the cytosolic (MVA pathway) and the fourth residue was incorporated *via* the MEP pathway. In the oil glands of peppermint, the MEP pathway serves IPP for both monoterpene and sesquiterpene and the MVA pathway remains blocked [58]. Chamomile sesquiterpene-labeling and quantitative $^{13}$C-NMR spectroscopy observed that two of the isoprene units of this metabolite were majorly formed through the MEP pathway, and the third unit derived from MVA as well as MEP pathways [59].

Laule *et al.* [60] reported that the MEP pathway can compensate for the MVA pathway, when there is a reduction in flux. But some reports based on tracer studies also suggest that the compartmentalization of the MVA and MEP pathways was not complete, and cross-talk of some metabolites happens [34, 61]. Hemmerlin *et al.* [62] found that DXP complemented growth inhibition by mevinolin (inhibitor of MVA pathway). With labeled DXP in a tracer study, it was found that sterols formed *via* the MVA pathway were also synthesized *via* the MEP pathway in the presence of mevinolin. Likewise, the growth inhibition by fosmidomycin (an inhibitor of DXR) could also be recovered by the MVA pathway [63]. The incorporation of labeled MVA into plastoquinone (plastidial isoprenoids) indicates the possibility of a specific transporter for isoprenoid intermediates between the plastids to the cytosol. Such a transporter has been reported that export isoprenoids across the plastidial envelope membrane [64].

## 4. SITE OF SYNTHESIS AND TRANSPORT OF SHIKONINS

Secondary metabolite accumulation in the cellular compartment may be toxic to the cell, hence these are sequestered intercellularly, intracellularly, and in an intra-tissue fashion [65]. Intra-tissue separation of nicotine is well characterized by its unique translocation; nicotine is synthesized in the roots and then translocated to the leaves, where it protects the plants from insects [66]. The biosynthetic site and transport of shikonins are poorly understood. Biosynthetic enzymes, after the prenylation step, are believed to be localized in membrane vesicles derived from ER, and shikonins are secreted out of the cells with lipids to form red granules that adhere to the cell walls [67]. The intracellular vesicles observed in shikonin-producing cells, where the putative shikonin precursors are located, are covered by a phospholipid monolayer [68].

One of the pathway's enzymes, PGT, was localized at the microsomal fraction of *L. erythrorhyzon* cells that contain specific vesicle membranes derived from the ER [69]. It has been suggested that all steps, including the coupling of PHB and GPP, take place in a special vesicle, which is also needed for the orderly biosynthetic reactions and the transport and secretion of the metabolite [69]. PHB-OG might be stored in the vacuoles for its protection from glucosidase before the initiation of shikonin biosynthesis and (Yazaki *et al.,* 1995). Once shikonin production is induced in the dark, PHB-OG is hydrolyzed to give PHB. PHB is immediately prenylated by geranyltrasferase [70] localized on ER membrane in the presence of GPP to form GHB [48]. PHB was found to be accumulated in the vacuoles of shikonin-free cells in the form of $\beta$-D-glucoside, PHB-OG (Yazaki *et al.*, 1986). Several intermediates of the shikonin biosynthesis, such as PHB, GHB, and GHQ, have been isolated from shikonin-free cell cultures of *L. erythrorhizon* grown in LS liquid medium [48].

## 5. PROSPECT OF SHIKONIN FOR USE AS A DRUG

With the increasing authenticity of ancient drugs through scientific validation and demonstrations these days, the medicinal properties of shikonins from the Boraginaceae family do have scientific evidence. Shikonin as a molecule is being shown as a promising candiate with a lot of beneficial effects implicated in its use. Its multiple target action is probably the best thing for the treatment of different ailments, for example, the antimicrobial properties of shikonin give an extra advantage to its wound healing properties. Shikonin's biological activity is assessed by observing cell viability, caspase-3 activity, generation of reactive oxygen species (ROS), and apoptotic marker expressions in AGS stomach cancer cells [71]. Shikonin's role as a wound healer, anti-inflammatory, antitumour, and anti-HIV activities is well reported [72 - 74].

Wang *et al.* [75] reported that the screening for anticancer shikonin derivatives is based on a cellular level to find compounds with stronger cytotoxicity. Though several compounds have been discovered with striking cytotoxicity *in vitro,* however, no selectivity was observed, and undoubtedly, the further outcomes have been disappointing because of their great damage to normal cells.

Numerous pharmacological properties of shikonin [83] are in listed in Table **1**.

Table 1. Shikonin pharmacological properties.

| Pharmacological Properties | Findings | Mechanism | Reference |
|---|---|---|---|
| Anti-cancer | Shikonin as a new therapeutic approach/agent for cancer chemotherapy | Shikonin induced the generation of ROS as well as caspase 3-dependent apoptosis. c-Jun-N-terminal kinases (JNK) activity was significantly elevated in shikonin-treated cells, thereby linking JNK to apoptosis. | [71] |
| | Shikonin as a potential novel alternative agent for the treatment of human prostate cancer. | Shikonin inhibits aggressive prostate cancer cell migration and invasion by reducing MMP-2/-9 expression *via* AKT/mTOR and ROS/ERK1/2 pathways. | [76] |

(Table 1) cont.....

| Pharmacological Properties | Findings | Mechanism | Reference |
|---|---|---|---|
| **Anti-inflammatory** | Shikonin's anti-inflammatory activity on two other classic mouse models | *In vitro,* authors demonstrated that shikonin inhibited TNF-α production in LPS-stimulated rat primary macrophages as well as NF-κB translocation from the cytoplasm to the nucleus. | [77] |
| **Wound healing effects** | Molecular basis of the wound healing by *L. erythrorhizon* and shikonin | The ethanol extracts of *L. erythrorhizon* and shikonin (100 nM) were able to promote cell proliferation in fibroblasts by up to 25% and decrease cell migration. Shikonin (1 μM) promoted wound healing in intestinal epithelial cells (IEC-18) through a mechanism that involved the increase of cell migration and TGFβ1 induction without increasing cell proliferation. | [78] [79] |
| **Antiallergic agent** | The dose dependent antiallergic effect was found. | Shikonin reduces histamine release mediated by anti-immunoglobulin E antibodies in basophils in a dose-dependent manner (IC50=2.6 μM). | [80] |
| **Antiviral activity** | The effects of shikonin against the HIV-1 receptor antagonist activity of multiple chemokines. | At nM concentrations, shikonin inhibited monocyte chemotaxis and calcium flux in response to a variety of chemokines. It downregulated surface expression and mRNA expression of CCR5, a primary HIV-1 co-receptor, in macrophages to a greater degree than the other receptors. | [81] [82] |

## CONCLUSION

Shikonin, a naphthoquinone pigment with so many important potential pharmacological properties, including anti-inflamatory, antibacterial, antifungal, antiparasitic, antivirals and others, has drawn the attention of researchers to develop drug and commercial products (cosmetics, dye, food additives, colorants, *etc.*). Understanding its biosynthesis is crucial for the modulation of biosynthetic pathways leading to high yield. Further, in-depth studies on pharmacological, toxicological and biochemical aspects will be important for this molecule to be used as an effective drug in the future.

## ACKNOWLEDGEMENTS

The authors duly acknowledge the molecular work on shikonins biosynthesis carried out during the doctoral programme of RSS at CSIR-IHBT, Palampur, H.P., India, and Bihar Agricultural University, Sabour, for support during the preparation of this book chapter.

# ABBREVIATIONS

**ACTH**   Acetoacetyl-CoA Thiolase

**HMGS**   3-Hydroxy-3-Methylglutaryl-CoA Synthase

**HMGR**   3-Hydroxy-3-Methylglutaryl-CoA Reductase

**MVK**   Mevalonate Kinase

**PMVK**   Phosphomevalonate Kinase

**MVDD**   Mevalonate Diphosphate Decarboxylase

**IPPI**   Isopentenyl Pyrophosphate Isomerase

**GDPS**   Geranyl Diphosphate Synthase

**DXS**   1-Deoxy-D-Xylulose 5-Phosphate Synthase

**DXR**   1-Deoxy-D-Xylulose 5-Phosphate Reductoisomerase

**MCT**   2-C-Methylerythritol 4-Phosphate Cytidyl Transferase

**CMK**   4-(Cytidine-5'-Diphospho)-2-C-Methylerythritol Kinase

**MDS**   2-C-Methylerythritol-2,4-Cyclophosphate Synthase

**HDS**   1-Hydroxy-2-Methyl-2-(E)-Butenyl 4-Diphosphate Synthase

**HDR**   1-Hydroxy-2-Methyl-2-(E)-Butenyl 4-Diphosphate Reductase

**PAL**   Phenylalanine Ammonia Lyase

**C4H**   Cinnamic Acid 4-Bydroxylase; 4-CL;]: 4-Coumaroyl-CoA Ligase

**PGT**   P-Hydroxybenzoate -M-Geranyltransferase

# REFERENCES

[1]     Papageorgiou, V.P.; Assimopoulou, A.N.; Couladouros, E.A.; Hepworth, D.; Nicolaou, K.C.; Nicolaou, K.C. The chemistry and biology of alkannin, shikonin, and related naphthazarin natural products. *Angew. Chem. Int. Ed.,* **1999**, *38*(3), 270-301.
        [http://dx.doi.org/10.1002/(SICI)1521-3773(19990201)38:3<270::AID-ANIE270>3.0.CO;2-0]
        [PMID: 29711637]

[2]     Sharma, R.A.; Singh, B.; Singh, D.; Chandrawat, P. Ethnomedicinal, pharmacological properties and chemistry of some medicinal plants of boraginaceae in india. *J. Med. Plants Res.,* **2009**, *3*, 1153-1175.

[3]     Kim, S.H.; Kang, I.C.; Yoon, T.J.; Park, Y.M.; Kang, K.S.; Song, G.Y.; Ahn, B.Z. Antitumor activities of a newly synthesized shikonin derivative, 2-hyim-DMNQ-S-33. *Cancer Lett.,* **2001**, *172*(2), 171-175.
        [http://dx.doi.org/10.1016/S0304-3835(01)00665-6] [PMID: 11566493]

[4]     Xiong, W.; Luo, G.; Zhou, L.; Zeng, Y.; Yang, W. *In vitro* and *in vivo* antitumor effects of acetylshikonin isolated from *Arnebia euchroma* (Royle) Johnst (Ruanzicao) cell suspension cultures. *Chin. Med.,* **2009**, *4*(1), 14.
        [http://dx.doi.org/10.1186/1749-8546-4-14] [PMID: 19594888]

[5]     Verpoorte, R. Metabolic engineering of plant secondary metabolism. In: *Metabolic Engineering of Plant Secondary Metabolism*; Verpoorte, R.; Alfermann, A.W., Eds.; Kluwer Academic Publishers: Dordrecht, **1999**.

[6]     Somerville, C.; Somerville, S. Plant functional genomics. *Science,* **1999**, *285*(5426), 380-383.
        [http://dx.doi.org/10.1126/science.285.5426.380] [PMID: 10411495]

[7]     Wink, M. Functions of plant secondary metabolites and their exploitation in biotechnology. A nnual plant reviews. Sheffield Academic Press: Sheffield, **1999**; Vol. 3, p. 362. a

[8]     Wink, M.; Waterman, P. Chemotaxonomy in relation to molecular phylogeny of plants. In: *Biochemistry of plant secondary metabolism. Annual Plant Reviews*; Wink, M., Ed.; Sheffield Academic Press: Sheffield, **1999**; pp. 300-341.

[9]     Bais, H. P.; Loyola-Vargas, V. M.; Flores, H. E.; Vivanco, J. M. Root specific metabolism: The biology and biochemistry of underground organs. *in vitro* cellular & developmental biology *Plant Sci.,* **2001**, *37*, 730-741.

[10]    Yazaki, K. Transporters of secondary metabolites. *Curr. Opin. Plant Biol.,* **2005**, *8*(3), 301-307. [http://dx.doi.org/10.1016/j.pbi.2005.03.011] [PMID: 15860427]

[11]    Boller, T.; Wiemken, A. Dynamics of vacuolar compartmentation. *Annu. Rev. Plant Physiol.,* **1986**, *37*(1), 137-164. [http://dx.doi.org/10.1146/annurev.pp.37.060186.001033]

[12]    Wiermann, R. Secondary plant products and cell and tissue differentiation. In: *The Biochemistry of Plants*; Academic Press: New York, **1981**; Vol. 7, pp. 85-116.

[13]    Martinoia, E.; Klein, M.; Geisler, M.; Bovet, L.; Forestier, C.; Kolukisaoglu, Ü.; Müller-Röber, B.; Schulz, B. Multifunctionality of plant ABC transporters : More than just detoxifiers. *Planta,* **2002**, *214*(3), 345-355. [http://dx.doi.org/10.1007/s004250100661] [PMID: 11855639]

[14]    Singh, R.S. Molecular Studies on Shikonin Biosynthesis in Arnebia euchroma *(Royle)* Johnston. PhD AmritsarGuru Nanak Deo University, **2011**.

[15]    Lichtenthaler, H.K.; Rohmer, M.; Schwender, J. Two independent biochemical pathways for isopentenyl diphosphate and isoprenoid biosynthesis in higher plants. *Physiol. Plant.,* **1997**, *101*(3), 643-652. a [http://dx.doi.org/10.1111/j.1399-3054.1997.tb01049.x]

[16]    Newman, J.D.; Chappell, J. Isoprenoid biosynthesis in plants: Carbon partitioning within the cytoplasmic pathway. *Crit. Rev. Biochem. Mol. Biol.,* **1999**, *34*(2), 95-106. [http://dx.doi.org/10.1080/10409239991209228] [PMID: 10333387]

[17]    Lange, B.M.; Rujan, T.; Martin, W.; Croteau, R. Isoprenoid biosynthesis: The evolution of two ancient and distinct pathways across genomes. *Proc. Natl. Acad. Sci.,* **2000**, *97*(24), 13172-13177. [http://dx.doi.org/10.1073/pnas.240454797] [PMID: 11078528]

[18]    Goldstein, J.L.; Brown, M.S. Regulation of the mevalonate pathway. *Nature,* **1990**, *343*(6257), 425-430. [http://dx.doi.org/10.1038/343425a0] [PMID: 1967820]

[19]    Pichersky, E.; Lewinsohn, E.; Croteau, R. Purification and characterization of *S*-linalool synthase, an enzyme involved in the production of floral scent in *Clarkia breweri. Arch. Biochem. Biophys.,* **1995**, *316*(2), 803-807. [http://dx.doi.org/10.1006/abbi.1995.1107] [PMID: 7864636]

[20]    Totté, N.; Charon, L.; Rohmer, M.; Compernolle, F.; Baboeuf, I.; Geuns, J.M.C. Biosynthesis of the diterpenoid steviol, an ent-kaurene derivative from *Stevia rebaudiana* Bertoni, *via* the methylerythritol phosphate pathway. *Tetrahedron Lett.,* **2000**, *41*(33), 6407-6410. [http://dx.doi.org/10.1016/S0040-4039(00)01094-7]

[21]    Gershenzon, J.; Croteau, R. Terpenoid biosynthesis: The basic pathway and formation of monoterpenes, sesquiterpenes and diterpenes. In: *Lipid Metabolism in Plants*; Moore, T.S., Jr, Ed.; CRC Press: Boca Raton, FL, **1993**; pp. 340-388.

[22]    McGarvey, D.J.; Croteau, R. Terpenoid metabolism. *Plant Cell,* **1995**, *7*(7), 1015-1026. [PMID: 7640522]

[23]   Bach, T.J. Some new aspects of isoprenoid biosynthesis in plants :A review. *Lipids,* **1995**, *30*(3), 191-202.
[http://dx.doi.org/10.1007/BF02537822] [PMID: 7791527]

[24]   Weissenborn, D.L.; Denbow, C.J.; Laine, M.; Lång, S.S.; Yang, Z.; Yu, X.; Cramer, C.L. HMG-GoA reductase and terpenoid phytoalexins: Molecular specialization within a complex pathway. *Physiol. Plant.,* **1995**, *93*(2), 393-400.
[http://dx.doi.org/10.1111/j.1399-3054.1995.tb02244.x]

[25]   Eisenreich, W.; Schwarz, M.; Cartayrade, A.; Arigoni, D.; Zenk, M.H.; Bacher, A. The deoxyxylulose phosphate pathway of terpenoid biosynthesis in plants and microorganisms. *Chem. Biol.,* **1998**, *5*(9), R221-R233.
[http://dx.doi.org/10.1016/S1074-5521(98)90002-3] [PMID: 9751645]

[26]   Flesch, G.; Rohmer, M. Prokaryotic hopanoids: The biosynthesis of the bacteriohopan skeleton. *Eur. J. Biochem.,* **1988**, *175*, 405-411.
[http://dx.doi.org/10.1111/j.1432-1033.1988.tb14210.x] [PMID: 3136017]

[27]   Eisenreich, W.; Bacher, A.; Arigoni, D.; Rohdich, F. Biosynthesis of isoprenoids *via* the non-mevalonate pathway. *Cell. Mol. Life Sci.,* **2004**, *61*(12), 1401-1426.
[http://dx.doi.org/10.1007/s00018-004-3381-z] [PMID: 15197467]

[28]   Zeidler, J.; Schwender, J.; Mueller, C.; Lichtenthaler, H.K. The non-mevalonate isoprenoid biosynthesis of plants as a test system for drugs against malaria and pathogenic bacteria. *Biochem. Soc. Trans.,* **2000**, *28*(6), 796-798.
[http://dx.doi.org/10.1042/bst0280796] [PMID: 11171212]

[29]   Rohdich, F.; Bacher, A.; Eisenreich, W. Isoprenoid biosynthetic pathways as anti-infective drug targets. *Biochem. Soc. Trans.,* **2005**, *33*(4), 785-791.
[http://dx.doi.org/10.1042/BST0330785] [PMID: 16042599]

[30]   Dubey, V.S.; Bhalla, R.; Luthra, R. An overview of the non-mevalonate pathway for terpenoid biosynthesis in plants. *J. Biosci.,* **2003**, *28*(5), 637-646.
[http://dx.doi.org/10.1007/BF02703339] [PMID: 14517367]

[31]   DellaPenna, D.; Pogson, B.J. Vitamin synthesis in plants: Tocopherols and carotenoids. *Annu. Rev. Plant Biol.,* **2006**, *57*(1), 711-738.
[http://dx.doi.org/10.1146/annurev.arplant.56.032604.144301] [PMID: 16669779]

[32]   Gomez-Roldan, V.; Fermas, S.; Brewer, P.B.; Puech-Pagès, V.; Dun, E.A.; Pillot, J.P.; Letisse, F.; Matusova, R.; Danoun, S.; Portais, J.C.; Bouwmeester, H.; Bécard, G.; Beveridge, C.A.; Rameau, C.; Rochange, S.F. Strigolactone inhibition of shoot branching. *Nature,* **2008**, *455*(7210), 189-194.
[http://dx.doi.org/10.1038/nature07271] [PMID: 18690209]

[33]   Umehara, M.; Hanada, A.; Yoshida, S.; Akiyama, K.; Arite, T.; Takeda-Kamiya, N.; Magome, H.; Kamiya, Y.; Shirasu, K.; Yoneyama, K.; Kyozuka, J.; Yamaguchi, S. Inhibition of shoot branching by new terpenoid plant hormones. *Nature,* **2008**, *455*(7210), 195-200.
[http://dx.doi.org/10.1038/nature07272] [PMID: 18690207]

[34]   Thiel, R.; Adam, K.P. Incorporation of [1- 13 c]1-deoxy- d -xylulose into isoprenoids of the liverwort conocephalum conicum. *Phytochemistry,* **2002**, *59*(3), 269-274.
[http://dx.doi.org/10.1016/S0031-9422(01)00453-8] [PMID: 11830134]

[35]   Rieder, C.; Jaun, B.; Arigoni, D. On the early steps of cineol biosynthesis in *eucalyptus globules. Helv. Chim. Acta,* **2000**, *83*(9), 2504-2513.
[http://dx.doi.org/10.1002/1522-2675(20000906)83:9<2504::AID-HLCA2504>3.0.CO;2-Z]

[36]   Luan, F.; Wüst, M. Differential incorporation of 1-deoxy-?-xylulose into (3S)-linalool and geraniol in grape berry exocarp and mesocarp. *Phytochemistry,* **2002**, *60*(5), 451-459.
[http://dx.doi.org/10.1016/S0031-9422(02)00147-4] [PMID: 12052510]

[37]   Fowler, D.J.; Hamilton, J.T.G.; Humphrey, A.J.; O'Hagan, D. Plant terpene biosynthesis. the

biosynthesis of linalyl acetate in mentha citrata. *Tetrahedron Lett.,* **1999**, *40*(19), 3803-3806.
[http://dx.doi.org/10.1016/S0040-4039(99)00532-8]

[38]   Nogués, I.; Brilli, F.; Loreto, F. Dimethylallyl diphosphate and geranyl diphosphate pools of plant
       species characterized by different isoprenoid emissions. *Plant Physiol.,* **2006**, *141*(2), 721-730.
       [http://dx.doi.org/10.1104/pp.105.073213] [PMID: 16461390]

[39]   Sando, T.; Takaoka, C.; Mukai, Y.; Yamashita, A.; Hattori, M.; Ogasawara, N.; Fukusaki, E.;
       Kobayashi, A. Cloning and characterization of mevalonate pathway genes in a natural rubber
       producing plant, *Hevea brasiliensis. Biosci. Biotechnol. Biochem.,* **2008**, *72*(8), 2049-2060.
       [http://dx.doi.org/10.1271/bbb.80165] [PMID: 18685207]

[40]   Alberts, A.W.; Chen, J.; Kuron, G.; Hunt, V.; Huff, J.; Hoffman, C.; Rothrock, J.; Lopez, M.; Joshua,
       H.; Harris, E.; Patchett, A.; Monaghan, R.; Currie, S.; Stapley, E.; Albers-Schonberg, G.; Hensens, O.;
       Hirshfield, J.; Hoogsteen, K.; Liesch, J.; Springer, J. Mevinolin: A highly potent competitive inhibitor
       of hydroxymethylglutaryl-coenzyme A reductase and a cholesterol-lowering agent. *Proc. Natl. Acad.
       Sci.,* **1980**, *77*(7), 3957-3961.
       [http://dx.doi.org/10.1073/pnas.77.7.3957] [PMID: 6933445]

[41]   Schwender, J.; Müller, C.; Zeidler, J.; Lichtenthaler, H.K. Cloning and heterologous expression of a
       cDNA encoding 1-deoxy- D -xylulose-5-phosphate reductoisomerase of *Arabidopsis thaliana*[1]. *FEBS
       Lett.,* **1999**, *455*(1-2), 140-144.
       [http://dx.doi.org/10.1016/S0014-5793(99)00849-2] [PMID: 10428488]

[42]   Singh, R.S.; Gara, R.K.; Bhardwaj, P.K.; Kaachra, A.; Malik, S.; Kumar, R.; Sharma, M.; Ahuja, P.S.;
       Kumar, S. Expression of 3-hydroxy-3-methylglutaryl-coa reductase, p-hydroxybenzoate-
       m-geranyltransferase and genes of phenylpropanoid pathway exhibits positive correlation with
       shikonins content in arnebia arnebia euchroma (royle) johnston. *BMC Mol. Biol.,* **2010**, *11*(1), 88.
       [http://dx.doi.org/10.1186/1471-2199-11-88] [PMID: 21092138]

[43]   Gaisser, S.; Heide, L. Inhibition and regulation of shikonin biosynthesis in suspension cultures of
       lithospermum. *Phytochemistry,* **1996**, *41*(4), 1065-1072.
       [http://dx.doi.org/10.1016/0031-9422(95)00633-8]

[44]   Stermer, B.A.; Bianchini, G.M.; Korth, K.L. Regulation of HMG-CoA reductase activity in plants. *J.
       Lipid Res.,* **1994**, *35*(7), 1133-1140.
       [http://dx.doi.org/10.1016/S0022-2275(20)39958-2] [PMID: 7964176]

[45]   Bach, T.J.; Boronat, A.; Campos, N.; Ferrer, A.; Wollack, K-U. Mevalonate biosynthesis in plants. In:
       *Biochemistry and Function of Sterols*; Parish, E.J.; Nes, W.D., Eds.; CRC Press: Boca Raton, FL,
       USA, **1997**; pp. 135-150.

[46]   Lange, B.M.; Severin, K.; Bechthold, A.; Heide, L. Regulatory role of microsomal 3-hydroxy-
       3-methylglutaryl-coenzyme A reductase for shikonin biosynthesis in Lithospermum erythrorhizon cell
       suspension cultures. *Planta,* **1998**, *204*(2), 234-241.
       [http://dx.doi.org/10.1007/s004250050252] [PMID: 9487727]

[47]   Schmid, H.V.; Zenk, M.H. P-hydroxybenzoic acid and mevalonic acid as precursors of the plant
       naphthoquinone alkannin. *Tetrahedron Lett.,* **1971**, *12*(44), 4151-4155.
       [http://dx.doi.org/10.1016/S0040-4039(01)97486-6]

[48]   Inouye, H.; Ueda, S.; Inoue, K.; Matsumura, H. Biosynthesis of shikonin in callus cultures of
       *Lithospermum erythrorhizon. Phytochemistry,* **1979**, *18*(8), 1301-1308.
       [http://dx.doi.org/10.1016/0031-9422(79)83012-5]

[49]   Yamamura, Y.; Sahin, F.P.; Nagatsu, A.; Mizukami, H. Molecular cloning and characterization of a
       cDNA encoding a novel apoplastic protein preferentially expressed in a shikonin-producing callus
       strain of Lithospermum erythrorhizon. *Plant Cell Physiol.,* **2003**, *44*(4), 437-446.
       [http://dx.doi.org/10.1093/pcp/pcg057] [PMID: 12721385]

[50]   Rani, A.; Singh, K.; Sood, P.; Kumar, S.; Ahuja, P.S. p-Coumarate: CoA ligase as a key gene in the
       yield of catechins in tea [Camellia sinensis (L.) O. Kuntze]. *Funct. Integr. Genomics,* **2009**, *9*(2), 271-

275.
[http://dx.doi.org/10.1007/s10142-008-0098-3] [PMID: 18931865]

[51]  Singh, K.; Kumar, S.; Rani, A.; Gulati, A.; Ahuja, P.S. Phenylalanine ammonia-lyase *(PAL)* and cinnamate 4-hydroxylase (C4H) and catechins (flavan-3-ols) accumulation in tea. *Funct. Integr. Genomics,* **2009**, *9*(1), 125-134.
[http://dx.doi.org/10.1007/s10142-008-0092-9] [PMID: 18679731]

[52]  Heide, L.; Tabata, M. Geranylpyrophosphate: P-hydroxybenzoate geranyltransferase activity in extracts of Lithospermum erythrorhizon cell cultures. *Phytochemistry,* **1987**, *26*(6), 1651-1655.
[http://dx.doi.org/10.1016/S0031-9422(00)82263-3]

[53]  Kleinig, H. The role of plastid in isoprenoid biosynthesis. *Annu. Rev. Plant Physiol. Plant Mol. Biol.,* **1989**, *40*(1), 39-59.
[http://dx.doi.org/10.1146/annurev.pp.40.060189.000351]

[54]  Lichtenthaler, H.K.; Schwender, J.; Disch, A.; Rohmer, M. Biosynthesis of isoprenoids in higher plant chloroplasts proceeds *via* a mevalonate-independent pathway. *FEBS Lett.,* **1997**, *400*(3), 271-274. b
[http://dx.doi.org/10.1016/S0014-5793(96)01404-4] [PMID: 9009212]

[55]  Chappell, J. Biochemistry and molecular biology of the isoprenoid biosynthetic pathway in plants. *Annu. Rev. Plant Physiol. Plant Mol. Biol.,* **1995**, *46*(1), 521-547.
[http://dx.doi.org/10.1146/annurev.pp.46.060195.002513]

[56]  Verpoorte, R. Secondary metabolism. In: *Metabolic engineering of plant secondary metabolism*; Verpoorte, R.; Alfermann, A.W., Eds.; Kluwer Academic Publishers: Dordrecht, **2000**; pp. 1-29.
[http://dx.doi.org/10.1007/978-94-015-9423-3_1]

[57]  Schwarz, K.M. Terpen-biosynthese in ginkgo biloba: Eine uberraschende geschichte, Ph.D. Zurich, Switzerland.Swiss Federal Institute of Technology, **1994**.

[58]  McCaskill, D.; Croteau, R. Monoterpene and sesquiterpene biosynthesis in glandular trichomes of peppermint *(Mentha x piperita)* rely exclusively on plastid-derived isopentenyl diphosphate. *Planta,* **1995**, *197*(1), 49-56.
[http://dx.doi.org/10.1007/BF00239938]

[59]  Adam, K.P.; Zapp, J. Biosynthesis of the isoprene units of chamomile sesquiterpenes. *Phytochemistry,* **1998**, *48*(6), 953-959.
[http://dx.doi.org/10.1016/S0031-9422(97)00992-8]

[60]  Laule, O.; Fürholz, A.; Chang, H.S.; Zhu, T.; Wang, X.; Heifetz, P.B.; Gruissem, W.; Lange, M. Crosstalk between cytosolic and plastidial pathways of isoprenoid biosynthesis in *Arabidopsis thaliana. Proc. Natl. Acad. Sci.,* **2003**, *100*(11), 6866-6871.
[http://dx.doi.org/10.1073/pnas.1031755100] [PMID: 12748386]

[61]  Arigoni, D.; Eisenreich, W.; Latzel, C.; Sagner, S.; Radykewicz, T.; Zenk, M.H.; Bacher, A. Dimethylallyl pyrophosphate is not the committed precursor of isopentenyl pyrophosphate during terpenoid biosynthesis from 1-deoxyxylulose in higher plants. *Proc. Natl. Acad. Sci.,* **1999**, *96*(4), 1309-1314.
[http://dx.doi.org/10.1073/pnas.96.4.1309] [PMID: 9990020]

[62]  Hemmerlin, A.; Hoeffler, J.F.; Meyer, O.; Tritsch, D.; Kagan, I.A.; Grosdemange-Billiard, C.; Rohmer, M.; Bach, T.J. Cross-talk between the cytosolic mevalonate and the plastidial methylerythritol phosphate pathways in tobacco bright yellow-2 cells. *J. Biol. Chem.,* **2003**, *278*(29), 26666-26676.
[http://dx.doi.org/10.1074/jbc.M302526200] [PMID: 12736259]

[63]  Fellermeier, M.; Kis, K.; Sagner, S.; Maier, U.; Bacher, A.; Zenk, M.H. Cell-free conversion of 1-deoxy-D-xylulose 5-phosphate and 2-C-methyl-D-erythritol 4-phosphate into $\beta$-carotene in higher plants and its inhibition by fosmidomycin. *Tetrahedron Lett.,* **1999**, *40*(14), 2743-2746.
[http://dx.doi.org/10.1016/S0040-4039(99)00361-5]

[64]    Bick, J.A.; Lange, B.M. Metabolic cross talk between cytosolic and plastidial pathways of isoprenoid biosynthesis: unidirectional transport of intermediates across the chloroplast envelope membrane *Arch Biochem Biophys,* **2003**, *415*(2), 146-154.

[65]    Yazaki, K.; Sugiyama, A.; Morita, M.; Shitan, N. Secondary transport as an efficient membrane transport mechanism for plant secondary metabolites. *Phytochem. Rev.,* **2008**, *7*(3), 513-524.
[http://dx.doi.org/10.1007/s11101-007-9079-8]

[66]    Hashimoto, T.; Yamada, Y. New genes in alkaloid metabolism and transport. *Curr. Opin. Biotechnol.,* **2003**, *14*(2), 163-168.
[http://dx.doi.org/10.1016/S0958-1669(03)00027-2] [PMID: 12732317]

[67]    Tsukada, M.; Tabata, M. Intracellular localization and secretion of naphthoquinone pigments in cell cultures of *L. erythrorhizon. Planta Med.,* **1984**, *50*(4), 338-341.
[http://dx.doi.org/10.1055/s-2007-969725] [PMID: 17340324]

[68]    Tabata, M. The mechanism of shikonin biosynthesis in lithospermum cell cultures. *Plant tissue culture letters,* **1996**, *13*(2), 117-125.
[http://dx.doi.org/10.5511/plantbiotechnology1984.13.117]

[69]    Yamaga, Y.; Nakanishi, K.; Fukui, H.; Tabata, M. Intracellular localization of p-hydroxybenzoate geranyltransferase, a key enzyme involved in shikonin biosynthesis. *Phytochemistry,* **1993**, *32*(3), 633-636.
[http://dx.doi.org/10.1016/S0031-9422(00)95147-1]

[70]    Mühlenweg, A.; Melzer, M.; Li, S.M.; Heide, L. 4-Hydroxybenzoate 3-geranyltransferase from *lithospermum erythrorhizon*: Purification of a plant membrane-bound prenyltransferase. *Planta,* **1998**, *205*(3), 407-413.
[http://dx.doi.org/10.1007/s004250050337] [PMID: 9640665]

[71]    Ko, H.; Kim, S.J.; Shim, S.H.; Chang, H.; Ha, C.H. Shikonin induces apoptotic cell death *via* regulation of p53 and nrf2 in ags human stomach carcinoma cells. *Biomol. Ther.,* **2016**, *24*(5), 501-509.
[http://dx.doi.org/10.4062/biomolther.2016.008] [PMID: 27257011]

[72]    Seto, Y.; Motoyoshi, S.; Nakamura, H.; Imuta, J.; Ishitoku, T.; Isayama, S. [Effect of shikonin and its derivatives, pentaacetylated shikonin (MDS-004) on granuloma formation and delayed-type allergy in experimental animals]. *pharmacy magazine,* **1992**, *112*(4), 259-271.
[http://dx.doi.org/10.1248/yakushi1947.112.4_259] [PMID: 1403659]

[73]    Wang, W.J.; Bai, J.Y.; Liu, D.P.; Xue, L.M.; Zhu, X.Y. [The antiinflammatory activity of shikonin and its inhibitory effect on leukotriene B4 biosynthesis]. *Yao Xue Xue Bao,* **1994**, *29*(3), 161-165.
[PMID: 8079645]

[74]    Kashiwada, Y.; Nishizawa, M.; Yamagishi, T.; Tanaka, T.; Nonaka, G.; Cosentino, L.M.; Snider, J.V.; Lee, K.H. Anti-AIDS agents, 18. sodium and potassium salts of caffeic acid tetramers from arnebia euchroma as anti-hiv agents. *J. Nat. Prod.,* **1995**, *58*(3), 392-400.
[http://dx.doi.org/10.1021/np50117a007] [PMID: 7775984]

[75]    Wang, R.; Yin, R.; Zhou, W.; Xu, D.; Li, S. Shikonin and its derivatives: A patent review *Expert Opin Ther Pat.,* **2012**, *22*(9), 977-997.
[http://dx.doi.org/10.1517/13543776.2012.709237]

[76]    Chen, Y.; Zheng, L.; Liu, J.; Zhou, Z.; Cao, X.; Lv, X.; Chen, F. Shikonin inhibits prostate cancer cells metastasis by reducing matrix metalloproteinase-2/-9 expression *via* AKT/mTOR and ROS/ERK1/2 pathways. *Int. Immunopharmacol.,* **2014**, *21*(2), 447-455.
[http://dx.doi.org/10.1016/j.intimp.2014.05.026] [PMID: 24905636]

[77]    Lu, L.; Qin, A.; Huang, H.; Zhou, P.; Zhang, C.; Liu, N.; Li, S.; Wen, G.; Zhang, C.; Dong, W.; Wang, X.; Dou, Q.P.; Liu, J. Shikonin extracted from medicinal chinese herbs exerts anti-inflammatory effect *via* proteasome inhibition. *Eur. J. Pharmacol.,* **2011**, *658*(2-3), 242-247.

[http://dx.doi.org/10.1016/j.ejphar.2011.02.043] [PMID: 21392503]

[78]    Hsiao, C.Y.; Tsai, T.H.; Chak, K.F. The molecular basis of wound healing processes induced by lithospermi radix: A proteomics and biochemical analysis. *Evid. Based Complement. Alternat. Med.,* **2012**, *2012*, 1-15.
[http://dx.doi.org/10.1155/2012/508972] [PMID: 23024692]

[79]    Andújar, I.; Ríos, J.L.; Giner, R.M.; Recio, M.C. Shikonin promotes intestinal wound healing *in vitro via* induction of TGF-β release in IEC-18 cells. *Eur. J. Pharm. Sci.,* **2013**, *49*(4), 637-641.
[http://dx.doi.org/10.1016/j.ejps.2013.05.018] [PMID: 23727294]

[80]    Takano-Ohmuro, H.; Yoshida, L.S.; Yuda, Y.; Morioka, K.; Kitani, S. Shikonin inhibits IgE-mediated histamine release by human basophils and Syk kinase activity. *Inflamm. Res.,* **2008**, *57*(10), 484-488.
[http://dx.doi.org/10.1007/s00011-008-8067-9] [PMID: 18830561]

[81]    Chen, X.; Yang, L.; Zhang, N.; Turpin, J.A.; Buckheit, R.W.; Osterling, C.; Oppenheim, J.J.; Howard, O.M.Z. Shikonin, a component of chinese herbal medicine, inhibits chemokine receptor function and suppresses human immunodeficiency virus type 1. *Antimicrob. Agents Chemother.,* **2003**, *47*(9), 2810-2816.
[http://dx.doi.org/10.1128/AAC.47.9.2810-2816.2003] [PMID: 12936978]

[82]    Min, B.S.; Miyashiro, H.; Hattori, M. Inhibitory effects of quinones on RNase H activity associated with HIV-1 reverse transcriptase. *Phytother. Res.,* **2002**, *16*(S1) 1, 57-62.
[http://dx.doi.org/10.1002/ptr.808] [PMID: 11933141]

[83]    Andújar, I.; Ríos, J.; Giner, R.; Recio, M. Pharmacological properties of shikonin :A review of literature since 2002. *Planta Med.,* **2013**, *79*(18), 1685-1697.
[http://dx.doi.org/10.1055/s-0033-1350934] [PMID: 24155261]

*Frontiers In Medicinal Chemistry*, 2023, *Vol. 10*, 249-261

# CHAPTER 9

# Fast Foods: Chemical Composition and Implications for Health

**Ruchi Kumari**[1] and **Ravi S. Singh**[2,*]

[1] *University Department of Home Science-Food and Nutrition, Tilka Manjhi Bhagalpur University, Bhagalpur-812 007, Bihar, India*

[2] *Department of Plant Breeding and Genetics, Bihar Agricultural University, Sabour, Bhagalpur, Bihar- 813210, India*

**Abstract:** With changing the scenarios of living style, professional work culture, and daily hectic routine, liberal and global thoughts are impacting our dietary patterns and normal food consumption. So the preference for foods is changing, and foods that can be ready in a shorter time, like "fast foods", are gaining popularity among the masses, especially young generations. The fast food business has become one of the fastest-growing industries across the globe. This growing trend of fast food consumption has also brought several health-associated issues, like obesity and heart-related problems. Therefore, health-conscious people do like to know the chemical ingredients embedded in fast foods as well as their packaging and storage. For this purpose, the chemistry relating to quality aspects of fast foods, including nutritional, physiological, sensory, flavor, microbiological and packaging, is very important for healthy consumption of fast food for a healthy life. In this book chapter, we have made efforts to bring updated information related to fast food, its chemical composition and implications for human health.

**Keywords:** Chemical composition, Calorie, Fast food, Indian fast food, Western fast food.

## 1. INTRODUCTION

With changing the scenarios of living style, professional work culture, and daily hectic routine, liberal and global thoughts are impacting our dietary patterns and normal food consumption. So the preference for food is changing, and foods that can be ready in a shorter time, like "fast foods", are gaining popularity among the masses, especially young generations. The fast food business has become one of the fastest-growing industries across the globe. The National Institute of Health

* **Corresponding author Ravi S. Singh:** Department of Plant Breeding and Genetics, Bihar Agricultural University, Sabour, Bhagalpur, Bihar- 813210, India; E-mail: ravissingh0202@gmail.com

**Ashok Kumar Jha & Ravi S. Singh (Eds.)**

(NIH, USA) defines fast food as quick and cheap alternatives to home meals. These foods are rich in saturated fat, sugar, salt and calories. As per the definition quoted at Wikipedia, fast food is food that is sold in a restaurant or store with pre-heated or pre-cooked ingredients and served to the customer in a package form for take-out/take-away. Bender and Bender's [1] definition of fast food is a universal term used for foods that can be produced in large quantities or mass production. Banerjee *et al.* [2] stated that fast food is a byproduct of technological advances in food processing, newly invented food additives and techniques for preservation. Though fast food saves time, it does not save us from consuming fats, sodium and preservatives.

Eating out in India has evolved from an occasion-driven activity to an everyday activity, and fast food has become a significant symbol of modern culture as it tends to satisfy customers in a relatively short time [3]. The emergence of the fast food industry has transformed global food culture in general, and particularly its effect can be seen in urban areas of India. In India, fast food culture emerged after independence and decades later due to the growth in the number of nuclear families as well as working parents, increasing per capita income as well as globalization. This culture further rose to prominence with the liberalization of the Indian economy after 1990. Reputed multi-national companies (MNCs) started their business in India, and the Indian market flooded with their outlets especially in the metro, even the presence can be seen in small cities, with some outlets functioning in shopping malls and other public areas. MNCs like Burger King, Pizza Hut, Domino's Pizza, McDonald's and KFC (Kentucky Fried Chicken) are serving several Western fast foods, including Burger, French fries, Pizza, Hamburgers, *etc.,* to satisfy the Indian consumer's taste buds [4].

India also has a long tradition of delicious foods with a variety of recipes that exist in every part of the country. Indian food included in the list of fast food are Alloo-tikki, Bhelpuri, Panipuri, Paav-bhaji, Chat, Pakora, Samosa, Kachaudi, Chole-Bhature, Idli, Dosa, Uttapam, *etc.*(Kumari 2020). Indian fast food depends on the cooking method. Indian fast foods are traditionally prepared by deep frying in fat [5]. There are enough data that suggest that fast foods have become an integral component of the diet in all sections of society. It was also found that youngsters often visit fast food channels just for the sake of fun and some change from daily routine eating [6]. Today, the fast food industry is adapted to Indian food requirements and is growing rapidly. As fast food is generally considered rich in calories, fat, sugar, and salt and poor in other nutrients, it has contributed to the rise of many non-communicable diseases and metabolic diseases such as obesity and overweight, type 2 diabetes mellitus, hypertension and heart-related issues, *etc.* In contrast to the classical way of qualitative and quantitative chemical analysis of foods, new ways and approaches are also being adopted that study the food and nutrition aspects on the line of other " omics" technologies such as metabolomics, genomics, transcriptomics, proteomics to enrich human health and knowledge. These "omics" approaches are helpful in understanding humans, food, microbe and the environment under the aegis of "Foodomics", a new multidisciplinary approach. It involves a range of aspects, from analysing the composition, quality, processing, safety and storage of foods to microbial interaction with pathogens and probiotics, to environmental safety and contamination, and to human clinical and nutrition aspects [7]. Foodomics unravels food-responsive gene regulation by integrating the study of nutrition, gene and omics. Further, foodomics is basically the study of chemical compounds present in food and their influence on gene expression by the application and integration of advanced omics technologies.

## 2. CHEMICALS USED AS FOOD ADDITIVES AND HEALTH ISSUES

Fast foods served in restaurants or stores are quickly ready and packaged for takeaway. These foods are energy rich foods with many things in higher concentration than the normal human requirement and considered nutritionally low grade for health point of view, for example, high content of sugar, fat, salt, protein and lower health friendly fiber, vitamin and mineral. Some of the chemicals such as sodium nitrite, sodium benzoate, azo-dicarbonamide (as a preservative), dimethyl-polysiloxane (as an anti-foaming agent), calcium caseinate (as an emulsifier), monosodium glutamate (as a flavor enhancer) often used in fast food, making these foods unsafe and unhealthy. Food packaging materials like wrappers usually contain phthalates, perfluoroalkyl and polyfluoroalkyl (PFAs), are reported to leach out of the wrapper and contaminate fast foods raising health issues, as these compounds are linked to infertility, diabetes, obesity and cancer. The chemistry of fast food additives, contaminants, agro-chemicals, together with their metabolism and toxicology decides the fate of the end product we consume. Food additives used to prolong the shelf life of foods and making more attractive are also sometimes a health concern. It is evident that too much fatty foods and sweets increase the insulin levels in the human body. Excess consumption of trans-fats due to deep frying can send mixed signals to the brain about hunger. Foods high in sugar and fat suppress the activity of a brain peptide called brain-derived neurotrophic factor that helps with learning and memory formation. Excess intake of fast foods increases calories that can interfere with the healthy production and functioning of brain synapses governing the function of learning and memory. Further, some of the fatty acids like omega-6 and omega-3 are essential for normal brain functions. A lower daily dose of these two increases the risk of dementia and other brain-related problems. Also, too much fast food intake leads to the loss of essential amino acids like tryptophan that increases feelings of depression. Even fast foods and processed foods increase childhood obesity, heart disease and diabetes and other chronic problems.

Chemical composition and structural changes in molecules during the preparation/processing of fast foods affect their quality. Many of the chemicals found in food occur naturally and include nutrients such as carbohydrates, protein, fat, fiber and a host of other elements and compounds, also fast foods enhanced with bioactive compounds like antioxidants, phytochemicals, and botanicals or bio-fortified foods are considered healthy. Some of the chemicals considered to be toxic to human health are part of fast foods, such as propylene glycol, tertiary butylhydroquinone (TBHQ), calcium sulfate, potassium bromate, phosphate additives, butylated hydroxytoluene (BHT), propylene glycol, *etc.*

## 2.1. Potassium Bromate

Potassium bromate is used as a food additive in recipes to improve the texture even after baking, if used in excess, some amounts remain in the baked product. This may be a carcinogen in humans since it has been shown to cause kidney, thyroid, and gastrointestinal cancer in animals (https://nj.gov/health/eoh/rtkweb/documents/fs/1559.pdf). The deleterious effect of potassium bromate administration on the renal and hepatic tissues of Swiss mice has also been reported [8] (Fig. **1**).

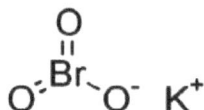

$$O^-\overset{\overset{\displaystyle O}{\|}}{Br}O^-\ \ K^+$$

**Fig. (1).** Potassium Bromate.

## 2.2. Propylene Glycol

The propylene glycol is a colorless synthetic compound used as an anti-caking substance considered to be generally safe for health. Several food products like ice cream, soft drinks, dressings, marinades, frostings, dairy products, *etc.,* use propylene glycol to preserve the texture by keeping foods moist and not letting drying out. It may cause toxicity if taken in higher amounts, but this still needs to be proven. The World Health Organization (WHO) has determined that 25 milligrams of propylene glycol for every kilogram of body weight is an acceptable ingestion amount. The most prominent danger propylene glycol may cause central nervous system depression, which can lead to decreased heart rate and slowed breathing [9] (Fig. **2**).

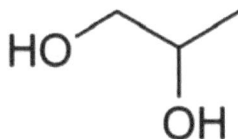

**Fig. (2).** Propylene glycol.

## 2.3. Tertiary Butyl Hydroquinone (TBHQ)

Fried meals and snacks found at fast-food restaurants are likely to contain the preservative tertiary butyl hydroquinone, or TBHQ, in order to prevent spoilage in oils and fats (usually animal fats). At concentrations less than 0.02%, TBHQ extends the shelf life of edible fats and oils [10]. However, studies indicated that TBHQ may lead to possible health complications. TBHQ exhibits antioxidative actions at concentrations that are lower than those which elicit adverse cellular effects; sublethal levels of TBHQ cause some adverse actions that may be clinically concerned [11] (Fig. **3**).

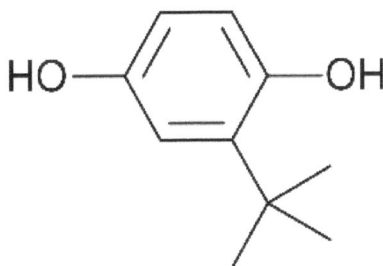

**Fig. (3).** Tertiary butylhydroquinone (TBHQ).

## 2.4. Calcium Sulfate

This is also an anti-caking substance and dough strengthener, used in rolls and baked items to add some calcium to foods. Calcium sulfate added directly to human food is generally recognized as safe (GRAS) by the U.S. Food and Drug Administration (FDA). But, high bolus intakes of sulfate ions may lead to gastrointestinal discomfort in some individuals [12] (Fig. **4**).

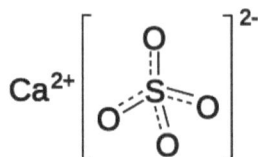

**Fig. (4).** Calcium Sulfate.

## 2.5. Phosphate Additives

Soda, flavored waters, packaged meat, processed cheese, and chicken nuggets are just a handful of the foods that are likely to contain this food additive, which derives from the mineral phosphorus and is designed to enhance flavor and act as an emulsifier. This is believed that high levels of phosphorus intake may be detrimental to bone, heart and kidneys [13].

## 2.6. Butylated Hydroxyl Toluene (BHT)

BHT is a synthetic chemical used to maintain the freshness of food, such as sandwich spreads, desserts, beverages, mayo, sauces, dry yeast, potato flakes, *etc.* If used in higher amounts in food, it may pose a risk to certain cancers. Butylated hydroxyl anisole (BHA) and butylated hydroxyl toluene (BHT) are widely used antioxidant food additives. They have been extensively studied for potential toxicities. Williams *et al.* [14] reviewed detailed experimental studies of genotoxicity and carcinogenicity and concluded that BHT does not pose a cancer hazard, but it may be anticarcinogenic at current levels of food additive use [14] (Fig. **5**).

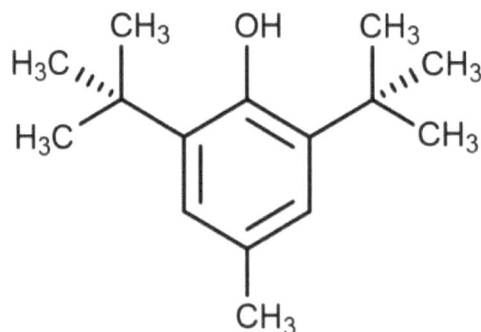

**Fig. (5).** Butylated hydroxytoluene.

## 2.7. Propyl Gallate

Propyl gallate is added in meat products, corn products, and mayonnaise as a food preservative to delay or check food spoilage and extend shelf life in oils. The various biological activity of propyl gallate is due to its free-radical scavenging ability, such as antimicrobial activity, enzyme inhibition, inhibition of the formation of nitrosamines, anesthesia, inhibition of neuromuscular response to chemicals, ionizing/ultraviolet radiation protection, antimutagenesis, anticarcinogenesis, antiteratogenesis, *etc* [15]. The studies on animal toxicity indicated that propyl gallate was slightly toxic when ingested, but no systemic effects were noted with dermal application [15] (Fig. **6**).

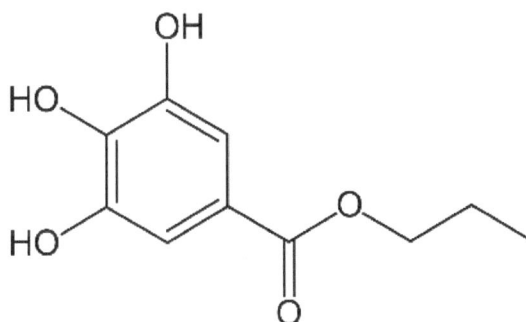

**Fig. (6).** Propyl gallate.

## 2.8. Phthalates

Phthalates are mainly used as plasticizers added to polyvinyl chloride plastics for softening effects. These can be found in any product that has contact with plastics during producing, packaging, or delivering, for example, take-home boxes, plastic containers, gloves, *etc.*, and these can cause health risks such as endocrine disruptors that disrupt hormonal balances [16, 17] (Fig. **7**).

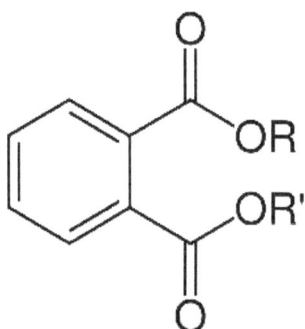

**Fig. (7).** Phthalates.

## 2.9. Fluorine

Per- and poly fluoro alkyl substances (also known as PFASs) are fluorine-based chemicals in fast-food packaging associated with cancer, fertility issues, low birth weight, and make poor immunity in the body [18, 19]. Generally used by most fast-food chains on the coating of containers and wrappers to prevent grease and water to come in contact with food containing fluorine in the form of PFAS (Fig. 8).

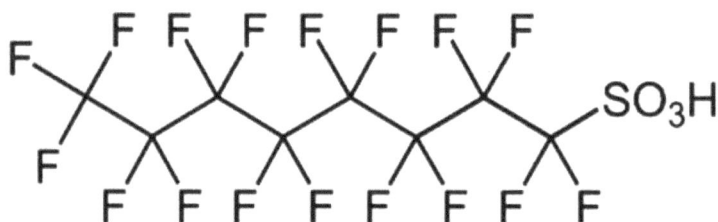

**Fig. (8).** Per- and polyfluoroalkyl substances (PFASs).

## 3. TRENDS OF FAST FOOD CONSUMPTION

Increasing fast food consumption and skipping of breakfast in diet is usually seen in the transition phase of adulthood. The normal balanced diet is being replaced by fast food, and this saga is not limited to young generations but also comprises people of all age-groups who ask the fast food in their day-to-day eating habits [4]. The changing mindset for food choices is the key force behind this.

The diversion in dietary behaviors from normal is a matter of concern for health, such as (1) weight gain, (2) increased blood pressure and decreased calcium absorption, (3) dental carries, and (4) fertility problems [5]. Consumption of fast food has an effect on social and mental health as well. In school days, there are a lot of educational challenges that require much attention to meet the nutritional balance (Table **1**). Poor nutritional habits can undermine the stamina and potentiality of learning, as well as deplete the strength that children need for making friends, interacting with family, participating in sports and games or simply feeling good about them.

## 4. REASONS FOR INCREASED FAST FOOD CONSUMPTION

- Changing lifestyle, high disposable income, professional work culture, and liberal and global thoughts are key divers letting consumers towards fast food.
- These impact dietary patterns and routine food consumption.
- Out of various foods consumed across the world, "fast food" is one that is becoming popular among the masses, especially young generations, thereby it is one of the fastest growing industries.
- Changing lifestyle leading to an increase in fast food consumption among teenagers.
- Mushrooming of fast food outlets impacts teenagers' food habits.
- Exposure to heavy advertisements by companies and restaurants of fast food products to attract teenagers towards fast food [4, 20, 21, 24].

**Table 1. Chemical content and nutritional datasheet of fast foods [7, 4] .**

| Food Items | Serving Size/100g | Total Calories | Total Fat (g) | Saturated Fat (g) | Trans Fat (g) | Carbohydrate (g) | Sodium (mg) |
|---|---|---|---|---|---|---|---|
| **Indian Fast Food** | | | | | | | |
| Aloo pakoda | 1 regular | 225 | 19 | | | 13 | |
| Bread pakoda | | 289 | | | 0 | 51 | 371 |
| Pani puri | 5 pieces | 270 | 12 | 1.5 | 0 | 33 | 410 |
| Chhole bhature | 281 g | | 27 | 4.1 | | 59 | 507 |
| Pavbhaji | 1 plate with ½ pav | 200 | 12 | 12 | - | 47 | 1,272 |
| Veg. Upama | 1 cup | 322 | 6 | - | - | 59 | 480 |
| Poha | 194 g | 360 | 6 | 1.1 | - | 69 | 446 |
| Plain paratha (sunfiower oil) | 1 piece (51.7gm) | 275 | 8 | 1 | - | 22 | 333 |
| Paneer paratha | 78 (gm) | 176 | 7.8 | 4.1 | - | 21 | 445 |

*(Table 1) cont.....*

| Food Items | Serving Size/100g | Total Calories | Total Fat (g) | Saturated Fat (g) | Trans Fat (g) | Carbohydrate (g) | Sodium (mg) |
|---|---|---|---|---|---|---|---|
| **Indian Fast Food** | | | | | | | |
| Aloo paratha | 1 piece | 162 | 5 | 1 | - | 26 | 33 |
| Idali | 1 piece (30 g) | 40 | 0.19 | 0.037 | - | 7.89 | 207 |
| Dosa | 1 piece (97 g) | 168 | 3.7 | 0.5 | 0 | 29 | 94 |
| **Western Fast food** | | | | | | | |
| Pizza | Large/94-146 | 200-390 | 7-19 | 3.5-7 | 0 | 25-38 | 340-800 |
| Burger/Hamburger | 100-209 | 250-470 | 9-19 | 3.5-7.0 | 0.5-1.0 | 31-54 | 520-1060 |
| French-fries | Regular/ 160-170 | 500-570 | 11-30 | 2-6 | 0-8 | 42-70 | 330-530 |
| Hot dog | 100 | 289 | 26 | 8 | - | 4.2 | 1090 |
| Chicken Sandwich | Premium-grilled /147-260 | 360-660 | 16-28 | 3.5-8 | 1-1.5 | 40-68 | 790-1860 |
| Fried Chicken/fish | Chicken Nuggets (6pc) / 96-218 | 250-630 | 15-41 | 3-6 | 1.5-4.5 | 15-47 | 670-1550 |
| Noodles | 100 | 138 | 2.1 | 0.4 | - | 25 | 5 |
| Chips | 100 | 536 | 35 | 11 | - | 53 | 8 |
| Chocolates | 100 | 545 | 31 | 19 | 0.1 | 61 | 24 |
| Ice-creams | 100 | 207 | 11 | 7 | | 24 | 80 |
| Pastries/Cake | 100 | 550 | 38 | 10 | - | 45 | 249 |
| Soft drinks | 100 | 40 | 0 | 0 | 0 | 11 | 4 |
| Bread roll | 100 | 310 | 6 | 1.4 | 1.8 | 52 | 467 |
| Salad | 100 | 152 | 10 | 1.6 | 0 | 15 | 203 |

## 5. CURBING FAST FOOD MENACE

Following suggestions may be considered based on various scientific reports [4, 5, 21 - 24]:

- Fast food should not be taken frequently, don't skip the regular diet.
- Fast food should be supplementary to the normal meal but not as an alternative, as it may impact health (BMI and obesity).
- Self-cooking is the best way, one can maintain proper hygiene, calorific, and nutritional values.
- Avoid cold drinks and other beverages rich in sugar and caffeine, along with fast foods.
- Eat fast food in the evening, not late at night or in the morning.

- Preference for fast food should be nutritive/calorific value, not on taste, convenience, price or as a status symbol.
- The size of fast food should be small or medium.
- Avoid spicy, oily, sugar and salt fast foods.
- Don't get attracted by promotional offers/advertisements of fast foods.
- It should be consumed as a refreshment.
- Check the nutritional/calorific label on fast food before consuming.
- Emphasis on educational knowledge or educational programme about fast foods through the regular syllabus, online e-content, journals, magazines, news-daily TV/radio, and public awareness campaigns.
- Imposing high taxes on fast foods to discourage consumption-a fat tax or surcharge has been placed upon fattening food, beverages or on overweight individuals.
- A fat tax aims to discourage unhealthy diets and offset the economic costs of obesity. In India, Kerala became the first state; in 2016 budgets, the government proposed a 14.5% 'fat tax' on burgers, pizzas and other junk foods served in branded restaurants, which officials from the quick service industry termed as 'detrimental' to consumption.

## CONCLUSION

It is important to decipher the chemicals (good or bad) that are embedded in fast foods making them delicious and chemically enhanced but also putting us at health risk, and to let the consumer know what they are actually consuming from a nutrition and health point of view. For this purpose, the chemistry relating to quality aspects of fast foods, including nutritional, physiological, sensory, flavor, microbiological and packaging, is very important for a healthy life. Furthermore, nowadays nutraceutical products also serve the purpose of medicine besides nutrition, which are known to provide physiological benefits/protection against chronic disease and are becoming popular among health conscious people.

## ACKNOWLEDGEMENTS

The authors thank the PG Department of Home Science-Food and Nutrition, Tilka Manjhi Bhagalpur University, Bhagalpur and Bihar Agricultural University, Sabour, for their support during the study.

## REFERENCES

[1]    Bender, A.; Bender, D. *A Dictionary of Food and Nutrition*; Oxford University Press: Oxford, **1995**.

[2]    Banerjee, S.; Joglekar, A.; Kundle, S. Consumer awareness about convenience food among working and non-working women. *Int. J. Sci. Res.,* **2013**, *2*(10), 2277-8179.

[3]    Narayan, B.; Prabhu, M. Examining fast-food consumption behaviour of students in Manipal University, India. *Afr. J. Hosp. Tour. Leis.,* **2015**, *4*(2), 1-9.

[4]     Kumari, R. *Comparative Study of Indian and Western Fast Food Consumption among Teenagers of Sabour Block, Bhagalpur*; Ph.D. thesis submitted to TilkaManjhi Bhagalpur University: Bhagalpur-812 005, India, **2020**.

[5]     Keshari, P.; Mishra, C. Growing menace of fast food consumption in India: Time to act. *Int. J. Community Med. Public Health,* **2016**, *3*(6), 1355-1362.
[http://dx.doi.org/10.18203/2394-6040.ijcmph20161600]

[6]     Goyal, A.; Singh, N.P. Consumer perception about fast food in India: An exploratory study. *Br. Food J.,* **2007**, *109*(2), 182-195.
[http://dx.doi.org/10.1108/00070700710725536]

[7]     Kumari, R.; Kumari, M.; Singh, R.S. Foodomics with perspective on nutritional and health aspects of fast food. In: *Recent Advances in Chemical sciences and Biotechnology*; Jha, A.K.; Kumar, U, Eds.; New Delhi Publication: New Delhi, **2018**; pp. 52-62.

[8]     Altoom, N.G.; Ajarem, J.; Allam, A.A.; Maodaa, S.N.; Abdel-Maksoud, M.A. Deleterious effects of potassium bromate administration on renal and hepatic tissues of Swiss mice. *Saudi J. Biol. Sci.,* **2018**, *25*(2), 278-284.
[http://dx.doi.org/10.1016/j.sjbs.2017.01.060] [PMID: 29472778]

[9]     Danger of drinking propylene glycol. Available from: https://sciencing.com/danger-inhalin--propylene-glycol-5499611.html (Retrieved on 07.04.2022)

[10]    Kashanian, S.; Dolatabadi, J.E.N. DNA binding studies of 2-tert-butylhydroquinone (TBHQ) food additive. *Food Chem.,* **2009**, *116*(3), 743-747.
[http://dx.doi.org/10.1016/j.foodchem.2009.03.027]

[11]    Kamemura, N.; Oyama, K.; Kanemaru, K.; Yokoigawa, K.; Oyama, Y. Diverse cellular actions of *tert*-butylhydroquinone, a food additive, on rat thymocytes. *Toxicol. Res.,* **2017**, *6*(6), 922-929.
[http://dx.doi.org/10.1039/C7TX00183E] [PMID: 30090553]

[12]    Calcium sulfate. Available from: https://healthjade.net/calcium-sulfate/ (retrieved on 08.04.2022)

[13]    Phosphorus and your diet. Available from: https://www.kidney.org/atoz/content/phosphorus (retrieved on 08.04.2022)

[14]    Williams, G.M.; Iatropoulos, M.J.; Whysner, J. Safety assessment of butylated hydroxyanisole and butylated hydroxytoluene as antioxidant food additives. *Food Chem. Toxicol.,* **1999**, *37*(9-10), 1027-1038.
[http://dx.doi.org/10.1016/S0278-6915(99)00085-X] [PMID: 10541460]

[15]    Anonymous final report on the amended safety assessment of propyl gallate. *Int. J. Toxicol.,* **2007**, *26*(3_suppl) 3, 89-118.
[http://dx.doi.org/10.1080/10915810701663176] [PMID: 18080874]

[16]    Benjamin, S.; Masaia, E.; Kamimura, N.; Takahashi, K.; Anderson, R. C.; Faisal, P. A. Phthalates impact human health: Epidemiological evidences and plausible mechanism of action. *J. Hazard. Mat.,* **2017**, *340*, 360-383.

[17]    Wang, Y.; Qian, H. Phthalates and their impacts on human health. *Healthcare,* **2021**, *9*(5), 603.
[http://dx.doi.org/10.3390/healthcare9050603] [PMID: 34069956]

[18]    Brown, J.B.; Conder, J.M.; Arblaster, J.A.; Higgins, C.P. Assessing human health risks from per- and polyfluoroalkyl substance (pfas)-impacted vegetable consumption: A tiered modeling approach. *Environ. Sci. Technol.,* **2020**, *54*(23), 15202-15214.
[http://dx.doi.org/10.1021/acs.est.0c03411] [PMID: 33200604]

[19]    Ojo, A.F.; Peng, C.; Ng, J.C. Assessing the human health risks of per- and polyfluoroalkyl substances: A need for greater focus on their interactions as mixtures. *J. Hazard. Mater.,* **2021**, *407*, 124863.
[http://dx.doi.org/10.1016/j.jhazmat.2020.124863] [PMID: 33373965]

[20]    Kumari, R.; Kumari, M. Principal component analysis for fast food consumption among teenagers of

sabour block in Bhagalpur, India. *Int. J. Curr. Microbiol. Appl. Sci.,* **2019**, *8*(8), 1675-1689.
[http://dx.doi.org/10.20546/ijcmas.2019.808.198]

[21]   Kumari, R.; Kumari, M. How much healthier is fast food? A survey on calorie status and life style diseases among teenagers of Sabour Block in Bhagalpur District of India. *Int. J. Appl. Home. Sci.,* **2020**, *7*(3-6), 44-50.

[22]   Kumari, R.; Kumari, M. Need of effective educational programme on fast food for awareness among teenagers of Sabour block in Bhagalpur district of India. *Int. J. Home Sci.,* **2020**, *6*(3), 254-263.

[23]   Kumari, R.; Kumari, M. Factors affecting the choice of fast food among teenagers of Sabour block in Bhagalpur district of India. *Pharma Innov.,* **2020**, *9*(10), 211-216.
[http://dx.doi.org/10.22271/tpi.2020.v9.i10c.5230]

[24]   Kumari, R.; Kumari, M. Quality aspects of fast foods and their consumption pattern among teenagers of rural-urban region of Sabour block in Bhagalpur district of India. *Pharma Innov.,* **2020**, *9*(4), 96-102.
[http://dx.doi.org/10.22271/tpi.2020.v9.i4b.4575]

# CHAPTER 10

# Implications of DNA-acting Agents as Anticarcinogenic Potential in Breast Cancer Therapeutics

**Lovely Sinha[1,*] and Ujjwal Kumar[2]**

[1] *Department of Pulmonary Medicine, All India Institute of Medical Sciences, Patna-801507, Bihar, India*

[2] *Research Associate, Department of Psychatry & Department of CFM, All India Institute of Medical Sciences, Deoghar - 814152, Jharkhand, India*

**Abstract:** Breast cancer is the most prevalent neoplasm diagnosed in women worldwide. There are many factors responsible for breast cancer susceptibility. Mutation in tumor suppressor genes *BRCA1* and *BRCA2* predispose women to the early onset of breast cancer. The *BRCA* genes are involved in multiple cellular processes in response to DNA damage, including checkpoint activation, gene transcription, and DNA repair. Several DNA-acting agents act as effective anticancer used for treating cancer disease. Certain groups of chemicals are known to affect specific phases of cell division, such as, Cyclophosphamide is the most potent and successful anticancer agent that acts by alkylating the N-7position of guanine to cause crosslinking of DNA's double helix, resulting in DNA breaks that interfere with the DNA replication and RNA transcription. This chapter deals with the classification of DNA-acting agents according to their modes of action.

**Keywords:** Breast Cancer, Cyclophosphamide, DNA-acting agent, DNA damage.

## 1. BACKGROUND

Breast cancer continues to be a leading healthcare problem and the most common cause of cancer deaths among women worldwide in the current scenario [1]. In recent years, the incidence rates of breast cancer have been high in more developed countries, whereas rates in less developed countries are low but increasing. The three most common cancers—breast, lung, and colorectal—together represent one-half of all new diagnoses, with breast cancer alone accounting for 30% of all new cancer diagnoses in women. According to the

* **Corresponding author Lovely Sinha:** Department of Pulmonary Medicine, All India Institute of Medical Sciences, Patna-801507, Bihar, India E-mail: lovely130297@gmail.com

**Ashok Kumar Jha & Ravi S. Singh (Eds.)**

Global Cancer Statistics 2020, the number of new deaths due to breast cancer has risen to 684,996 (6.9%), more than the number reported in earlier years [2]. In fact, India has seen a drastic increase in breast cancer, and the death rate is higher in rural areas despite lower incidences of breast cancer compared to urban cities, indicating variation in disease susceptibility and clinical outcomes [3].

Cancer is a multistep process that involves cumulative genetic and epigenetic alterations, including the activation of oncogenes and the dysfunction of tumor suppressor genes [4]. *BRCA1* and *BRCA2* are tumor suppressor genes that control cell growth and cell death and also show inherited mutations in women with breast cancer. The estimated lifetime risk for females who carry *BRCA1* and *BRCA2* gene mutations is about 65% of total breast cancer cases. Those who have already developed breast cancer are at an increased risk for secondary malignancy compared to non-carriers and their families of *BRCA1* & *BRCA2* mutations [5].

Genetic changes are involved in the origin of breast cancer, as well as in various other human cancers. Epigenetic changes in DNA may be caused by a number of mutagens to which the individual is exposed through lifestyle or environmental factors such as heavy metal contamination, but they also represent physical and chemical changes in the DNA. Numerous factors are attributed to causing breast cancer. These factors include chemical substances (such as tobacco, asbestos, industrial waste, groundwater arsenic contamination, and pesticides), diet (saturated fat, red meat, overweight), ionizing radiation, pathogens, etc. Both genetic and environmental factors affect breast cancer risks, but the molecular pathophysiology of gene-environment interactions is complex [6, 7].

Long-term exposure to environmental pollutants (*e.g.*, fossil fuel combustion products and cooking oils in the home, heavy metals, and occupational respiratory carcinogens) has a significant effect on influencing breast cancer incidence and mortality [8]. Carcinogenic residues of environmental pollutants halt the cell cycle events and cause DNA damage. The cell cycle is the progression of events that ensures the generation of two daughter cells from one parental cell. It is described in four major phases: the First gap phase (G1), DNA synthesis stage (S), the Second gap phase (G2), and the Mitosis phase (M), respectively. The time period that a cell remains in the G1 phase depends on the tissue type and whether it is a normal or tumor cell. If the cell is a proliferating cell, it will quickly move into the synthesis phase (S). During this phase, the DNA is replicated, and at the end of the S phase, two copies of DNA are present in the cell. The next phase is the G2 phase, where preparations are largely made for the final cell cycle phase, the M phase or the mitosis phase. There are two major control checkpoints in the cell cycle. One of these is at the G1/S stage when cells commit to replicate, while the second is at the G2/M stage, when cells commit to divide [9]. Of these two major points in the cell cycle, the G1/S stage is of major importance in understanding cancer and chemotherapy.

## 2. DNA ACTING AGENTS

Chemicals specific for DNA synthesis inhibition and others that modify the structure are also known. It is understood that the mechanism could be different, but the ultimate results may be the same, for example, the inhibition of cell division or alteration of gene expressions in the growing cell population or differentiating cells [7]. These compounds act as anticancer or antineoplastic agents that are useful in the treatment of cancer.

These compounds can be broadly classified into a few groups:

a. Nucleic acid base analogues
b. Nucleoside antibiotics
c. Alkylating agents
d. Nitroso compounds

## 2.1. Nucleic Acid Base Analogues

Purines and pyrimidines are basic components of nucleic acids. In both normal and altered growth of living systems, these universal components are involved in cellular functions and multiplication. A base analogue should be sufficiently similar to one of the four normal bases of DNA or ribonucleic acid (RNA) so that it can be incorporated into DNA during replication or into RNA during transcription by competing with the endogenous ones. Such a substance should be able to alter base pairing in the template strand. However, if a base analogue has more than one mode of hydrogen bonding, it could be mutagenic. Most of the analogues can participate in many reactions of their normal counterparts and may act on multiple loci [10]. However, it has become increasingly clear that there are qualitative differences that can be utilized as a rational approach to cancer chemotherapy. Nucleic acid base analogues can be categorized into two classes:

### 2.1.1. Purine Analogues

These analogues are structurally and functionally similar to naturally occurring purines like adenine and guanine. Examples include 6-mercaptopurine, 6-azathiopurine, 6-methylthiopurine, 6-thioguanine, Allopurinol, *etc.* [10].

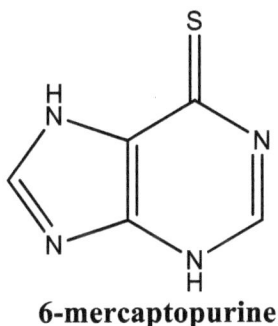

**6-mercaptopurine**

## 2.1.2. Pyrimidine Analogues

These analogues are similar to naturally occurring pyrimidines, both structurally and functionally. Examples include 5-azacytidine, 5-azauridine, 5-azafluorouridine, 5-bromo-2-deoxyuridine, arabinosyl cytosine, *etc* [10].

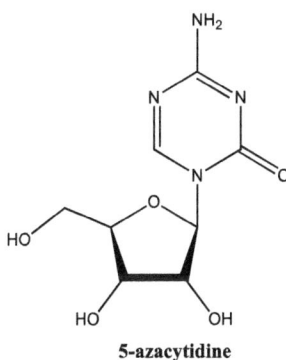

5-azacytidine

## 2.2. Nucleoside Antibiotics

The antibiotics that can resemble nucleosides in their structure have been termed nucleoside antibiotics. They can fall into two major groups.

### 2.2.1. Amino Acid Linked Compounds

Amino acid-linked compounds are another class of compounds that interfere with protein synthesis in various biological systems. These compounds do not function as structural analogues of nucleosides. Examples of amino acid-linked compounds include puromycin, lysylamino adenosine, homocitrullyl amino adenosine, blastidin, *etc* [10].

These compounds disrupt protein synthesis by targeting specific steps or components of the translation process, ultimately leading to the inhibition of protein production in cells.

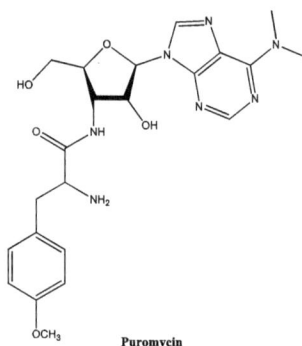

**Puromycin**

## 2.2.2. Adenosine-like Compounds

Adenosine-like compounds, unlike amino acid-linked compounds, do not contain amino acids. However, with a few exceptions, they are converted into nucleotide derivatives in cells and participate in many reactions similar to adenosine and its nucleotides. These adenosine-like antibiotics can be considered as both structural and functional analogues of nucleic acid components. Examples of adenosine-like compounds include tubermycin, cordycepin, showdomycin, and others [10].

These compounds exhibit similarities in structure and function to adenosine and its nucleotides, allowing them to interact with nucleic acid components and potentially interfere with cellular processes related to nucleic acid metabolism or protein synthesis.

## 2.3. Alkylating Agents

Alkylating agents are a class of compounds that carry one, two, or more alkyl groups in reactive forms. These agents have complex actions on DNA. They are known to react with purine bases, particularly guanine at the N-7 atom. Bifunctional alkylating agents, which have two alkyl reactive groups, can lead to cross-linking between the opposite strands of DNA molecules. Alkylation of purines at position N-7 can also result in the formation of unstable quaternary nitrogens. This can cause the alkylated purines to separate from the deoxyribose, creating a gap that may interfere with DNA replication or lead to the incorporation of incorrect bases. Additionally, the phosphate group in DNA can be alkylated, forming unstable phosphate triesters that can hydrolyze the sugar and phosphate, ultimately breaking the DNA chain.

The action of alkylating agents on DNA leads to abnormal base pairing and inhibition of cell division, eventually resulting in cell death. Alkylating anticancer drugs are effective during all phases of the cell cycle and are used to treat a wide variety of cancers. However, it's important to note that long-term use of alkylating agents can promote mutagenic and carcinogenic characteristics [11, 12]. Examples of alkylating agents include nitrogen mustard, melphalan, chlorambuol, cyclophosphamide, and arecoline, among others.

## 2.4. Nitroso Compounds

Nitroso compounds have been proven to be carcinogenic. For their carcinogenic activity and chromosome-breaking effects, it is necessary for the molecule to have at least one alkyl group. Additionally, the presence of oxygen is required for their carcinogenic effects. It is believed that alkylating agents formed through enzyme-catalyzed oxidative dealkylation are responsible for these effects [10]. Examples of nitroso compounds include N-nitroso-N-methylurethane, N-methylphenylnitrosamine, N-hydroxyphenylnitrosamine ammonium, and nitrosoguanidine [10, 13].

Considering the significant alteration in DNA structure and function caused by these chemicals, we have conducted investigations on the effects of cyclophosphamide, a potent DNA-acting agent, on the cell growth and differentiation of breast cancer patients.

## 3. CHEMICALS

### 3.1. Cyclophosphamide

Cyclophosphamide (CP) is a cyclic phosphoramide ester and is widely recognized as one of the most potent DNA-acting agents utilized in immunosuppressive and antineoplastic treatments [14, 15]. It was first reported by Arnold Bourseaux and Norbert Brock in 1958 [16 - 18]. CP, classified as a nitrogen mustard compound, belongs to the group of cytostatic alkylating agents. Its mechanism of action involves the alkylation of the N-7 position of guanine in DNA, leading to the formation of crosslinks within the double helical structure, as shown in Fig. (**1**). This process ultimately results in DNA breaks, which impede DNA synthesis and RNA transcription [18].

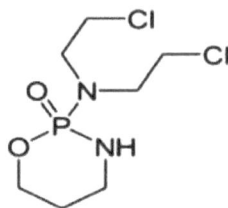

**Fig. (1).** Chemical Structure of Cyclophosphamide.

### 3.1.1. Biochemistry

IUPAC Name: 2-[Bis(2-chloroethyl)amino]tetrahydro-2H-1, 3, 2-oxazaphospho rine 2-oxide.

Common name (synonyms): AstaB518; Clafen; Endoxan; Mitoxan.

Molecular formula: $C_7H_{15}C_{12}N_2O_2P$. Description of properties are given in Table **1**.

**Table 1. Physical and chemical properties of Cyclophosphamide.**

| Properties | Value |
|---|---|
| Appearance | Odorless, fine white crystalline powder |
| Melting Point | 49.5-53°C |
| Boiling Point | 336°C |
| Density | 1.479 g/cm3 |
| Solubility | Soluble in chloroform, dioxane, and glycols; slightly soluble in benzene, carbon tetrachloride; very slightly soluble in ether and acetone |
| Partition Coefficient | 0.63 |
| pKa | 4.5-6.5 |

### 3.1.2. Uses

Cyclophosphamide has found wide application in the treatment of various diseases [19 - 21]. It has been used in the management of ovarian cancer, breast cancer, prostate cancer, lupus erythematosus, lung cancer, multiple sclerosis, Hodgkin's lymphoma, thrombocytopenic purpura, rheumatoid arthritis, idiopathic pulmonary fibrosis, Wegener granulomatosis, polyarteritis nodosa, and anemia [22]. At lower doses, Cyclophosphamide can function as an anti-angiogenic agent or an immune stimulator. It is also employed for the mobilization of hematopoietic stem cells (HSCs) from the bone marrow into the peripheral blood. In transplantation, Cyclophosphamide is utilized as an immunosuppressive agent to prevent graft rejection in renal, hepatic, and cardiac transplants. However, its use as an anti-cancer drug is limited due to its associated side effects [23].

### 3.1.3. Metabolic Activity

Cyclophosphamide undergoes metabolic activation in the liver by cytochrome P-450 enzymes. The major metabolite formed is 4-Hydroxy-cyclophosphamide, which is in equilibrium with its tautomer, aldophosphamide. Aldophosphamide spontaneously breaks down to produce the active compound phosphoramide mustard and acrolein. Phosphoramide mustard is responsible for the anti-tumor effects of cyclophosphamide, while acrolein is responsible for the development of hemorrhagic cystitis, a side effect observed during treatment [24 - 26].

The alkylating activity of cyclophosphamide and its metabolites leads to the formation of highly reactive carbonium ions, which can react with DNA/RNA and proteins. This results in the disruption of nucleic acid function, including changes in nucleotide base mispairs and cross-linking of DNA/DNA or DNA/protein. These effects inhibit DNA synthesis and can lead to DNA mutations, which have implications for carcinogenicity, cytotoxicity, teratogenicity, and reproductive toxicity following chronic exposure to cyclophosphamide [27].

Given the potential health risks associated with cyclophosphamide, it is crucial to prioritize safety measures when working with this compound. Personal protective equipment should be used, proper handling and storage procedures should be followed, and established safety protocols should be adhered to in order to minimize the risk of exposure and ensure the well-being of individuals involved. The classification of cyclophosphamide as a reportable hazardous chemical by the Institutional Biosafety Committee reflects the importance of recognizing and addressing the potential hazards associated with its use.

### 3.1.4. Mechanism of Action

The mechanism of action of Cyclophosphamide (CP) involves its metabolic activation and the formation of active metabolites. The initial step is the hydroxylation of the cyclophosphamide ring, resulting in the formation of 4-Hydroxycyclophosphamide (4-OH-CP) and its tautomer, aldophosphamide. These metabolites spontaneously break down to produce phosphoramide mustard (PM), a bifunctional alkylating agent, and acrolein.

Phosphoramide mustard acts as an alkylating agent and forms covalent bonds with DNA, particularly at the N-7 position of guanine bases. This leads to the formation of cross-links between DNA strands, resulting in the inhibition of DNA replication and RNA transcription. The cross-linking of DNA strands interferes with the normal structure and function of DNA, ultimately leading to cell death.

Acrolein, another metabolite of CP, can induce toxicity in the urinary system. It has been implicated in the development of hemorrhagic cystitis, which is characterized by inflammation and bleeding in the bladder. Acrolein can also have additional cytotoxic effects on cells.

N-dechloroethylation is another important metabolic pathway of CP. It generates N-dechloro-ethylated metabolites and chloroacetaldehyde (CAA) as a byproduct. CAA has the potential to cause nephrotoxicity, which refers to kidney toxicity.

To counteract the cytotoxic effects of these metabolites, the body employs aldehyde dehydrogenases (ALDHs) that catalyze the conjugation of the metabolites with glutathione (GSH) *via* GSHS-transferases. This conjugation process helps in neutralizing the cytotoxic effects of the metabolites and facilitating their elimination from the body.

It is important to note that the exact mechanisms and pathways of CP metabolism and action are complex and may vary depending on factors such as individual variability and co-administration of other drugs.

## 4. GENETIC EFFECT OF CYCLOPHOSPHAMIDE

### 4.1. Effect on Various Somatic Cells by Cyclophosphamide

The exposure of various somatic cells to cyclophosphamide (CP) has been found to have mutagenic and genotoxic effects. These effects include:

a. *Gene Mutations*: CP has the ability to induce mutations in the genetic material of somatic cells. This can result in changes in the DNA sequence, leading to altered gene function or expression.

b. *Chromosome Aberrations*: CP exposure can cause structural abnormalities in chromosomes, such as deletions, duplications, translocations, and inversions. These aberrations can disrupt normal genetic processes and potentially lead to cell dysfunction or malignancy.

c. *Micronuclei Formation*: CP has been shown to induce the formation of micronuclei in somatic cells. Micronuclei are small, extra nuclear structures that contain fragments or whole chromosomes that were not properly incorporated into the daughter nuclei during cell division. The presence of micronuclei is an indicator of genotoxic damage and can be associated with chromosomal instability and an increased risk of genetic abnormalities.

d. *Sister Chromatid Exchanges*: CP exposure can lead to sister chromatid exchanges (SCEs) in somatic cells. SCEs occur when DNA strands from sister chromatids break and exchange genetic material. These exchanges can result in genetic rearrangements and potentially contribute to the development of genetic disorders or cancer.

Studies conducted in different organisms, such as rats, mice, Chinese hamsters, and fruit flies, have provided evidence of CP-induced chromosomal damage, micronuclei formation, and gene mutations. These observations support the mutagenic and carcinogenic properties of CP [26, 29].

It is important to note that the mutagenic and genotoxic effects of CP can have significant implications for human health, particularly in individuals exposed to the drug for extended periods or at high doses. Therefore, appropriate safety measures and monitoring should be implemented to minimize the risks associated with CP exposure (Fig. **2**).

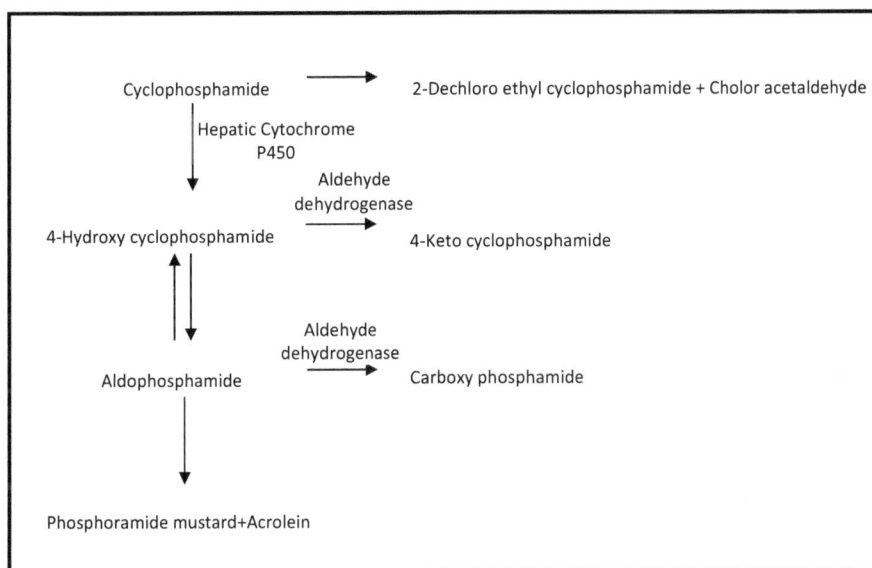

**Fig. (2).** Metabolism of cyclophosphamide with enzymatic bioactivation in the vertical and horizontal directions in the inactivation processes.

## 4.2. DNA Damage By Cyclophosphamide

Cyclophosphamide (CP) is known to induce DNA damage, which plays a central role in its teratogenic, mutagenic, and antineoplastic effects. Various studies have investigated the impact of cyclophosphamide on DNA in mammalian cells derived from somatic cells and germ cells [29].

One of the mechanisms through which CP exerts its cytotoxicity is by cross-linking cellular DNA. Research has shown that CP exposure leads to the formation of interstrand and DNA-protein cross-links, while single-strand breaks are not observed [24, 25]. Prior to affecting RNA or protein synthesis, CP inhibits embryonic DNA synthesis [26]. Additionally, CP influences cell cycle progression by causing G0/G1 and S phase arrest, resulting in the accumulation of cells in the G0/G1 phase compared to the control group. Higher concentrations of CP dose-dependently inhibit G0/G1, S phase, and G2/M phase [27].

Phosphoramide mustard, which is a bifunctional alkylating agent produced through CP metabolism, contributes to cytotoxic action by inducing DNA cross-linking [28]. It binds to the N-7 position of guanine and the phosphate backbone of DNA [29, 30]. This leads to the formation of a mixture of interstrand and DNA-protein cross-links, along with cell enlargement. Studies have shown that incubation of intact cells or isolated nuclei with phosphoramide mustard significantly increases the amount of cross-linked DNA [31].

Acrolein, another metabolite of CP, has been reported to bind to proteins, forming DNA adducts and basic sites, and causing DNA single-strand breaks (SSB) [32]. Biochemical and biological experiments in Saccharomyces cerevisiae suggest that non-activated CP has a weak but detectable ability to cause DNA strand breaks. However, activated CP induces both DNA strand breaks and interstrand cross-links [33].

Numerous studies confirm that CP is a DNA-damaging agent during spermatogenesis. Exposure of rat spermatocytes to CP results in synaptic failure, fragmentation of the synaptonemal complex, and altered centromeric DNA sequences [34]. Prolonged CP exposure leads to a significant increase in both cross-links in spermatozoal nuclei and DNA single-strand breaks, with the cross-links primarily attributed to DNA-DNA linkages. As there is no DNA repair during spermiogenesis, this stage produces dysfunctional germ cells due to genome damage [35].

Higher concentrations of CP in lymphocytes also cause nucleosomal DNA fragmentation [36]. A study conducted on peripheral mononuclear blood cells from fifteen ovarian carcinoma patients who received cyclophosphamide therapy detected DNA strand breaks and DNA cross-links [37].

In brief, CP induces various types of DNA damage, including DNA cross-links, DNA-protein cross-links, DNA adducts, and DNA strand breaks. These DNA lesions contribute to the cytotoxic and mutagenic effects of cyclophosphamide, emphasizing the significance of understanding the mechanisms of DNA damage and implementing appropriate safety measures when working with this compound.

## 4.3. Chromosomal Damage by Cyclophosphamide

In somatic cells, it has been shown in a variety of cultured cells exposed to CP produce gene mutations, chromosomal aberrations, micronuclei and sister chromatid exchanges. The dose-dependent frequency of the induced types of chromosomal abnormalities has been found in unfertilized metaphase II-oocytes after induced ovulation against the alkylating agent CP. In another experiment, the chromosomal abnormalities were studied in the treated epidydimal spermatozoa from male rats with CP by using fluorescent *in-situ* hybridization (FISH) assay. The reviewed literature results showed that CP disrupts meiotic events before the pachytene stage. The double size of various abnormalities such as disomy, nullisomy and diploidy spermatozoa were seen when compared to normal cells [30]. Those Patients who were receiving CP chemotherapy were studied for acute cytogenic effect on the peripheral blood lymphocytes by chromosomal aberration and micro nuclei assay. The results of this study showed the highest incidence of micronuclei as well as the highest level of chromosomal damage [31]. Women's breast cancer cells by chemotherapy along with cyclophosphamide in peripheral blood lymphocytes were cultured to determine the frequencies of sister chromatid exchanges (SCE) and chromosomal aberrations (CA). The number of patients were varying from one to three for SCE and two to five for CA [32]. Even working medical staffs are continuously exposed to cytostatic agents such as CP also has chromosomal aberration. Long-term occupational exposure to these drugs increases the chromosome and chromatid breaks [33]. In another study, synaptonemal complex damage occurs when a male rat is exposed to CP, and this damage is more as compared to meiotic metaphase chromosomal damage [34]. In the rat exposed to CP along with oxidative stress, chromosome aberration occurred as translocation in bone marrow cells [35]. In another study, pregnant rats were exposed to CP on the 12th day of gestation. For cytogenetic analysis, the pups were collected and the liver was dissected. A variety of abnormal chromosomal features, such as gaps, chromatid & chromosomal breaks, acentric fragments, centromeric breakage, chromatin bodies and aneuploidy, were observed in the dispersed metaphase plates [36]. The Animal model was also used to examine the effect of CP on chromosome. The fifth instar nymphs of grasshopper were treated with CP at different concentrations. Based on the analysis of the 42-hour timepoint, chromatid and chromosome breaks were the most prevalent chromosome aberration observed. Additionally, CP increases the number of chromosome aberrations per cell in a different dose and time dependent manner [37].

## 4.4. Mutagenicity and Apoptosis Due to Cyclophosphamide

Cyclophosphamide (CP) exhibits mutagenic properties primarily through its active metabolite, phosphoramide mustard. This metabolite forms mono- and bifunctional guanine adducts, leading to a wide range of mutations. Studies have demonstrated that nitrogen mustards, including CP, can induce various types of mutations, such as base substitutions at G.C and A.T base pairs, intragenic and multi-locus deletions, and chromosomal rearrangements [38]. In particular, CP has been shown to induce A.T-T.A transversions and adenine adducts in the *supF* gene of the shuttle plasmid *pZ189* during replication in human cells [39]. CP and its analogs have also exhibited mutagenic activity in bacterial assays, such as *E. coli* and *Salmonella typhimurium*, following biotransformation using isolated rodent liver homogenates [40]. These mutagenic effects are characterized by back mutations in nature.

Furthermore, CP has been found to induce apoptosis in mature human lymphocytes in *in vivo* settings. Apoptosis, or programmed cell death, is characterized by specific morphological changes and nucleosomal DNA fragmentation. The quantification of fragmented DNA can be achieved through 3'-OH end labeling [41]. The concentration of CP administered has been shown to play a role in inducing apoptosis in lymphocytes.

Overall, the mutagenicity of CP is primarily attributed to its active metabolite phosphoramide mustard, which forms guanine adducts leading to a variety of mutations. Additionally, CP has been observed to induce apoptosis in lymphocytes, characterized by DNA fragmentation and morphological changes. These findings highlight the genotoxic effects of CP and emphasize the importance of understanding its mutagenic potential and implementing appropriate safety precautions during its use.

## 5. ABSORPTION, DISTRIBUTION AND ELIMINATION OF CYCLO PHOSPHAMIDE

Cyclophosphamide exhibits good absorption when taken orally, with peak concentrations reached within 1-3 hours. Its bioavailability ranges from 85% to 100%. When administered intravenously, the drug is rapidly absorbed into the bloodstream. Cyclophosphamide is distributed throughout the body, with a volume of distribution of approximately 30-50 liters, which is similar to the total body water volume. However, only a limited amount of cyclophosphamide and its metabolites penetrate into body fluids.

Metabolites such as Carboxy and DC Cyclophosphamide are not typically found in cerebrospinal fluid, while PM (phosphoramide mustard) and

Cyclophosphamide can be detected. The elimination of cyclophosphamide and its metabolites primarily occurs through the urine within 24 hours after the start of treatment. Carboxycyclophosphamide is the major metabolite excreted in the urine. Hepatic metabolism plays a major role in the elimination of cyclophosphamide from the body, although a small fraction is eliminated through renal excretion as unchanged drug in the urine. Less than 20% of the administered dose is eliminated unchanged in the urine, while approximately 30-60% of the total cyclophosphamide dose is eliminated renally as metabolites. A small fraction of the dose is eliminated *via* feces and expired air.

The plasma half-life of cyclophosphamide varies between 5-9 hours, with a large concentration range. In children and young adults, the half-life is shorter compared to adults. The total systemic clearance of cyclophosphamide ranges from 4-5 L/h, with the majority of clearance being non-renal. During the first day after the dose, the plasma half-life of cyclophosphamide in humans is approximately 5 hours [42].

## 6. TERATOGENECITY

Spermatogenic cells, which undergo rapid division, differentiation, and nuclear remodeling during spermiogenesis, are highly susceptible to the toxic effects of chemotherapeutic drugs [43 - 45]. Among these drugs, alkylating agents such as cyclophosphamide, busulfan, and ifosfamide are known to cause significant damage to spermatogenic cells. These agents work by alkylating the guanine residues of DNA, leading to the formation of intra and interstrand DNA links, as well as single and double-strand breaks [46, 47]. Consequently, apoptosis in germ cells is increased.

*In vitro* studies have shown that exposure to cyclophosphamide (CP) can result in chromosomal breakage, sister chromatid exchange, DNA damage, and reduced telomere function by altering telomerase activities in spermatogonial cells [48]. Moreover, studies in rats have revealed that CP treatment alters the expression of genes involved in stress response in germ cells, nuclear matrix proteins in spermatozoa, and the basic proteome and chromatin structure of spermatozoa. CP also interferes with meiotic progression in spermatocytes and the maturation of sperm in the epididymis.

These findings highlight the teratogenic effects of cyclophosphamide on spermatogenic cells, emphasizing the potential for DNA damage, apoptosis, and disruption of normal sperm development and maturation. The impact on fertility and reproductive outcomes underscores the importance of considering the potential risks and implementing appropriate strategies for fertility preservation in individuals undergoing cyclophosphamide treatment.

## 7. LIMITATIONS

Cyclophosphamide, an oxazaphosphorine used in chemotherapy, has certain limitations that restrict its application. One of the major limitations is its urotoxicity, particularly the development of hemorrhagic cystitis (HC), which becomes dose-limiting without adequate uroprotection [48]. HC occurs due to the metabolites of cyclophosphamide, including phosphoramide mustard and acrolein, which can alkylate DNA and modify proteins. The activation of cyclophospha-

mide by cytochrome P450 in the liver, and to a lesser extent in the lung, generates reactive oxygen species such as superoxide anions [49].

Besides cytochrome P450, other enzymes like prostaglandin H synthase and horseradish peroxidase can also metabolize cyclophosphamide to active compounds, potentially through a free radical mechanism. Lipoxygenases, present in blood cells, lungs, brain, and spleen, can co-oxidize cyclophosphamide as well [50]. The metabolites generated from cyclophosphamide, especially reactive oxygen species, are highly reactive and can modify components of both malignant and healthy cells. Consequently, cyclophosphamide has been associated with cardiotoxicity, nephrotoxicity, liver damage, and lung damage [51].

The direct contact of acrolein, one of the metabolites, with the urothelium leads to urothelial damage characterized by edema, ulceration, neovascularization, hemorrhage, and necrosis. To mitigate these toxic effects, cytoprotection of healthy tissues is crucial. Antioxidants are substances that can protect cells from the damage caused by unstable molecules called free radicals. By interacting with free radicals and stabilizing them, antioxidants inhibit some of the damage caused by these reactive species. This can be particularly beneficial in reducing the risk of cancer development, as free radical damage has been implicated in cancer progression [52].

In brief, the limitations of cyclophosphamide include urotoxicity, the potential for inducing cardiotoxicity, nephrotoxicity, liver damage, and lung damage. The generation of reactive metabolites, such as acrolein and phosphoramide mustard, and the associated production of reactive oxygen species contribute to these limitations. The use of cytoprotective measures, such as antioxidants, can help mitigate the adverse effects on healthy tissues and improve the therapeutic index of cyclophosphamide treatment.

## CONCLUSION AND FUTURE PERSPECTIVE

In conclusion, although many drugs have been developed for pharmaceutical use, their mechanisms of action are still not fully understood. Breast cancer remains a significant challenge for women, and there is a pressing need to understand drug mechanisms and target DNA synthesis inhibition for effective treatment. Various DNA-acting agents have been discovered and utilized in cancer treatment. This study sheds light on the different types of clinically used DNA-acting agents that have the potential to be effective in treating breast cancer.

Moving forward, it is essential to identify cancer predisposition genes that can serve as early diagnostic markers, along with the development of targeted DNA-acting drugs. Early detection of cancer predisposition genes can aid in identifying individuals at higher risk and implementing preventive measures or early intervention strategies.

Moreover, an alternative approach to address this issue is the design of DNA sequence-specific drugs. These drugs would be capable of recognizing specific sequences of DNA bases and selectively blocking their expression. However, developing such drugs is a complex task that requires extensive research and understanding of the intricate mechanisms involved.

In the future, continued research efforts are needed to unravel the detailed mechanisms of action of DNA-acting agents, discover new therapeutic targets, and improve treatment outcomes for breast cancer. Additionally, advancements in personalized medicine and genomics can contribute to tailoring treatment approaches based on individual genetic profiles, leading to more effective and targeted therapies for breast cancer patients.

# REFERENCES

[1] Bray, F.; Ferlay, J.; Soerjomataram, I.; Siegel, R.L.; Torre, L.A.; Jemal, A. Global cancer statistics 2018: GLOBOCAN estimates of incidence and mortality worldwide for 36 cancers in 185 countries. *CA Cancer J. Clin.,* **2018**, *68*(6), 394-424.
[http://dx.doi.org/10.3322/caac.21492] [PMID: 30207593]

[2] Sung, H.; Ferlay, J.; Siegel, R.L.; Laversanne, M.; Soerjomataram, I.; Jemal, A.; Bray, F. Global cancer statistics 2020: GLOBOCAN estimates of incidence and mortality worldwide for 36 cancers in 185 countries. *CA Cancer J. Clin.,* **2021**, *71*(3), 209-249.
[http://dx.doi.org/10.3322/caac.21660] [PMID: 33538338]

[3] Malvia, S.; Bagadi, S.A.; Dubey, U.S.; Saxena, S. Epidemiology of breast cancer in Indian women. *Asia Pac. J. Clin. Oncol.,* **2017**, *13*(4), 289-295.
[http://dx.doi.org/10.1111/ajco.12661] [PMID: 28181405]

[4] Jones, P.A.; Laird, P.W. Cancer-epigenetics comes of age. *Nat. Genet.,* **1999**, *21*(2), 163-167.
[http://dx.doi.org/10.1038/5947] [PMID: 9988266]

[5] Mehrgou, A.; Akouchekian, M. The importance of BRCA1 and BRCA2 genes mutations in breast cancer development. *Med. J. Islam. Repub. Iran,* **2016**, *30*, 369.
[PMID: 27493913]

[6] Darvishi, K.; Sharma, S.; Bhat, A.K.; Rai, E.; Bamezai, R.N.K. Mitochondrial DNA G10398A polymorphism imparts maternal Haplogroup N a risk for breast and esophageal cancer. *Cancer Lett.,* **2007**, *249*(2), 249-255.

[http://dx.doi.org/10.1016/j.canlet.2006.09.005] [PMID: 17081685]

[7]     Parkin, D.M. International variation. *Oncogene,* **2004**, *23*(38), 6329-6340.
        [http://dx.doi.org/10.1038/sj.onc.1207726] [PMID: 15322508]

[8]     Lewtas, J. Air pollution combustion emissions: Characterization of causative agents and mechanisms
        associated with cancer, reproductive, and cardiovascular effects. *Mutat. Res. Rev. Mutat. Res.,* **2007**,
        *636*(1-3), 95-133.
        [http://dx.doi.org/10.1016/j.mrrev.2007.08.003] [PMID: 17951105]

[9]     Newton, H.B., Ed. *Handbook of brain tumor chemotherapy, molecular therapeutics, and
        immunotherapy*; Academic Press, **2018**.

[10]    Roy-Burman, P. *Analogues of nucleic acid components: Mechanisms of action*; **2012**, Vol. 25.

[11]    Murray, D.; Meyn, R.E. Enhancement of the DNA cross-linking activity of nitrogen mustard by
        misonidazole and diethyl maleate in a mouse fibrosarcoma tumor *in vivo. Cancer Res.,* **1984**, *44*(1),
        91-96.
        [PMID: 6690065]

[12]    Davidson, D. Davidson's The Biochemistry of the nucleic acids.'ILnman and Hall,London, **1976**, pp.
        297-305.

[13]    Magee, P.N.; Barnes, J.M. Carcinogenic nitroso compounds. *Adv. Cancer Res.,* **1967**, *10*, 163-246.
        [http://dx.doi.org/10.1016/S0065-230X(08)60079-2] [PMID: 4862936]

[14]    Fraiser, L.H.; Kanekal, S.; Kehrer, J.P. Cyclophosphamide toxicity. *Drugs,* **1991**, *42*(5), 781-795.
        [http://dx.doi.org/10.2165/00003495-199142050-00005] [PMID: 1723374]

[15]    Moore, M.J. Clinical pharmacokinetics of cyclophosphamide. *Clin. Pharmacokinet.,* **1991**, *20*(3), 194-
        208.
        [http://dx.doi.org/10.2165/00003088-199120030-00002] [PMID: 2025981]

[16]    Fereidan-Esfahani, M.; Tobin, W.O. Cyclophosphamide in treatment of tumefactive multiple sclerosis.
        *Mult. Scler. Relat. Disord.,* **2021**, *47*, 102627.
        [http://dx.doi.org/10.1016/j.msard.2020.102627] [PMID: 33246262]

[17]    Mitchell, C.D.; D'Angio, G.J. Does cyclophosphamide (CPM) improve survival rates in patients with
        solid tumors? *Am. J. Clin. Oncol.,* **1986**, *9*(4), 277-280.
        [http://dx.doi.org/10.1097/00000421-198608000-00001] [PMID: 3751964]

[18]    Carter, S.K.; Livingston, R.B. Cyclophosphamide in solid tumors. *Cancer Treat. Rev.,* **1975**, *2*(4),
        295-322.
        [http://dx.doi.org/10.1016/S0305-7372(75)80010-7] [PMID: 766966]

[19]    Brock, N.; Hohorst, H.J. Metabolism of cyclophosphamide. *Cancer,* **1967**, *20*(5), 900-904.
        [http://dx.doi.org/10.1002/1097-0142(1967)20:5<900::AID-CNCR2820200552>3.0.CO;2-Y] [PMID:
        6024299]

[20]    Harahap, Y.; Tanujaya, A.T.; Nurahman, F.; Vianney, A.M.; Purwanto, D.J. Determination of $O^6$-
        Methylguanine in dried blood spot of breast cancer patients after cyclophosphamide administration.
        *Heliyon,* **2021**, *7*(7), e07558.
        [http://dx.doi.org/10.1016/j.heliyon.2021.e07558] [PMID: 34337181]

[21]    Maccubbin, A.E.; Caballes, L.; Riordan, J.M.; Huang, D.H.; Gurtoo, H.L. A cyclophosphamide/DNA
        phosphoester adduct formed *in vitro and in vivo. Cancer Res.,* **1991**, *51*(3), 886-892.
        [PMID: 1988129]

[22]    Zhu, M.X.; Zhao, J.Y.; Chen, G.A.; Guan, L. Early embryonic sensitivity to cyclophosphamide in
        cardiac differentiation from human embryonic stem cells. *Cell Biol. Int.,* **2011**, *35*(9), 927-938.
        [http://dx.doi.org/10.1042/CBI20110031] [PMID: 21561436]

[23]    Madondo, M.T.; Quinn, M.; Plebanski, M. Low dose cyclophosphamide: Mechanisms of T cell
        modulation. *Cancer Treat. Rev.,* **2016**, *42*, 3-9.

[http://dx.doi.org/10.1016/j.ctrv.2015.11.005] [PMID: 26620820]

[24] Stork, C.M.; Schreffler, S.M. *Cyclophosphamide. Encyclopedia of Toxicology,* 3rd; Elsevier Science & Technology, **2014**, pp. 1111-1113.

[25] Yule, S.M.; Price, L.; McMahon, A.D.; Pearson, A.D.J.; Boddy, A.V. Cyclophosphamide metabolism in children with non-Hodgkin's lymphoma. *Clin. Cancer Res.,* **2004**, *10*(2), 455-460.
[http://dx.doi.org/10.1158/1078-0432.CCR-0844-03] [PMID: 14760065]

[26] Panigrahy, S.K.; Jatawa, S.; Tiwari, A. Therapeutic use of cyclophosphamide and its cytotoxicaction: A challenge for researchers. *J. Pharm. Res.,* **2011**, *4*(8), 2755-2757.

[27] Mirkes, P.E. Cyclophosphamide teratogenesis: A review. *Teratog. Carcinog. Mutagen.,* **1985**, *5*(2), 75-88.
[http://dx.doi.org/10.1002/tcm.1770050202] [PMID: 2859667]

[28] Zhang, J.; Tian, Q.; Zhou, S.F. Clinical pharmacology of cyclophosphamide and ifosfamide. *Curr. Drug Ther.,* **2006**, *1*(1), 55-84.
[http://dx.doi.org/10.2174/157488506775268515]

[29] Anderson, D.; Bishop, J.B.; Garner, R.C.; Ostrosky-Wegman, P.; Selby, P.B. Cyclophosphamide: Review of its mutagenicity for an assessment of potential germ cell risks. *Mutat. Res.,* **1995**, *330*(1-2), 115-181.
[http://dx.doi.org/10.1016/0027-5107(95)00039-L] [PMID: 7623863]

[30] Barton, T.S.; Wyrobek, A.J.; Hill, F.S.; Robaire, B.; Hales, B.F. Numerical chromosomal abnormalities in rat epididymal spermatozoa following chronic cyclophosphamide exposure. *Biol. Reprod.,* **2003**, *69*(4), 1150-1157.
[http://dx.doi.org/10.1095/biolreprod.103.016261] [PMID: 12773405]

[31] Kopjar, N.; Garaj-Vrhovac, V.; Milas, I. Acute cytogenetic effects of antineoplastic drugs on peripheral blood lymphocytes in cancer patients chromosome aberrations and micronuclei. *Tumori,* **2002**, *88*(4), 300-312.
[http://dx.doi.org/10.1177/030089160208800412] [PMID: 12400982]

[32] Silva, L.M.; Takahashi, C.S.; Carrara, H.H.A. Study of chromosome damage in patients with breast cancer treated by two antineoplastic treatments. *Teratog. Carcinog. Mutagen.,* **2002**, *22*(4), 257-269.
[http://dx.doi.org/10.1002/tcm.10019] [PMID: 12111710]

[33] Nikula, E.; Kiviniitty, K.; Leisti, J.; Taskinen, P.J. Chromosome aberrations in lymphocytes of nurses handling cytostatic agents. *Scand. J. Work Environ. Health,* **1984**, *10*(2), 71-74.
[http://dx.doi.org/10.5271/sjweh.2355] [PMID: 6382593]

[34] Backer, L. C.; Gibson, J. B. Synaptonemal complex damage in relation to meiotic chromosome aberrations after exposure of male mice to cyclophosphamide. *Mut. Res. / Environ. Mutag. Rel. Sub.,* **1988**, *203*, 317-330.

[35] Bykovskaia, N.V.; Diuzhikova, N.A.; Vaĭdo, A.I.; Lopatina, N.G.; Shvartsman, P.Ia. Frequency of chromosome aberrations induced by stress and cyclophosphane in bone marrow cells of rats selected for the threshold of nervous system excitability. *Genetika,* **1994**, *30*(9), 1224-1228.
[PMID: 8001806]

[36] Ajit kumar, S.; Gajendra, S. Cyclophosphamide induced chromosomal aberrations and associated congenital malformations in rat. *In vitro* cell dev bio. *Animal,* **1998**, *34*, 751-752.

[37] Ren, Z.; Ma, E.; Guo, Y. Chromosome aberration assays for the study of cyclophosphamide and Bacillus thuringiensis in Oxya chinensis (Orthoptera: Acrididae). *Mutat. Res. Genet. Toxicol. Environ. Mutagen.,* **2002**, *520*(1-2), 141-150.
[http://dx.doi.org/10.1016/S1383-5718(02)00199-7] [PMID: 12297154]

[38] Povirk, L.F.; Shuker, D.E. DNA damage and mutagenesis induced by nitrogen mustards. *Mutat. Res. Rev. Genet. Toxicol.,* **1994**, *318*(3), 205-226.
[http://dx.doi.org/10.1016/0165-1110(94)90015-9] [PMID: 7527485]

[39]  Wang, P.; Bauer, G.B.; Bennett, R.A.O.; Povirk, L.F. Thermolabile adenine adducts and A.cntdot.T base pair substitutions induced by nitrogen mustard analogs in an SV40-based shuttle plasmid. *Biochemistry,* **1991**, *30*(49), 11515-11521.
[http://dx.doi.org/10.1021/bi00113a005] [PMID: 1660721]

[40]  Ellenberger, J.; Mohn, G. Mutagenic activity of cyclophosphamide, ifosfamide, and trofosfamide in different genes of Escherichia coli and Salmonella typhimurium after biotransformation through extracts of rodent liver. *Arch. Toxicol.,* **1975**, *33*(3), 225-240.
[http://dx.doi.org/10.1007/BF00311275] [PMID: 1096853]

[41]  Pette, M.; Gold, R.; Pette, D.F.; Hartung, H.P.; Toyka, K.V. Mafosfamide induces DNA fragmentation and apoptosis in human T-lymphocytes A possible mechanism of its immunosuppressive action. *Immunopharmacology,* **1995**, *30*(1), 59-69.
[http://dx.doi.org/10.1016/0162-3109(95)00005-E] [PMID: 7591714]

[42]  Fleming, R. A. An overview of cyclophosphamide and ifosfamide pharmacology. *Pharmac. J. Human. Pharma. Drug. Ther.,* **1997**, *17*(5P2), 146S-154S.

[43]  Drumond, A.L.; Meistrich, M.L.; Chiarini-Garcia, H. Spermatogonial morphology and kinetics during testis development in mice: A high-resolution light microscopy approach. *Reproduction,* **2011**, *142*(1), 145-155.
[http://dx.doi.org/10.1530/REP-10-0431] [PMID: 21521798]

[44]  Meistrich, M.L.; Finch, M.; da Cunha, M.F.; Hacker, U.; Au, W.W. Damaging effects of fourteen chemotherapeutic drugs on mouse testis cells. *Cancer Res.,* **1982**, *42*(1), 122-131.
[PMID: 7198505]

[45]  Codrington, A.M.; Hales, B.F.; Robaire, B. Spermiogenic germ cell phase-specific DNA damage following cyclophosphamide exposure. *J. Androl.,* **2004**, *25*(3), 354-362.
[http://dx.doi.org/10.1002/j.1939-4640.2004.tb02800.x] [PMID: 15064312]

[46]  Qiu, J.; Hales, B.F.; Robaire, B. Effects of chronic low-dose cyclophosphamide exposure on the nuclei of rat spermatozoa. *Biol. Reprod.,* **1995**, *52*(1), 33-40.
[http://dx.doi.org/10.1095/biolreprod52.1.33] [PMID: 7711181]

[47]  Colvin, O.M. An overview of cyclophosphamide development and clinical applications. *Curr. Pharm. Des.,* **1999**, *5*(8), 555-560.
[http://dx.doi.org/10.2174/1381612805666230110214512] [PMID: 10469891]

[48]  Giraud, B.; Hebert, G.; Deroussent, A.; Veal, G.J.; Vassal, G.; Paci, A. Oxazaphosphorines: New therapeutic strategies for an old class of drugs. *Expert Opin. Drug Metab. Toxicol.,* **2010**, *6*(8), 919-938.
[http://dx.doi.org/10.1517/17425255.2010.487861] [PMID: 20446865]

[49]  Weber, G. F.; Weber, G. F. DNA damaging drugs. *Molec. therap. cancer.,* **2015**, 9-112.

[50]  Stankiewicz, A.; Skrzydlewska, E. Amifostine antioxidant effect on serum of rats treated with cyclophosphodamide. *Pol. J. Environ. Stud.,* **2005**, *14*(3), 341-346.

[51]  Ogino, M. H.; Tadi, P. *Cyclophosphamide*; StatPearls Publishing: Treasure Island (FL), **2020**.

[52]  Assreuy, A.M.S.; Martins, G.J.; Moreira, M.E.F.; Brito, G.A.C.; Cavada, B.S.; Ribeiro, R.A.; Flores, C.A. Prevention of cyclophosphamide-induced hemorrhagic cystitis by glucose-mannose binding plant lectins. *J. Urol.,* **1999**, *161*(6), 1988-1993.
[http://dx.doi.org/10.1016/S0022-5347(05)68870-2] [PMID: 10332487]

# CHAPTER 11

# *Aloe Vera*-A Medicinal Plant as Potential Therapeutic Agents for Liver Cancer

**Lovely Sinha**[1,*], **Ghanshyam Kumar Satyapal**[1] and **Shailendra Kumar**[2]

[1] *Department of Biotechnology, School of Earth Biological & Environmental Sciences, Central University of South Bihar, Gaya, India*

[2] *Human Molecular Genetics Laboratory, Department of Pathology/Lab Medicine, All India Institute of Medical Sciences, Patna, India*

**Abstract:** Liver cancer is the sixth most commonly diagnosed cancer and the fourth leading cause of cancer death worldwide. Research over the last two decades has revealed that medicinal plants have been used for the treatment of various neoplastic diseases. *Aloe vera* is a ubiquitously naturally occurring and drought-resisting herbal medicinal plant. Some reports suggest that Aloe vera possesses wound and burn healing activities and anti-inflammatory as well as immunomodulatory effects. There are no direct studies available on the role of the Aloe vera extract and its active ingredient like aloe-emodin that modulates antiaging and anticancer activities, particularly on immune cells as well as liver cancer cells. *Aloe vera* has many bioactive compounds and pharmacological properties that may show an important role in liver cancer prevention and treatment through the enhancement of regeneration, antiaging activity, antioxidant activity, anticancer activity and modulation of genetic pathways. Here, we discuss the study of the anticancer effect and modulation of expression of various genes in response to *Aloe vera* in liver cancer.

**Keywords:** Aloe-vera, Anti-cancer, Anti-aging, Liver cancer.

## 1. INTRODUCTION

### 1.1. Overview

Cancer is responsible for one in eight deaths and is a major public health problem worldwide [1-2]. According to estimates from World Health Organization (WHO) in 2015, cancer is the first or second leading cause of death before the age of 70 years in 91 of 172 countries, and third or fourth rank in an additional 22 countries. In 2019, 1,762,450 new cancer cases and 606, 880 cancer deaths are

---

* **Corresponding author Lovely Sinha:** Department of Biotechnology, School of Earth Biological & Environmental Sciences, Central University of South Bihar, Gaya, India; E-mail: lovely130297@gmail.com

**Ashok Kumar Jha & Ravi S. Singh (Eds.)**

projected to occur in the United States [3]. Now a days, a higher mortality rate due to liver cancer or Hepatocellular carcinoma (HCC) worldwide may be attributed to aggressive cancer cell growth and increases global health challenges [6]. It may arise as a result of chemical or biological damage to normal cells in a multistep process that involves changes at the initiation level followed by promotion and progression, which lead to malignancy [4].

Globally, liver cancer ranks third in terms of cancer mortality. This malignancy occurs more often among men than women, with the highest incidence rates reported in East Asia [5]. It is predicted that liver cancer will rank sixth among the most frequently diagnosed diseases and fourth among the leading causes of cancer-related death worldwide in 2018. The two to three times rate of mortality and incidence are higher among men in most world regions. Liver cancer is the leading cause of cancer death among men in 20 countries, in part because of its high fatality rate [3]. Due to improved clinical practices in the developed world, there has been a constant increase in 5 years survival rates from 3% to 18% for liver and intrahepatic bile duct cancer from 1975 to 2011. For 2018, the estimated cases of liver and intrahepatic bile duct cancer were 42,220 (30,610 Males and 11,610 Females), and estimated deaths were 30,200 (20,540 Males and 9,660 Females) in the United States. This poses a socio economic toll, and there is a need to further enhance research efforts in finding new promising therapeutic entities against longer cancer cell survival and enormous growth [6]. Different methods like surgery, radiotherapy, chemotherapy, hormone therapy, photo-dynamic therapy, immunotherapy, monoclonal antibodies therapy, gene therapy, *etc.,* are used currently, single or in a combination of two or more, for the treatment of cancer. The most common mode of treatment for cancer includes radiotherapy, chemotherapy and surgery. But nowadays, current treatment modalities are failing because of serious side effects and merely extend the patient's lifespan by a few years only. Considering these drawbacks, efforts have focused on identifying new molecular targets that would allow limited cancer treatment side effects. Thus, there is a need to utilize alternative concepts or approaches to the prevention of human cancer. In this regard, we targeted the herbal products that have been implicated in cancer prevention and that promote human health without recognizable side effects.

Plants have been used for the treatment of various diseases of human beings and animals since time immemorial. Briefly, Aloe vera is a ubiquitously naturally occurring and drought-resisting herbal plant. Aloe vera has its many bioactive compound and pharmacological properties and it may show an important role in liver cancer prevention and treatment through the enhancement of regeneration, antiaging activity, antioxidant activity, anticancer activity and modulation of genetic pathways [7]. A natural constituent of Aloe vera leaves Aloe-emodin has been reported to be nontoxic for normal cells but possesses specific toxicity for neuroectodermal tumor cells [7, 8, 9]. Aloe-emodin has been reported to induce apoptotic cell death in H460 cells. The expression of PKA, PKC, Bcl-2, caspase-3 and p38 was involved in aloe-emodin induced apoptosis of H460 cells. The signaling order in the aloe-emodin induced cell death pathway may be PKA, PKC, Bcl-2, caspase-3 and then p38. P38 clearly is an important determinant of apoptotic death induced by aloe-emodin [10]. Moreover, the reactive oxygen species (ROS) is one of the causes of cancer progression. The imbalance between the production and accumulation of ROS which further results failure of cells to maintain normal physiological redox-regulated functions. This, in turn, leads to DNA damage, unregulated cell signaling, change in cell motility, cytotoxicity, apoptosis, and cancer initiation [11]. Low molecular weight fraction (LMWF) obtained from Aloe vera extract induced disruption of intercellular junctions, and it inhibited the production of reactive oxygen species [12]. It has been reported that there is an increased generation of ROS and oxidative stress associated with cancerous cells in comparison to normal cells and results in stimulation of cellular proliferation, mutations, genetic instability and cell death. Aloe vera has several bioactive compounds including aloe-emodin that can reduce ROS and thus, it can be used for potential biomedicines in cancer treatment. The current study is focused to investigate the anticancer effect of aloe vera in liver cancer as a medicinal therapeutic agent. This review provides an update on the modulation of expression of various genes in response to Aloe vera in liver cancer.

## 2. LIVER CANCER

Hepatocellular carcinoma (HCC) or Liver Cancer is one of the most frequent cancers among humans, with 0.25–1 million newly diagnosed cases each year. It is developed due to various factors, including chronic hepatitis-B infection, chronic hepatitis-C infection, exposure to aflatoxin-beta, cirrhosis of the liver, oral contraceptives, cigarette smoking, *etc*. It is essential to understand how the liver works in order to understand liver cancer thoroughly. Physiological processes such as metabolism, secretion, and storage are regulated by the liver. Unfortunately, numerous toxicants attack it. Throughout tumor progression and its inhibition through chemotherapy, the host system's biological and histological parameters will reflect the numerous pathological changes, particularly pertaining to the liver, which is known to be the major organ affected in carcinogenesis [13]. The liver is the second largest organ and the largest gland in human beings. It is found in the upper belly, the internal form of the human being, its function is to absorb and remove waste from the blood. In the liver, there can be a mass of tissue called a tumor or growth in the presence of additional waste cells. Benign or malignant tumors may occur.

## 3. ALOE VERA AND ITS ACTIVE INGREDIENTS

Aloe vera (Aloe barbadensis Miller) Fig. (**1**) belongs to the Liliaceal family and is a perennial succulent. It resembles cactus and grows in hot, dry climates. Aloe vera is one of the most versatile medicinal plants and has many phytoconstituents that show phytopharmacological properties like antitumor and antioxidant activity, anti-inflammatory activity, hypoglycemic and hypolipidemic activity, wound healing activity, antimutagenic activity, immunomodulatory activity, gastroprotective activity, antifungal activity, *etc* [7, 14].

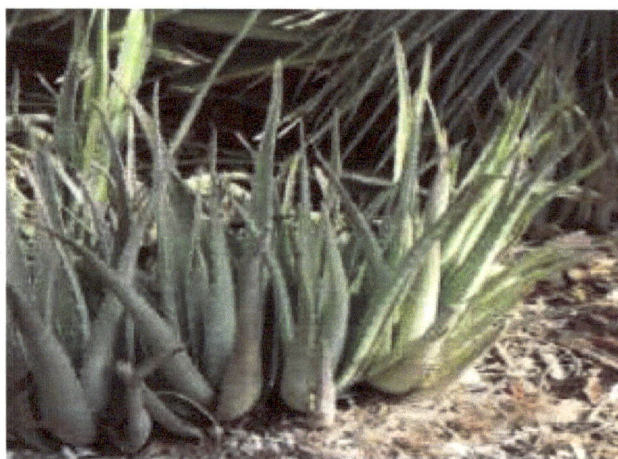

**Fig. (1).** Aloe Vera plant.

The Aloe vera gel also increases the level of hyaluronic acid and dermatan sulphate in granulation tissue. For the generation of new tissue, there is a requirement for oxygen and metabolites during angiogenesis. It has been observed that Aloe vera increases the blood supply after its intake treatment [15]. This suggests increased oxygen access due to Aloe vera phytoconstituents. Aloe vera contains 75 potentially active constituents: vitamins, enzymes, minerals, sugars, lignin, saponins, salicylic acids and amino acids [16 - 18]. Aloe vera 's phytoconstituents are primarily glycoproteins, anthraquinones, saccharides, and low molecular weight substances. Aloe vera extract has low molecular weight compounds that were shown to inhibit the release of reactive oxygen species from human neutrophils and suggested to influence the immune response of the individual. Low molecular weight fraction (LMWF) obtained from Aloe vera extract induced disruption of intercellular junctions and it inhibited the production of reactive oxygen species [23]. Its phytoconstituents may also have a great role in removing wrinkles and rejuvenating the face, and it may be beneficial to delay aging.

Acute Hepatic necrosis resembles an acute, toxic inflammatory response which can be induced by Reactive oxygen species and free-radical-mediated reactions. Anthraquinones act as antioxidants and radical scavengers. Aloe vera, like anthraquinone and aloe-emodin, reduces such inflammatory response and liver necrosis that occur by carbon tetrachloride and lipid peroxidation. Although various research findings suggest that Aloe vera's phytoconstituents are likely to be associated with reduced cancer risks having anti-carcinogenic properties [7, 15].

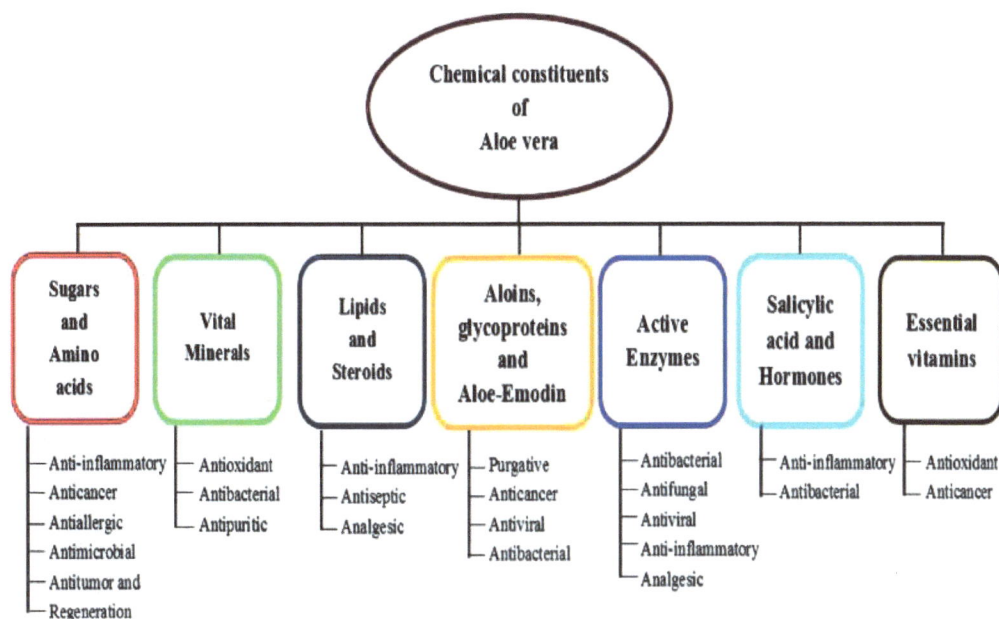

**Fig. (2).** Constituents of *Aloe vera* and its biological properties [15].

Aloe vera contains super carbohydrates, which provide protection against cancer, particularly liver cancer, by preventing its genesis, regressing its growth and inhibiting its metastasis (Fig. **2**). Acemannan is a polysaccharide extracted from root, pulp, leaves or aerial parts of Aloe vera and it stimulates the immune system and possesses significant anticancer activity. Other bioactive compounds, Emodin and lectins, also exhibit strong anticancer property and also enhance immune response by activating macrophages and releasing cytokines such as interferon, interleukin and tumor necrosis factor. It has been reported that Aloe-emodin inhibits cancer cell growth and spread of stomach cancer and various sarcomas, including leukemia, by inducing apoptosis. In addition, the antioxidant properties of Aloe vera reduce the side effects of chemotherapy and radiotherapy [19, 20, 21].

The current trend to identify natural products as new cancer preventative agents to overcome side effects is based on a conceptual basis and understanding of their mechanisms of action in carcinogenesis. Our study analyzed the cytotoxic potential of aloe-emodin, a hydroxyl anthraquinone naturally present in the leaves of Aloe vera (Fig. **3**). Some reports described the selective *in vitro* and *in vivo* killing of neuroectodermal tumor cells by aloe-emodin, the anticancer activity of which is based on apoptotic cell death, promoted by a drug uptake process specific to a tumor cell that may present opportunities for new anticancer agents [23].

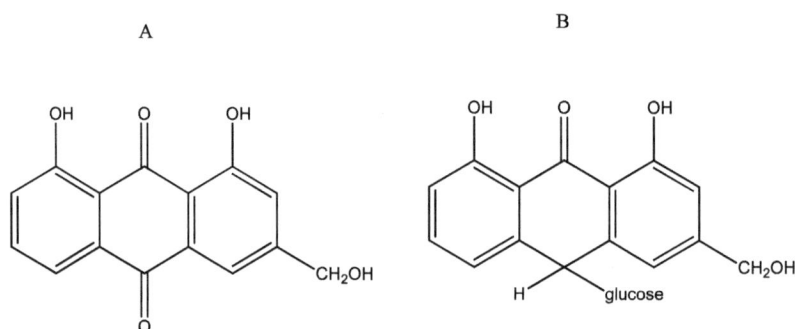

Fig. (3). Chemical structure of A. Aloe-emodin (1, 8-dihydroxy-3-hydroxymethyl-9, 10-anthracenedionez) and B. Aloin (10–19, 59-anhydroglucosyl-aloe-emodin-9-anthrone) [22].

Aloe vera has also been reported to have antibacterial and anti-inflammatory actions. We therefore investigated the effect of aloe-emodin and Aloe vera gel extract supplementation in induced chemical hepatocarcinogenesis in the human. The major bioactive compounds of phenolics were found to be flavonoid groups such as quercetin and kaempferol [24]. These flavonoid groups of Aloe vera also have anticancer properties.

In different constituents of Aloe vera extract, our study targeted aloe-emodin that belongs to anthraquinone and has selective anticancer activity against several cancers like neuroectodermal tumors. Aloe-emodin (1, 8-dihydroxy-3-(hydroxymethyl) - anthraquinone) is an active component from the root and rhizome of Rheum palmatum that has been reported to exhibit antitumor effects through an unknown mechanism. Aloe-emodin (40M)-induced apoptosis of H460 cells involves modulation of cAMP-dependent protein kinase, protein kinase C, Bcl-2, caspase-3 and p38 protein expression. In the regulation of apoptosis, various signals such as cAMP-dependent protein kinase, protein kinase C, Bcl-2, caspase-3 and p38 are involved in cell death. Their relationship has been investigated by aloe-emodin [10]. Some reports also suggested that aloe-emodin induced apoptosis in human liver cancer cells HepG2 and Hep3B through different apoptotic mechanisms [25]. Also, some reported study shows the cytotoxic and genotoxic activities initiation on human hepatocellular carcinoma (HepG2) cells in response of Aloe vera extract through induction of apoptotic pathway [26].

Aloe vera gel prepared from small fractions contains lectin-like substances that promote normal human cell growth like human fibroblasts. Yagi *et al.* reported on the cell proliferation activity of a 29 kDa glycoprotein composed of two 14 kDa subunits. This was found to enhance the proliferation of baby hamster kidney cells and normal human dermal fibroblasts [21, 26]. From the above knowledge, I conclude that further understanding of these individual components and their effects is essential if Aloe vera is to be successfully developed for therapeutic purposes.

## CONCLUSION

Hepatocellular carcinoma (HCC) is the most common primary liver cancer, which is associated with conditions resulting in chronic liver injury mainly caused by a hepatitis virus infection, alcohol intoxication, *etc.* Current treatment modalities, including surgery and liver transplantation, offer limited survival benefits. One of the greatest challenges in cancer therapy is to achieve a high therapeutic effect by maximizing the desired reactions and minimizing the underside effects. Considering these drawbacks, we targeted the herbal products that have been implicated in cancer prevention and that promote human health without recognizable side effects. Already it had been reported that Aloe vera and its bioactive compound Aloe-emodin have anti-oxidant, wound healing, antiaging and anticancer properties. The genes can be targeted as a novel therapeutic approach in response to herbal drugs for the treatment of cancer. Further understanding the mechanisms of modulation of gene regulation in response to Aloe vera would certainly have important implications for research on and management of human cancers.

The cytotoxic effect of Aloe vera in several human cancers and its proliferative effect in most normal cells suggest that Aloe vera might serve as good anticancer drugs. In contrast, most anti-cancer treatments often exhibit serious toxicity and disturb normal and malignant cells alike. To reduce this ill effect, we have scrutinized the herbal method that may bring new insight into many serious clinical problems which we have to face in aging societies.

# REFERENCES

[1]     Lopez, A.D.; Mathers, C.D.; Ezzati, M.; Jamison, D.T.; Murray, C.J.L. Global and regional burden of disease and risk factors, 2001: Systematic analysis of population health data. *Lancet,* **2006**, *367*(9524), 1747-1757.
[http://dx.doi.org/10.1016/S0140-6736(06)68770-9] [PMID: 16731270]

[2]     Siegel, R.L.; Miller, K.D.; Jemal, A. Cancer statistics, 2019. *CA Cancer J. Clin.,* **2019**, *69*(1), 7-34.
[http://dx.doi.org/10.3322/caac.21551] [PMID: 30620402]

[3]     Bray, F.; Ferlay, J.; Soerjomataram, I.; Siegel, R.L.; Torre, L.A.; Jemal, A. Global cancer statistics 2018: Globocan estimates of incidence and mortality worldwide for 36 cancers in 185 countries. *CA Cancer J. Clin.,* **2018**, *68*(6), 394-424.
[http://dx.doi.org/10.3322/caac.21492] [PMID: 30207593]

[4]     Dhanasekaran, M.; Baskar, A.A.; Ignacimuthu, S.; Agastian, P.; Duraipandiyan, V. Chemopreventive potential of epoxy clerodane diterpene from tinospora cordifolia against diethylnitrosamine-induced hepatocellular carcinoma. *Invest. New Drugs,* **2009**, *27*(4), 347-355.
[http://dx.doi.org/10.1007/s10637-008-9181-9] [PMID: 18853103]

[5]     Altekruse, S.F.; McGlynn, K.A.; Reichman, M.E. Hepatocellular carcinoma incidence, mortality, and survival trends in the United States from 1975 to 2005. *J. Clin. Oncol.,* **2009**, *27*(9), 1485-1491.
[http://dx.doi.org/10.1200/JCO.2008.20.7753] [PMID: 19224838]

[6]     Sadaf, N.; Kumar, N.; Ali, M.; Ali, V.; Bimal, S.; Haque, R. Arsenic trioxide induces apoptosis and inhibits the growth of human liver cancer cells. *Life Sci.,* **2018**, *205*, 9-17.
[http://dx.doi.org/10.1016/j.lfs.2018.05.006] [PMID: 29738779]

[7]     Joseph, B.; Raj, S.J. Pharmacognostic and phytochemical properties of aloe veralinn an overview. *Int. J. Pharm. Sci. Rev. Res.,* **2010**, *4*(2), 106-110.

[8]     Fenig, E.; Nordenberg, J.; Beery, E.; Sulkes, J.; Wasserman, L. Combined effect of aloe-emodin and chemotherapeutic agents on the proliferation of an adherent variant cell line of merkel cell carcinoma. *Oncol. Rep.,* **2004**, *11*(1), 213-217.
[http://dx.doi.org/10.3892/or.11.1.213] [PMID: 14654928]

[9]     Wasserman, L.; Avigad, S.; Beery, E.; Nordenberg, J.; Fenig, E. The effect of aloe emodin on the proliferation of a new merkel carcinoma cell line. *Am. J. Dermatopathol.,* **2002**, *24*(1), 17-22.
[http://dx.doi.org/10.1097/00000372-200202000-00003] [PMID: 11803275]

[10]    Yeh, F.T.; Wu, C.H.; Lee, H.Z. Signaling pathway for aloe-emodin-induced apoptosis in human H460 lung nonsmall carcinoma cell. *Int. J. Cancer,* **2003**, *106*(1), 26-33.
[http://dx.doi.org/10.1002/ijc.11185] [PMID: 12794753]

[11]    Fu, P.P.; Xia, Q.; Hwang, H.M.; Ray, P.C.; Yu, H. Mechanisms of nanotoxicity: Generation of reactive oxygen species. *Yao Wu Shi Pin Fen Xi,* **2014**, *22*(1), 64-75.
[PMID: 24673904]

[12]    Avila, H.; Rivero, J.; Herrera, F.; Fraile, G. Cytotoxicity of a low molecular weight fraction from *Aloe vera(Aloe barbadensis Miller* gel. *Toxicon,* **1997**, *35*(9), 1423-1430.
[http://dx.doi.org/10.1016/S0041-0101(97)00020-2] [PMID: 9403965]

[13]    Lin, S.Y.; Elledge, S.J. Multiple tumor suppressor pathways negatively regulate telomerase. *Cell,* **2003**, *113*(7), 881-889.
[http://dx.doi.org/10.1016/S0092-8674(03)00430-6] [PMID: 12837246]

[14]    Kumar, S.; Yadav, J.P. Ethnobotanical and pharmacological properties of *Aloe vera*: A review. *J. Med. Plants Res.,* **2014**, *8*(48), 1387-1398.

[15]    Keyhanian, S.; Stahl-Biskup, E. Phenolic constituents in dried flowers of *aloe vera(Aloe barbadensis)* and their *in vitro* antioxidative capacity. *Planta Med.,* **2007**, *73*(6), 599-602.
[http://dx.doi.org/10.1055/s-2007-967202] [PMID: 17520524]

[16]   Govind, P. Some important anticancer herbs: A review. *I. Res. J. Pharamacy,* **2011**, *2*, 45-53.

[17]   Vogler, B.K.; Ernst, E. *Aloe vera*: A systematic review of its clinical effectiveness. *Br. J. Gen. Pract.,* **1999**, *49*(447), 823-828.
[PMID: 10885091]

[18]   Surjushe, A.; Vasani, R.; Saple, D.G. *Aloe vera*: A short review. *Indian J. Dermatol.,* **2008**, *53*(4), 163-166.
[http://dx.doi.org/10.4103/0019-5154.44785] [PMID: 19882025]

[19]   McAnalley, B.H.; Carpenter, R.H.; McDaniel, H.R. Administration of acemannan. US5106616, **1992**.

[20]   Pecere, T.; Gazzola, M.V.; Mucignat, C.; Parolin, C.; Vecchia, F.D.; Cavaggioni, A.; Basso, G.; Diaspro, A.; Salvato, B.; Carli, M.; Palù, G. Aloe-emodin is a new type of anticancer agent with selective activity against neuroectodermal tumors. *Cancer Res.,* **2000**, *60*(11), 2800-2804.
[PMID: 10850417]

[21]   Sharma, N.; Vashist, H.; Kumar, A. Reputation of herbal drugs in treatments of liver cancer. *Int. J. Pharm.,* **2018**, *3*(3).

[22]   Kuo, P.L.; Lin, T.C.; Lin, C.C. The antiproliferative activity of aloe-emodin is through p53-dependent and p21-dependent apoptotic pathway in human hepatoma cell lines. *Life Sci.,* **2002**, *71*(16), 1879-1892.
[http://dx.doi.org/10.1016/S0024-3205(02)01900-8] [PMID: 12175703]

[23]   Chemical structure of AE (1, 8-dihydroxy-3-hydroxymethyl-9, 10-anthracenedione; A) and aloin (10–19, 59-anhydroglucosyl-aloe-emodin-9-anthrone; B.)

[24]   Agarry, O.O.M.T.; Bello, M. Comparative antimicrobial activities activities of *Aloe vera* gel and leaf. *Afr. J. Biotechnol.,* **2005**, *4*(12), 1413-1414.

[25]   Choi, S.; Chung, M.H. A review on the relationship between *Aloe vera* components. *Seminars in integrative medicine,* WB Saunders **2003**, *1*, 53-62.

[26]   Choi, S-W.; Son, B-W.; Son, Y-S.; Park, Y-I.; Lee, S-K.; Chung, M-H. The wound-healing effect of a glycoprotein fraction isolated from *aloe vera*. *Br. J. Dermatol.,* **2001**, *145*(4), 535-545.
[http://dx.doi.org/10.1046/j.1365-2133.2001.04410.x] [PMID: 11703278]

# SUBJECT INDEX

## A

Abdominal cramps 198
Abnormal calcium signaling 210
Acid(s) 5, 38, 41, 59, 68, 70, 95, 156, 181,
　　182, 183, 188, 189, 217, 237, 264, 284
　abscisic 237
　acetic 41
　Acetylsalicylic 59
　betulinic 181, 189
　boric 5, 38
　citric 5
　hyaluronic 284
　hydrolysate 188
　hydrolysis 183
　hydrolysis products 182
　phosphonic 95
　propanoic 156
　Retinoic 68
　ribonucleic 264
　salicylic 284
　shikimic 217
　triterpene 189
　valproic 70
Action 197, 253, 286
　anti-inflammatory 286
　antidepressant 197
　antioxidative 253
Activity 27, 29, 168, 170, 219, 269, 275, 281,
　　282, 284
　alkylating 269
　anti-tumor 168
　antiaging 281, 282
　antimutagenic 284
　antiparasitic 219
　antiproliferative 27, 29, 170
　immunomodulatory 284
　telomerase 275
Acute myeloid leukemia (AML) 162
Acyclic nucleoside phosphonates (ANPs) 85,
　　88, 112
Agar 24, 40

　dilution method 24
　disc diffusion method 40
Agents 12, 83, 206, 251, 268, 283
　anti-angiogenic 268
　anti-foaming 251
　anticorrosive 206
　oxidizing 12
　synthetic effective chemotherapy 83
　therapeutic 283
Akt signaling pathway 167
Alzheimer disorder 67
Alzheimer's disease 53, 193, 194, 210
Analgesic 38, 59
　activities 38
　agent 59
Angina 68
Angiogenesis 164, 284
Anthracyclines antibiotics 163
Anti-Alzheimer's Activity 194
Anti-cancer activity 61, 169
Anti-diabetic 31
　activity 31
　effects 31
Anti-HBV activity 101
Anti-HIV activities 94, 105, 114, 127, 240
Anti-inflammatory 18, 33, 34, 38, 54, 241,
　　284
　activity 18, 33, 34, 38, 241, 284
　effects 34, 54
Anti-microbial agents 18
Anti-parkinson activity 194
Anti-proliferative activity 27
Anti-stress activity 26
Anti-stroke activity 195
Anti-tubercular activity 21, 23, 24, 25, 26
Anti-tumor 61, 162
　agent 162
　immunity 61
Antiallergic agent 241
Antibacterial activity 19, 20, 35, 36, 38, 40, 42
Anticancer activity 31, 281, 282, 286
Anticonvulsant activity 196